"This book will make a tremendous difference to the millions of people
who suffer unnecessarily from mental health problems.
Nutritional medicine is the future."
Dr. Hyla Cass, *Assistant Clinical Professor of Psychiatry,*
UCLA School of Medicine

"This excellent book gives us a most powerful weapon
in our fight against mental disease."
Dr. Abram Hoffer, *psychiatrist*

"This ... ad it."

"If you ... ood the
und ... you

"We n ... aponry
again ... ll be a
good ... better

G ... in

"This boo ... t is about
as useful ... food can
make ... fact?

"If you ... lertness,
this boo ... better!
This ... ght,

About the Author

Patrick Holford began his academic career in experimental psychology. While at York University he became interested in the biochemistry of mental illness. His research led him to two pioneers in the field: Dr. Carl Pfeiffer from Princeton's Brain Bio Center, and Dr. Abram Hoffer, former director of psychiatric research for Saskatchewan, Canada. Both claimed that nutritional therapy gave outstanding results in treating mental health problems. He became their student and later, that of twice Nobel prize winner Dr Linus Pauling.

In 1984 Patrick Holford founded the Institute for Optimum Nutrition (ION). A charitable and independent educational trust for furthering education and research in nutrition, ION is now one of the most respected training colleges for clinical nutritionists.

At ION he researched the role of nutrition in intelligence, culminating in a landmark trial in 1987 proving that nutritional supplementation can raise IQ. He also researched nutritional approaches to depression, schizophrenia, and eating disorders, and developed a method for assessing a person's optimal nutrition requirements that has been tested on more than 100,000 people.

Since 1997 he has written twenty popular books, now translated into seventeen languages. The first, *The Optimum Nutrition Bible*, has sold over a million copies worldwide.

Backed by more than twenty years of research and clinical experience, Patrick Holford is committed to bringing this radical, new, and proven approach to mental health to those who need it. In the UK he now directs the Mental Health Project, which aims to establish out-patient clinics and halfway houses to help in the recovery of people with mental health problems (see page 360).

Other books by Patrick Holford

The Optimum Nutrition Bible
100% Health
Beat Stress and Fatigue
Say No to Cancer
Say No to Heart Disease
Say No to Arthritis
Improve Your Digestion
Balancing Hormones Naturally (with Kate Neil)
Boost Your Immune System (with Jennifer Meek)
Supplements for Superhealth
The Optimum Nutrition Cookbook (with Judy Ridgway)
The 30-Day Fatburner Diet
Six Weeks to Superhealth
Natural Highs (with Dr. Hyla Cass)

The definition of insanity:

to keep doing the same things
and expect different results.

OPTIMUM NUTRITION

FOR THE MIND

PATRICK HOLFORD

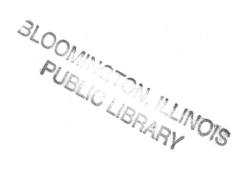
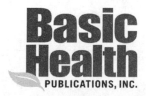

Basic Health
PUBLICATIONS, INC.

Mental health is a complex affair. While all the nutrients and herbs referred to in this book have been proven safe, those seeking help are advised to consult a qualified clinical nutritionist or health professional who can run the necessary tests and is informed about drug-nutrient interactions. The recommendations given in this book are solely intended as education and information, and should not be taken as medical advice. Neither the author nor the publisher accept liability for readers who choose to self-prescribe. *All supplements should be kept out of reach of infants and young children.*

The information contained in this book is based upon the research and personal and professional experiences of the author. It is not intended as a substitute for consulting with your physician or other health care provider. Any attempt to diagnose and treat an illness should be done under the direction of a health care professional.

The publisher does not advocate the use of any particular health care protocol but believes the information in this book should be available to the public. The publisher and author are not responsible for any adverse effects or consequences resulting from the use of the suggestions, preparations, or procedures discussed in this book. Should the reader have any questions concerning the appropriateness of any procedures or preparation mentioned, the author and the publisher strongly suggest consulting a professional health care advisor.

Published by
Basic Health Publications, Inc.
8200 Boulevard East • North Bergen, NJ 07047 • 1-201-868-8336

Published by arrangement with Judy Piatkus (Publishers) Limited, London, England

Library of Congress Cataloging-in-Publication Data
Holford, Patrick.
  Optimum nutrition for the mind / Patrick Holford.
    p. cm.
  Includes bibliographical references and index.
  ISBN 1-59120-105-5
1. Brain—Popular works. 2. Nutrition—Popular works. 3. Mental illness—Nutritional aspects—Popular works. 4. Nootropic agents—Popular works. 5. Dietary supplements—Popular works. I. Title.
QP376.H68   2004
153—dc22
                                        2003026903

Edited by Barbara Kiser • Text design by Paul Saunders
Cover design by Mike Stromberg

Printed in the United States of America

10 9 8 7 6 5 4 3 2 1

CONTENTS

Foreword   xi

Acknowledgments   xiv

Guide to Abbreviations and Measures   xv

A Note on Notes, Recommended Reading, and Resources   xv

Part 1—FOOD FOR THOUGHT   1

1. You Think What You Eat   2
2. The Five Essential Brain Booster Foods—Check Yourself Out   8
3. Complex Carbohydrates—The Best Brain Food   14
4. Smart Fats—The Architects of Higher Intelligence   22
5. Phospholipids—Your Memory's Best Friends   33
6. Amino Acids—The Alphabet of Mind and Mood   37
7. Intelligent Nutrients—The Brain's Master Tuners   45

Part 2—PROTECTING YOUR BRAIN   53

8. The Brain Agers—Oxidants, Alcohol, and Stress   54
9. Sugar and Stimulants Make You Stupid   61
10. Avoiding Brain Pollution   68
11. Brain Allergies   77

Part 3—IMPROVING YOUR IQ, MEMORY, AND MOOD   87

12. How to Boost Your Intelligence   88
13. Enhancing Your Memory   93
14. Beating the Blues   105
15. Balancing Out Hormonal Mood Swings   119

16. Unwinding Anxiety with Natural Relaxants   127
17. Solving Sleeping Problems   135

Part 4—WHAT IS MENTAL ILLNESS?   143

18. Understanding Mental Illness   144
19. Getting the Right Diagnosis   150
20. What's Your Problem?   157
21. The Dangers of Drugs and How to Get Off Them   169

Part 5—SOLVING DEPRESSION, MANIC DEPRESSION, AND SCHIZOPHRENIA   177

22. Overcoming Depression   178
23. Mood Swings and Manic Depression   190
24. Demystifying Schizophrenia   200
25. Schizophrenia Can Be Cured   204

Part 6—MENTAL HEALTH IN THE YOUNG   219

26. Learning Difficulties, Dyslexia, and Dyspraxia   220
27. The Attention Deficit Disaster   226
28. Answers for Autism   238
29. The Way Up from Down's Syndrome   250
30. Diet, Crime, and Delinquency   256
31. Beating Addictions   263
32. Overcoming Eating Disorders   272
33. Fits, Convulsions, and Epilepsy   278

Part 7—MENTAL HEALTH IN OLD AGE   285

34. Putting the Brakes on Parkinson's Disease   286
35. Preventing Age-Related Memory Decline   293
36. Say No to Alzheimer's Disease   301
37. Smart Drugs and Hormones   312

Part 8—ACTION PLAN FOR MENTAL HEALTH   **321**

38. Finding Help   322
39. The Brain-Friendly Diet in a Nutshell   326
40. Brain-Friendly Supplements   328

    Last Word   330

REFERENCES AND RESOURCES   **331**

    References   332
    Recommended Reading   356
    Useful Addresses   359

    Index   369

FOREWORD

No one can question the massive adaptive stress all human beings are facing as we enter the twenty-first century. As the pace of life accelerates, with cellphones, email, and instant news, there are a number of big questions at hand. Can we cope? Do we have the brains to adapt? In many cases, the answer is no. Fatigue, anxiety, sleeping problems, mood swings, memory problems, and the blues are the hallmarks of our age. Those even less well adapted become mentally ill. ADHD, autism, schizophrenia, and suicide are all on the increase. How can we stay mentally sharp and happy in our hectic times?

When the needs are very great, the solution may be just around the corner. The needs of the majority, and especially the mentally ill, are enormous—and they are not being met. But the solution is, in fact, already visible and developing rapidly. Patrick Holford, a skillful and insightful writer and nutritionist, has provided the necessary information in this excellent and important book. If the methods he outlines were widely practiced, they would go a long way toward meeting the problems of our modern mental health crises. People suffering from mental illnesses, who today receive too little help, will find this book just what they need to take to their mental health providers to show them highly safe and successful treatments, backed by considerable research.

Recently King County, in the state of Washington, passed legislation making its state institutions accountable for the treatment of the mentally ill. Its new mission is to vastly improve the recovery rates of its patients. This book contains the very information needed to persuade its psychiatrists that only by following orthomolecular or nutritional psychiatry will they be able to reach recovery rates that are greater than 10 percent. Tranquilizer use alone helps well under 10 percent of schizophrenic patients to fully recover.

I have been practicing psychiatry for the past fifty years and have seen it develop from our use of one vitamin, B_3, to treat schizophrenia, to its present state, which is much more comprehensive and applicable to a large variety of psychiatric conditions. My clinical observations fully confirm what Patrick Holford describes so well in this book.

Optimum Nutrition for the Mind fulfills a major modern need for information about the causes, prevention, and treatment of diseases, including psychiatric disorders, which today make up the massive wave of illness that is sweeping the globe. At the same time, "affluent malnutrition" is spreading across all the high-tech nations. Is it a coincidence, or is such malnutrition triggering the massive deterioration in our nations' health?

About half the population of Canada, the United States, and the United Kingdom suffer from one or more degenerative disease such as schizophrenia, the bipolar psychoses, depression, anxiety, Alzheimer's disease, arthritis, diabetes, neurological disease, obesity, immune deficiency, addictions, cancer, cardiovascular disease, and so on. It is difficult to pick up a daily paper without some reference to the serious health crises facing our nations. In some of the wealthiest countries, like the United States and Canada, governments are more and more concerned about the costs of heathcare and disease treatment and are making strenuous but mostly futile efforts to control costs—without any attempt to really reduce them by getting their people well.

We do know what should be done. We must provide information to the public and to the healing professions that will halt the continual spread of disease due to malnutrition. This is another area where Patrick Holford's book will be a key element. As a student and follower of Dr. Carl Pfeiffer, one of the pioneers in nutritional medicine, Holford has followed the development of this new field assiduously, and it shows.

At the beginning of the orthomolecular era it was very difficult for physicians to enter the field. There were a small number of very good books that specialized in certain aspects of the entire program. Some went very heavily into the question of hypoglycemia and carbohydrate metabolism. Some dealt much more with the allergic reactions that can create almost any psychiatric syndrome. Some emphasized the vitamins, some the minerals. But most of the publishers were small, with small advertising budgets, and these books were never promoted very well. Only within the past ten years have we had books that covered the whole field.

This book is one of the better ones because of its wide coverage of every aspect of orthomolecular practice, with descriptions of all the syndromes with which psychiatrists must deal. For interested physicians, this makes it much easier to enter the field, as they can find the information they need in one or two books.

We desperately need doctors to transform their practices as quickly as possible in order to slow the ever-increasing rate of disease development. The curve that relates prevalence of serious chronic illness against time is not linear. It is curvilinear upward, and if unchecked we will see over 75 percent of our populations suffer from one or more serious chronic illnesses in the next decade or two. *Optimum Nutrition for the Mind* gives us a most powerful weapon in our fight against mental disease. It is also essential reading for anyone wanting to stay in top mental health throughout life, free from depression, memory decline, and, even worse, senility.

Abram Hoffer M.D., Ph.D.

Dr. Abram Hoffer, former Director of Psychiatric Research in Saskatchewan, Canada, ran the first ever double-blind controlled trial in the history of psychiatry, in the 1950s, proving the power of vitamins in treating schizophrenia. Even though his ideas were attacked and ridiculed, he has persevered, and now in his eighties, he continues to help hundreds of people with mental health problems get better through optimum nutrition.

ACKNOWLEDGMENTS

This book would not have been possible without the help, support, and research of many people. First, I would like to thank Dr. Abram Hoffer and the late Dr. Carl Pfeiffer with all my heart. I consider these great men my mentors, the first pioneers of a badly needed mental health revolution, from whom I have learned so much about mental health and nutrition. I am indebted to both for their contributions to various chapters of this book, posthumously in the case of Dr. Carl Pfeiffer.

I am also deeply indebted to Shane Heaton, both for his help with the research, editing, and moral support, and for his contributions in Chapters 26, 27, and 28. Many thanks also to Dr. Geoffrey and Lucille Leader for their contributions to Chapter 34 on Parkinson's disease, to Imogen Caterer for her help with Chapters 23, 29, and 33, to Tuula Tuormaa for her help with the sections on allergies, to Dr. Alex Richardson for all her help and invaluable research on essential fats, and to Dr. Hyla Cass for keeping me up to date with new and interesting research. I am also indebted to Sarah Carolides, Amanda Moore, and Carolyn Bird for generously sharing their research, and to the graduates of the Institute for Optimum Nutrition, the front line troops, who are putting this essential knowledge into practice for the benefit of those who suffer from mental health problems. Finally, I would like to thank my staff—Bebe, Cath, and Murali—and my publisher Piatkus, especially Gill, Penny, and Barbara on editorial, as well as Philip, Jana, and Judy for their support, encouragement, and enthusiasm.

Guide to Abbreviations and Measures

Most vitamins are measured in milligrams or micrograms. Vitamins A, D, and E are also measured in international units (IU), a measurement designed to standardize the various forms of these vitamins, which have different potencies.

1 gram (g) = 1,000 milligrams (mg) = 1,000,000 micrograms (mcg)

1 mcg or retinal (1 mcg RE) = 3.3 IU of vitamin A
1 mcg RE of beta-carotene = 6 mcg of beta-carotene
100 IU of vitamin D = 2.5 mcg
100 IU of vitamin E = 67 mg

A Note on Notes, Recommended Reading, and Resources

In each part of the book, you'll find numbered references. These refer to notes gathered in the References section that starts at the back of the book on page 331. The research papers listed here are there for those readers who want to study this subject in depth. I also refer to books and websites that are more oriented to the layperson throughout this book. Details of these can be found in Recommended Reading (page 356) and, Useful Addresses (page 359) at the back of the book. Many of these books and research papers are available at the Institute for Optimum Nutrition library in Putney, London.

PART 1

FOOD FOR THOUGHT

How you think and feel is directly affected by what you eat. This idea may seem strange, yet the fact is that eating the right food has been proven to boost your IQ, improve your mood and emotional stability, sharpen your memory, and keep your mind young. In this part of the book, you will discover the Five Brain Foods that will keep you in tip-top mental health.

Chapter 1

YOU THINK WHAT YOU EAT

How sharp is your mind, how balanced is your mood, how consistent is your energy, how happy are you—and what, if anything, do these qualities have to do with what you eat? These are some of the questions we set out to answer in Britain's biggest-ever health survey, involving 22,000 people and conducted by our website, www.mynutrition.co.uk, in 2001. Here's what we found:

- 76 percent of people are often tired

- 58 percent suffer from mood swings

- 52 percent feel apathetic and unmotivated

- 50 percent suffer from anxiety

- 47 percent have difficulty sleeping

- 43 percent have poor memories or difficulty concentrating

- 42 percent suffer from depression.

Does this sound like anybody you know? Welcome to the twenty-first century. Despite improvements in diet and better standards of living, the average human today is clearly one exhausted creature. What's going on, and what's going wrong?

Our minds and bodies have been shaped over millions of years of evolution. Our species, *Homo sapiens*, learned to adapt to changing climates, to changing food supplies, and to a changing world. But it takes time to adapt, and change can be painful. Right now we have a problem. Humanity is struggling to adapt to life in a phase that makes the Industrial Revolution seem like child's play. Our physical environment is changing, for instance. We have invented some 10 million new chemicals, thousands of which are added to our food, are found in common household products, and are in the water we drink and the air we breathe.

Our psychological environment is changing even faster. This layer of our environment consists of concepts of who we are, who we're with, and what we do. Memories of times and places. Thoughts and feelings. All these make up the fabric of our psychological world. You can't see it or touch it, but it is no less real. We tell the story of our life across a matrix of time and space.

Yet in the last fifty years, our whole experience of time and space has changed fundamentally. What we could do in a week, we can do in a day. The distance we would have covered in a day we can cover in an hour. You want to speak to a friend? Pick up your mobile. You want to send a letter? Write an email and get a reply in ten minutes. You want to go somewhere? Jump on a plane. We no longer live in towns and cities, we live in the world. Global news reaches us in under an hour. We can even fly almost anywhere in a day. Every culture is exposed to every other culture.

But this cross-culturalization is placing untold strains on us, from America to Afghanistan, Africa, and eastern Europe. Many of us are struggling to survive, let alone thrive in the new millennium. Putting the squeeze on time and space isn't making us happy.

The High Cost of Living

So these are exceptionally challenging times. Some of us are rising to the challenge, but most of us are struggling to keep up and are living with tiredness, anxiety, stress, depression, and sleeping problems. Too many people are suffering from mental health problems ranging from attention deficit disorder to Alzheimer's disease, depression, and schizophrenia. In fact, the world over there's been a massive rise in the incidence of mental health problems, especially among young people. Suicide, violence, and depression are on the increase, according to the World Health Organization. Mental health problems, they say, are fast becoming the number one health issue this century, with one in ten people suffering at any point in time, and one in four people suffering at some point in their life.[1]

Having worked with thousands of people with these problems and researched their underlying causes, I've come to the conclusion that most can be prevented, and in many cases reversed, by a fundamentally new approach to mental well-being.

This has nothing to do with today's therapeutic front runners, drugs, or psychotherapy. By "drugs" I include the staggering array we prescribe for ourselves—from caffeine to chocolate. We've all been down this road. Tired? Choose caffeine, sugar, or a cigarette. We drink 1.5 billion caffeinated drinks a week in Britain, including tea, coffee, and cola, and we eat 6 million kilos of sugar and 2 million kilos of chocolate every week. We also smoke 1.5 billion cigarettes in that time. Anxious or depressed? Have a drink. We drink 120 million alcoholic drinks a week—and smoke 10 million cannabis joints. And if things get really bad? Go to the doctor for a prescribed drug. In Britain we're popping 532 million tranquilizers, 463 million sleeping pills, and 823 million antidepressants every year. All of these work to some extent, but at what cost, in terms of side effects and dependence?

Meanwhile, psychotherapy is becoming increasingly popular. More people are now seeking professional help, and more and more frequently, with at least 10 million visits a year. Alternatively, you can do a life-changing course, read a self-help book, or change your state of mind through yoga or meditation. All of these can help, if you've got the time.

But aren't we forgetting something? Any intelligent person can recognize that our diets have changed radically in the last 100 years, along with our environment. When you consider that the body and brain are entirely made from molecules derived from food, air, and water, and that simple molecules like alcohol can fundamentally affect the brain, isn't it unlikely that changes in diet and the environment have had no effect on our mental health?

I believe, and present evidence in this book, that most of us are not achieving our full potential for mental health, happiness, alertness, and clarity because we are not achieving optimum nutrition for the mind. I also believe that a significant proportion of mentally unwell people do not need drugs or do not respond as well as they could to psychotherapy because the primary cause of their problem is neither a lack of drugs, nor only a lack of psychological insight or support, but also a chemical imbalance brought on by years of inadequate nutrition and exposure to pollutants and environmental toxins.

As Einstein said, "The problems we have created cannot be solved at the same level of thinking we were at when we created them." We need a new way of thinking about mental health that includes the role of nutrition and the chemical environment and how these affect the way we think and feel.

Mind and Body Are Not Separate

One of the most limiting concepts in the human sciences is the idea that the mind and the body are separate. Try asking an anatomist, a psychologist, and a biochemist where the mind begins and the body ends. It is a stupid question, and yet that is exactly what modern science has done by separating psychology from anatomy and physiology.

But, it's not just the scientists who live by this false distinction. It's us. When you're having difficulty concentrating, when your mood is low, when you struggle to find a memory, do you consider that you may be poorly nourished? Why not? Every one of these states—your thinking, feeling, mental energy, and focus—happen across a network of interconnecting brain cells, each one of which depends on an optimal supply of nutrients to work efficiently. Consider these experiments:

- We measured the IQ scores of ninety schoolchildren and then gave thirty of them a high-dose multivitamin, thirty a dummy pill and thirty nothing. After eight months we reevaluated their IQ. Only those children on the vitamins had a staggering increase in their non-verbal IQ of over ten points![2] Since our study, published more than a decade ago, fifteen other studies have confirmed that supplements boost children's IQ. The effect is real.

- Dr. Thomas Crook from the Memory Assessment Clinic in Maryland in the United States gave 149 people with age-related memory impairment a daily dose of 300 mg of a nutrient called phosphatidyl serine. When they were tested after twelve weeks, their memory had improved to the level of those twelve years younger.[3]

- Dr. Bernard Rimland from California compared the results of 1,591 hyperactive children treated with drugs to those of 191 hyperactive children given nutritional supplements. The nutritional approach was eighteen times more effective.[4] Yet, despite this, drug prescriptions for children are almost doubling every year.

- Dr. Carl Birmingham from the Eating Disorders Clinic in Vancouver, Canada, gave people with anorexia a zinc supplement or a placebo. Those taking zinc increased their body weight twice as rapidly as those given the dummy pills.[5]

- Dr. Abram Hoffer from Canada has treated 5,000 people diagnosed with schizophrenia with high-dose multinutrients, especially large doses of vitamin B_3 and vitamin C. His published forty-year follow-up reports reveal a 90 percent cure rate—defined as free of symptoms, able to socialize with family and friends, and paying income tax.[6] Despite this lifetime of research and results, Hoffer's approach to schizophrenia has been largely sidelined.

- Dr. Poldinger and colleagues from Basel University in Switzerland gave depressed patients either a state-of-the-art SSRI antidepressant or a nutrient called 5-HTP. 5-HTP outperformed the drug on every measure, resulting in greater improvements in their depression, anxiety, and insomnia, and no side effects.[7] This is in sharp contrast to the estimated one suicide every day caused directly by adverse reactions to this class of antidepressant drug (see Chapter 21).

- Bernard Gesch, director of the charity Natural Justice, gave prison inmates supplements of vitamins, minerals, and essential fats, or placebos, and demonstrated a dramatic 35 percent decrease in aggressive acts only in those taking the supplements.[8]

The evidence is there if you look for it. You can change how you think and feel by changing what you put into your mouth. However you feel now, as you follow the guidelines in this book, you will notice gradual improvements in your mind and mood.

You don't have to be clinically depressed, anxious, unable to concentrate, hyperactive, or losing your memory or your mind to benefit from this book. Optimum nutrition can sharpen up your mood and your mind even if you feel "all right." Feeling just "all right" isn't all right. You should, and can, feel alert, energetic, happy, and unstressed, with a clear mind and a sharp intelligence.

Optimum Nutrition and Psychotherapy Work Wonders

Of course, improving our mental health isn't only about nutrition. While, sadly, most psychotherapists ignore the role of nutrition and the brain's chemistry on how we think and feel, let's not make the same mistake of omission. I believe the solution for the mental health problems that plague our society lies in the combination of optimum nutrition and good psychological support, which includes a place you can call home, being treated with respect and dignity, and counseling.

The combination of optimum nutrition and psychotherapy works wonders for a wide variety of mental health problems, from depression to schizophrenia—and it works much better than drugs. Most of the psychiatrists I work with find that while drugs can be lifesaving in the short-term, they become unnecessary with the right combination of nutrients and psychological support.

We Need a Radical New Approach Based on Science

With mental health problems rising at such a pace, we need a new way of thinking about the state of our minds. As Marcel Proust said, "The real act of discovery consists, not in finding new lands, but in seeing with new eyes." We need to wake up to the fact that changes in nutrition, and chemical imbalances, underlie probably the majority of mental health problems. You can't just psychoanalyze away deficiencies in essential fats, vitamins, minerals, and other key brain nutrients. We must think our way out of the box and wake up to the fact that chemistry directly affects how we think and feel.

This means a new basis for both diagnosing and treating problems, and a new way of living and eating that supports our mental health, rather than eroding it. I believe we already have solutions to most forms of mental illness. We just have to look with new eyes. This book is dedicated to that vision.

In summary, we can now say with confidence that:

- Most people are achieving well below their full potential for intelligence, memory, concentration, emotional balance, and happiness.

- The right combination of nutrients works better than drugs, and without the side effects.

- Psychotherapy works best if you're optimally nourished.

- Most mental health problems can be solved or, at least, considerably relieved with the right nutrition, together with the right psychological support and guidance.

Chapter 2

THE FIVE ESSENTIAL BRAIN BOOSTER FOODS— CHECK YOURSELF OUT

Whether you're in good shape or are currently dealing with a mental health problem, there are five essential foods you need to tune up your brain.

- **Balance your glucose**—it's fuel for the brain.

- **Essential fats**—these keep your brain "well oiled."

- **Phospholipids**—these memory molecules give "oomph" to the brain.

- **Amino acids**—these are the brain's messengers.

- **Intelligent nutrients**—these include vitamins and minerals that "fine tune" your mind.

Knowing a few simple facts about your amazing brain shows you why these foods are so important for your mind. Every day we have around 6,000 thoughts. Most of them are repeats! Every single thought you think is represented by a "ripple" of activity across the network of nerves called your brain.

Here's how it works:

What we call the brain is a network of neurons—special nerve cells that connect to other neurons. You've got 100 billion neurons, each connecting to thousands of others. To get an idea of just how complex that is, let's look at the Amazon rain forest. The Amazon stretches for 2,700,000 square miles and it contains about 100 billion trees. So there are as many cells in our brain as trees in the entire Amazon rainforest, and as many connections as leaves!

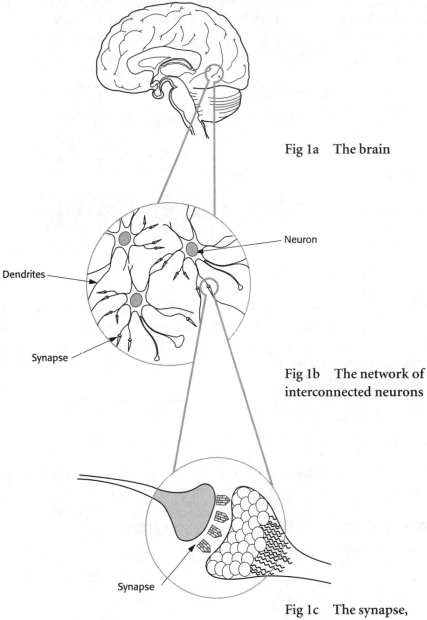

Fig 1a   The brain

Fig 1b   The network of interconnected neurons

Fig 1c   The synapse, where two cells meet

The connections between neurons are called dendrites. Where one dendrite meets another neuron, there's a gap, like the "spark" gap in a spark plug. This gap is called a synapse, and it's across this gap that messages are sent from one neuron to another.

The message is sent from a sending station and received in a receiving station, called a receptor. These sending and receiving stations are built out of **essential fats**, found in fish and seeds; **phospholipids**, present in eggs and organ meats; and **amino acids**, the raw material of protein.

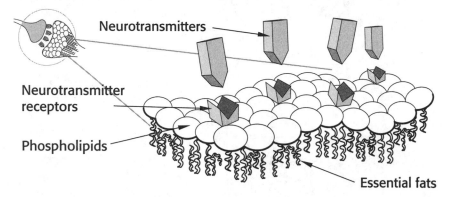

Fig 1d   Close-up of a receptor

The message itself, the neurotransmitter, is in most cases made out of amino acids. Different amino acids make different neurotransmitters. For example, the neurotransmitter serotonin, which keeps you happy, is made from the amino acid tryptophan. adrenaline and dopamine, which keep you motivated, are made from phenylalanine.

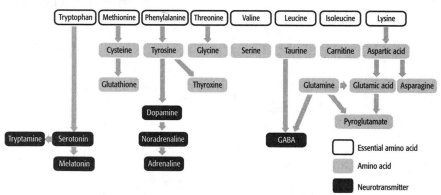

Fig 1e   Neurotransmitters are made from amino acids

Turning an amino acid into a neurotransmitter is no simple job. Enzymes in the brain that depend on **intelligent nutrients** do it. These include vitamins, minerals, and special amino acids.

You are not only what you eat. How you think and feel depends on what you eat! You can check out whether you are getting enough of these essential brain foods using the Brain Food Check below.

Brain Food Check

In each section there are ten questions. Check the box for "yes." If you tick five or more in the "yes" column, the chances are you're not getting enough of this essential brain food factor.

Glucose Check

☐ Do you usually eat white bread, rice, or pasta instead of brown/whole-grain?

☐ Do you crave certain foods such as carbohydrates?

☐ Do you have tea, coffee, sugary foods or drinks, or cigarettes at regular intervals during the day?

☐ Do you usually eat fruit, vegetables, or other carbohydrates without protein foods at the same time?

☐ Do you sometimes skip meals, especially breakfast?

☐ Do you wake unrefreshed or need something to get you going in the morning, like tea, coffee, or a cigarette?

☐ Do you often feel drowsy during the day?

☐ Do you sometimes lose concentration?

☐ Do you get dizzy or irritable if you don't eat often?

☐ Do you avoid exercise because you don't have the energy?

Fat Check

☐ Do you eat oily fish (salmon, trout, sardines, herring, mackerel, or fresh tuna) less than once a week?

☐ Do you eat seeds or their cold-pressed oils less than three times a week?

☐ Do you eat meat or dairy products most days?

☐ Do you eat processed or fried foods (such as ready meals, chips, crisps) three or more times a week?

☐ Do you have dry or rough skin or a tendency to eczema?

☐ Do you have a poor memory or difficulty concentrating?

☐ Do you suffer from PMS or breast tenderness?

☐ Do you suffer from water retention?

☐ Do you suffer from dry, watery, or itchy eyes?

☐ Do you have inflammatory health problems such as arthritis?

Phospholipid Check

☐ Do you eat fish (especially sardines) less than once a week?

☐ Do you eat fewer than three eggs per week?

☐ Do you eat liver, soy/tofu, or nuts less than three times per week?

☐ Do you take less than 5 g of lecithin each day?

☐ Is your memory declining?

☐ Do you sometimes go looking for something and forget what it was you were looking for?

☐ Do you find it hard to do calculations in your head?

☐ Do you sometimes have difficulty concentrating?

☐ Do you have a tendency toward depression?

☐ Are you a "slow learner"?

Amino Acid Check

☐ Do you eat less than one portion of protein-rich foods (meat, dairy, fish, eggs, tofu) each day?

☐ Do you eat fewer than two servings of vegetable sources of protein (beans, lentils, quinoa, seeds, nuts, whole grains, and so on) each day?

☐ If you're vegetarian, do you rarely combine different protein foods such as those mentioned above?

☐ Are you very physically active, or do you work out a lot?

☐ Do you suffer from anxiety, depression, or irritability?

☐ Are you frequently tired or lack motivation?

☐ Do you sometimes lose concentration or have poor memory?

☐ Do you have very low blood pressure?

☐ Do your hair and nails grow slowly?

☐ Are you constantly hungry, and do you frequently get indigestion?

Intelligent Nutrient Check

☐ Do you eat fewer than five servings of fresh fruits and vegetables (excluding potato) every day?

☐ Do you eat fewer than one portion of dark green vegetable a day?

☐ Do you eat fewer than three portions of fresh or dried tropical fruit a week?

☐ Do you eat seeds (such as pumpkin, sunflower, tahini) or unroasted nuts fewer than three times a week?

☐ Are you currently not taking a multivitamin/mineral supplement every day?

☐ Do you usually eat white bread, rice, or pasta instead of brown/whole grain?

☐ Do you consume more than one unit of alcohol most days?

☐ Do you suffer from anxiety, depression, or irritability?

☐ Do you suffer from muscle cramps?

☐ Do you have white marks on more than two fingernails?

The Gut-Brain Connection

It used to be thought that all our thinking is done by neurons in the brain. We now know that the digestive system contains 100 million neurons and produces as many neurotransmitters as the brain. The gut, for example, produces two-thirds of the body's serotonin, the "happy" neurotransmitter. So in essence, you're feeding two brains. Every time you eat something, it sends signals to the brain because the gut and the brain are in permanent communication. This is why the right foods can make you happy, and the wrong foods can make you feel anxious or depressed.

The following five chapters tell you how to feed your brain the right food to make it sing!

Chapter 3

COMPLEX CARBOHYDRATES— THE BEST BRAIN FOOD

The most important nutrient of all for the brain and nervous system is glucose, the fuel they run on. We humans are solar-powered. We use plants to collect the sun's energy for us in the form of glucose. The plants absorb hydrogen and oxygen (H_2O—water) from the soil, and carbon and oxygen (CO_2— carbon dioxide) from the air, and combine these atoms together using the sun's energy to make carbohydrate (COH).

We then digest the carbohydrate down into glucose and deliver this into both our brain and body cells. The glucose is then "burned" within our cells, liberating the sun's energy, which is what keeps us alive.

Your brain consumes more glucose than any other organ. In a sedentary day your brain can consume up to 40 percent of all the carbohydrates you eat. That's why you get hungry after exams! Any imbalance in the supply of glucose to the brain may cause you to experience fatigue, irritability, dizziness, insomnia, excessive sweating (especially at night), poor concentration and forgetfulness, excessive thirst, depression and crying spells, digestive disturbances, and blurred vision.

Basically, the more carbohydrates you eat and the more regularly you eat them, the healthier you are and the better your brain works. But it's not quite that simple. Some carbohydrates are better at fueling the body properly than others.

Research at the Massachusetts Institute of Technology found a massive 25 percent difference between the IQ scores of children who were in the top fifth of the population for consumption of refined carbohydrates, compared with children who were in the bottom fifth.[9] So staying away from white bread, processed cereals, and sugar seems to be crucial to having a higher IQ. But that's not all. To maximize mental performance, you need an *even* supply of glucose to the brain. This has been well proven by Professor David Benton at Swansea University, who has found that dips in blood sugar are directly associated with poor attention, poor memory, and aggressive behavior.[10]

So what kind of carbohydrates will fit the bill?

Food for Fuel

Although we can make energy from protein, fat, and carbohydrates, carbohydrate-rich foods are the best kind of fuel. This is because when fat and protein are used to make energy, there is a buildup of toxic substances in the body. Carbohydrates are the only "smokeless" fuel.

But they need to be "slow-releasing," too. Complex carbohydrates like whole grains, vegetables, beans, or lentils, or simpler carbohydrates such as fruit, take longer to digest than refined carbohydrates. So when you eat, say, brown rice, your body does exactly what it's designed to do. It digests it and releases its potential energy steadily and gradually.

Why Refined Is Bad

What's so bad about refined carbohydrates, though? By overprocessing carbohydrates, we are in essence cheating nature by isolating the sweetness in the food and discarding the rest. All forms of concentrated sugar—white sugar, brown sugar, malt, glucose, honey, and syrup—are "fast-releasing" sugars, causing a rapid increase in blood sugar levels. The way the body responds to a sudden onslaught of sugar in the blood is to take it out into the cells. If they don't need more fuel, the sugar is put into storage, first as "glycogen" in muscles and the liver, then as fat. Most concentrated forms of sugar are also devoid of vitamins and minerals, unlike natural sources such as fruit. White sugar has had around 90 percent of its vitamins and minerals removed. Without vitamins and minerals, our metabolism becomes inefficient, contributing to poor energy levels, concentration, and weight control.

Fruit principally contains a simple sugar, fructose. This needs no digesting, so it can enter the bloodstream quickly, like glucose. However, it is classified as "slow-releasing." This is because the body has to convert fructose to glucose, a process that slows down its effect on the body.

Some fruits, such as grapes and dates, contain pure glucose and are therefore faster-releasing. Apples, on the other hand, are mainly fructose and so are slow-releasing. Bananas contain both, and raise blood sugar levels quite speedily. But all fresh fruit contains fiber, which slows down the release of the sugars it contains.

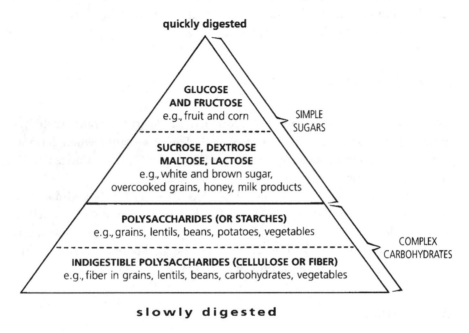

quickly digested

GLUCOSE
AND FRUCTOSE
e.g., fruit and corn   SIMPLE
SUGARS

SUCROSE, DEXTROSE
MALTOSE, LACTOSE
e.g., white and brown sugar,
overcooked grains, honey, milk products

POLYSACCHARIDES (OR STARCHES)
e.g., grains, lentils, beans, potatoes, vegetables   COMPLEX
CARBOHYDRATES

INDIGESTIBLE POLYSACCHARIDES (CELLULOSE OR FIBER)
e.g., fiber in grains, lentils, beans, carbohydrates, vegetables

slowly digested

Fig 2   The sugar family

Refined carbohydrates such as white bread, white rice, or processed cereals have an effect similar to that of refined sugar. The process of refining or even cooking starts to break down complex carbohydrates into simple carbohydrates, in effect predigesting them. When you eat them, you get a rapid increase in blood sugar level and a corresponding surge in energy. The surge, however, is followed by a drop as the body scrambles to balance your blood sugar level.

Foods that Keep Blood Sugar Even

But how do you know which foods are fast- or slow-releasing? The measure of a food's fast- or slow-releasing effect is linked to how high it raises your blood sugar, and this can be worked out on a scale called the glycemic index (or GI for short). This compares the effect on your blood sugar of various foods against pure glucose (see Figure 3). The curve created by glucose is given a value of 100, and other foods are scored in relation to this. So if the effect of eating a food is measured and shown by a curve with half the area of that of glucose, its GI score is 50. The amount of food tested obviously affects how high the blood sugar level will go. Here, we've used a normal serving size of a food to indicate its relative effect on your blood sugar.

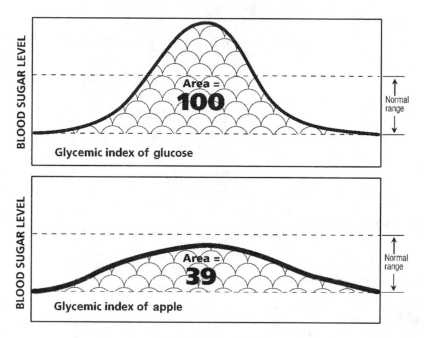

Fig 3   Measuring the glycemic index of a food

The chart below gives the GI score of an average serving of common foods. Check out what you eat for breakfast. If you start your day with raisins and puffed rice cereal, both of which have a high GI score, you're setting yourself up for a rapid burn-out. But kick off with oat flakes, sweetened with a chopped apple—both of which are slow-releasing—and your energy and concentration will last for longer.

Generally, foods with a GI score below 50 are great to include in your diet, while those with a score above 70 should be avoided or mixed with a low-scoring food. Those with a score hovering between 50 and 70 should be eaten infrequently and only with a low-scoring food. For example, bananas are quite high, with a score of 62. Oat flakes and skimmed milk are low, with a score of 49 and 32, respectively. So having a bowl of oat flakes with skimmed milk and half a banana for breakfast would help to keep your blood sugar level on an even keel, while eating cornflakes (scoring 80) with raisins (scoring 64) would be bad news.

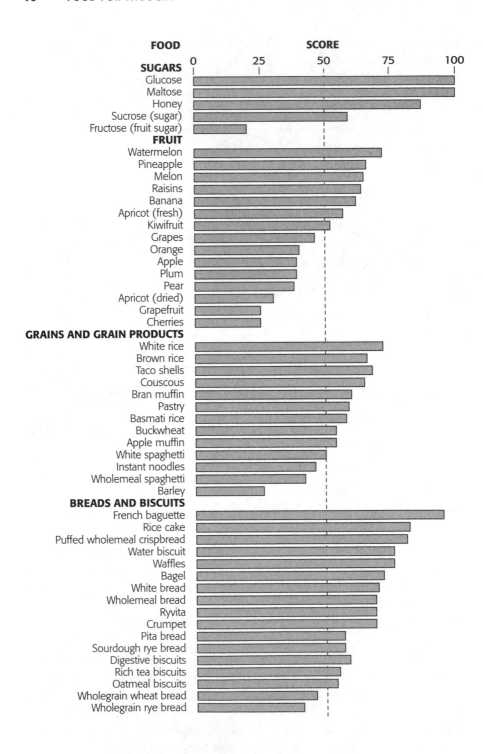

Fig 4   Glycemic index of foods

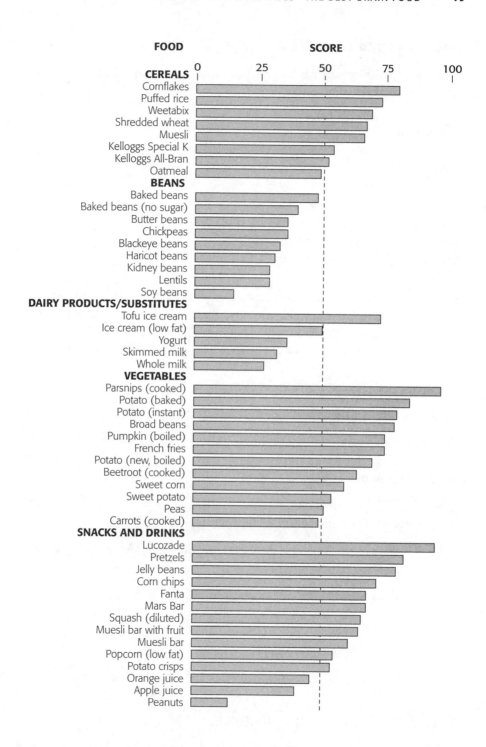

FOOD   **SCORE**

CEREALS
Cornflakes
Puffed rice
Weetabix
Shredded wheat
Muesli
Kelloggs Special K
Kelloggs All-Bran
Oatmeal
BEANS
Baked beans
Baked beans (no sugar)
Butter beans
Chickpeas
Blackeye beans
Haricot beans
Kidney beans
Lentils
Soy beans
DAIRY PRODUCTS/SUBSTITUTES
Tofu ice cream
Ice cream (low fat)
Yogurt
Skimmed milk
Whole milk
VEGETABLES
Parsnips (cooked)
Potato (baked)
Potato (instant)
Broad beans
Pumpkin (boiled)
French fries
Potato (new, boiled)
Beetroot (cooked)
Sweet corn
Sweet potato
Peas
Carrots (cooked)
SNACKS AND DRINKS
Lucozade
Pretzels
Jelly beans
Corn chips
Fanta
Mars Bar
Squash (diluted)
Muesli bar with fruit
Muesli bar
Popcorn (low fat)
Potato crisps
Orange juice
Apple juice
Peanuts

Bad News and Good News Foods

Here's a few examples of what to eat, and what not to eat, to keep your blood sugar level and brain in good balance:

Instead of	Eat
White toast and jam	Brown toast and baked beans
Cornflakes with honey	Oatmeal with raisins
Croissants & baguettes	Wholegrain rye breads
White rice	Wholemeal spaghetti
Chocolate bars	Raw vegetable crudités
Bananas	Apples or oranges
Crackers or rice cakes	Oatcakes

It's best to decrease the sugar content of your diet slowly. Gradually get used to less sweetness. For example, sweeten cereal with fruit. Dilute fruit juices until they're half juice, half water. Avoid foods with added sugar. Limit dried fruit. Eat fast-releasing fruits like bananas with slow-releasing carbohydrates such as oats.

The Protein Connection

You can further balance your blood sugar by eating some protein with carbohydrates. This has been proven to "slow-release" the carbohydrate you are eating even more effectively.

Here's how:

- Eat some seeds or nuts when you have fruit.

- Eat the seeds of the fruit when you eat fruit. For example, eat the apple core or make a watermelon juice by blending the fruit and seeds.

- Add seeds or nuts to your carbohydrate-based breakfast cereal.

- Eat some salmon or chicken with brown basmati rice.

- Eat tofu with wholemeal pasta.

- Have some cottage cheese on oatcakes, or hummus with rye bread.

Stay Away from Sugar Substitutes

While they won't raise your blood sugar levels, most sugar substitutes are not exactly good for you. Aspartame, the most widely used, is particularly bad for those with mental health problems. A study of the effects of aspartame on patients with depression was halted by the Institutional Review Board in the United States because of the severity of reactions in individuals with mood disorder. Sixty-three percent experienced memory loss with aspartame (compared to none on the placebo), 75 percent an increase in nausea, 25 percent an increase in temper, and 37 percent worsened depression. Among the controls who did not have mood disorders, 20 percent experienced memory loss after taking aspartame, and 40 percent experienced nightmares.[11]

In summary, here are some general guidelines to ensure you get enough slow-releasing carbohydrates, the best brain fuel:

- Eat whole foods—whole grains, lentils, beans, nuts, seeds, fresh fruit and vegetables—and avoid refined, white, and overcooked foods.

- Eat five or more servings of fruits and vegetables per day. Choose dark green, leafy, and root vegetables such as watercress, carrots, sweet potatoes, broccoli, Brussels sprouts, spinach, green beans, or peppers, raw or lightly cooked. Choose fresh fruit such as apples, pears, berries, melon, or citrus fruit. Have bananas in moderation. Dilute fruit juices and only eat dried fruits infrequently in small quantities, preferably soaked.

- Eat four or more servings of whole grains such as rice, millet, rye, oats, whole wheat, corn, or quinoa in cereal, breads, and pasta.

- Avoid any form of sugar and foods with added sugar.

- Combine protein foods with carbohydrate foods by eating cereals and fruit with nuts or seeds and ensuring you eat starch foods (potato, bread, pasta, or rice) with fish, lentils, beans, or tofu.

Chapter 4

SMART FATS—THE ARCHITECTS OF HIGHER INTELLIGENCE

Your brain is 60 percent fat, if you take out all the water. This fatty tissue does need replenishing, but it's crucial to know which fats will feed your brain the best.

Some fats are not only good for you, they are absolutely vital for mental health. Not only do you need them to stay free from disease—and depression, dyslexia, attention deficit disorder, fatigue, memory problems, Alzheimer's disease and schizophrenia have all been linked to deficiency—you also need them in optimal amounts if you want to maximize your intelligence.

Our ability to perform in this world depends upon a balance of mental, emotional, and physical intelligence. Mental intelligence we are well aware of, with IQ tests that determine a person's ability to make intellectual connections and deal with complex concepts. But emotional intelligence is no less important. Your "EQ" is a measure of your ability to respond emotionally to situations in an appropriate and sensitive way. If you lose your temper easily and oscillate between depression and hyperactivity, lacking emotional balance and perspective, there's room for improvement—however "bright" you are.

Then there's physical intelligence. Your "PQ" is all about your brain-body coordination. For example, a lot of children diagnosed with attention deficit disorder are clumsy by nature and have trouble with skills such as handwriting, reading, and taking notes in class.

Each type of intelligence is affected by our intake of "essential" fats known as omega-3 and omega-6. Animals low in essential fats perform poorly on mental intelligence tasks, showing poor memory. Children deficient in essential fat levels have more learning difficulties, while children who are breastfed have higher IQs at age eight than bottle-fed babies, which is thought to be due to the higher levels of essential fats in breast milk.

The bottom line is that fat, at least the right kind, is good for you. As well as improving your mental health, the essential fats reduce the risk of cancer, heart disease, allergies, arthritis, eczema, and infections.

Good Fats, Bad Fats

Conclusive research now clearly shows that the amount and type of fat consumed during fetal development, infancy, childhood, adolescence, adulthood, old age—and indeed every day of your life—has a profound effect on how you think and feel. The brain and nervous system are totally dependent on a family of fats. These include:

- Saturated and monounsaturated fat

- Cholesterol

- Omega-3 (polyunsaturated) fat—especially EPA and DHA

- Omega-6 (polyunsaturated) fat—especially GLA and AA.

The first two types can be made in the body. The omega fats, however, have to be obtained through diet.

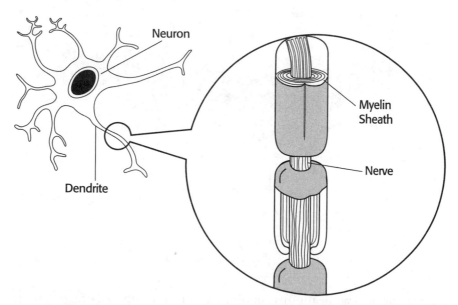

Fig 5 Close-up of a neuron

To understand why these fats are so important, let's take a closer look at a brain cell. If you remember from Chapter 2, the making of intelligence involves the careful connecting up of billions of nerve cells, each one of which links to as many as 20,000 others. The "messengers," neurotransmitters, deliver their messages across connection points called synapses into receptor sites. These receptor sites are contained within the myelin sheath, a membrane surrounding every neuron in the brain. It's a bit like a layer of insulation around an electrical wire and is roughly 75 percent fat. But what kind of fat?

The myelin sheath is made out of phospholipids (more on these in the next chapter) that each have a saturated and unsaturated fatty acid attached (see figure below). The unsaturated fatty acid (bent) is usually an omega-3 or omega-6 fat. It is this balance that seems to be critical for the brain's structure and function. So for brain health, both omega-3 and omega-6 fat families must be present in your diet.

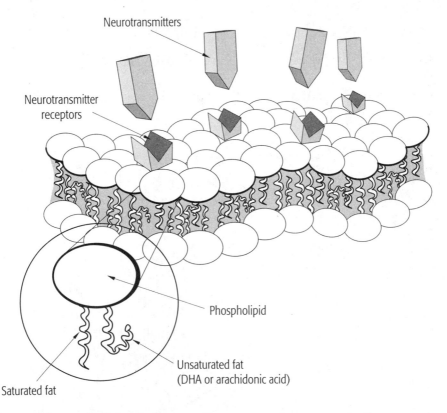

Neurotransmitters

Neurotransmitter receptors

Phospholipid

Unsaturated fat
(DHA or arachidonic acid)

Saturated fat

Fig 6 The myelin sheath surrounding neurons is composed of phospholipids and fats

Are You Fat Deficient?

If you are fat-phobic, you are depriving yourself of essential, health-giving nutrients. The same is true if you eat too much "hard" fat, either from saturated fat found in dairy products or meat, or damaged fats found in processed or fried foods and some margarines. In fact, unless you go out of your way to eat the right kind of fat-rich foods, or supplement essential fats, the chances are you're missing out. Most people in the West are eating too much saturated "killer" fats and are undernourished in essential, healing fats. Check yourself out on this questionnaire, scoring 1 for each "yes" answer.

Essential Fats Check

☐ Do you have difficulty learning?

☐ Do you have a poor memory or difficulty concentrating?

☐ Do you have poor coordination or impaired vision?

☐ Do you have dry, unmanageable hair or dandruff?

☐ Do you have dry or rough skin or a tendency to eczema?

☐ Do you have brittle, easily frayed, or soft nails?

☐ Are you often thirsty?

☐ Do you suffer from PMS or breast tenderness?

☐ Do you suffer from dry, watery, or itchy eyes?

☐ Do you have inflammatory health problems such as arthritis?

☐ Do you have high blood pressure or high blood lipids?

If you have answered "yes" to more than four questions, you are very likely deficient in essential fats. Check that your diet contains enough seeds, seed oils, and fish.

Ultimately, the most precise way to know your fat status is to have a blood test. This gives you a complete breakdown of all the essential fats and what you're lacking. These tests are available through clinical nutritionists.

Fat Figures

How much fat do you need to eat? It is best to consume no more than 20 percent of overall calories as fat. The current average in Britain is around 40 percent. In countries with a low incidence of fat-related diseases, like Japan, Thailand, and the Philippines, people consume only about 15 percent of their total calorie intake as fat. For example, Japanese people eat 40 g of fat a day. British people eat 140 g of fat a day.

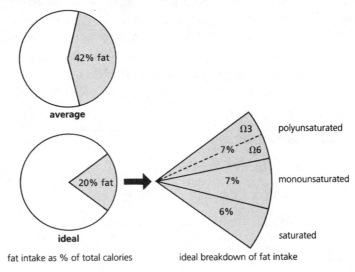

fat intake as % of total calories   ideal breakdown of fat intake

Fig 7   What we eat vs. what we need

Most authorities now agree that, of our total fat intake, no more than one-third should be saturated (hard) fat, and at least one-third should be polyunsaturated oils providing the two essential fat families, omega-3 and omega-6. (More on these in a minute.) These two essential fat families also need to be roughly in balance—in other words, 1:1, which is the ratio our pre-Industrial Revolution ancestors achieved. Nowadays, an average balance is more like 1:20 in favor of omega-6. It may be not just gross deficiency in these fats, but also the gross imbalance between the two types, that is contributing to the mental and other health problems we see today.

Most people are deficient in both omega-6 and omega-3 fats. In addition, a high intake of saturated fats and damaged polyunsaturated fats, known as "trans" fats, stops the body from making good use of the little essential fat the average person does eat in a day.

Fantastic Fats: The Essential Omega

By now you'll have gathered how important the omega fat families are to mental and emotional health. Let's delve deeper, first taking a closer look at the essential fats so many of us lack—the omega-3s.

The Omega-3s

Why is the modern-day diet likely to be more deficient in omega-3 fats than in omega-6s? It's all because the grandmother of the omega-3 family, alpha-linolenic acid, and her metabolically active grandchildren EPA (eicosapentaenoic acid) and DHA (docosahexaenoic acid), are more unsaturated and so more prone to damage by cooking, heating, and food processing. In fact, the average person today eats a mere one-sixth of the omega-3 fats found in the diet of people living in 1850. This decline is partly due to food choices, but mainly to food processing.

Omega-3 fats are not only important because they are part of myelin. It's from these fats that the body and brain make **prostaglandins**, extremely active hormonelike substances. More and more functions of prostaglandins are being found every year, but for now we know that they relax blood vessels and so lower blood pressure, help to maintain water balance in the body, boost immunity, decrease inflammation and pain, and help insulin to work—which is good for blood sugar balance. In the brain they regulate the release and performance of neurotransmitters, and low levels are known to be involved in various conditions, including depression and schizophrenia. You'll see evidence throughout this book that shows how omega-3 fats improve learning, behavioral problems, attention deficit disorder, depression, and schizophrenia.

As these fats get converted in the body to more "active" substances, they become more unsaturated, and generally the word referring to them gets longer. Take oleic acid—that's one degree of unsaturation. Then there's linoleic—two degrees of unsaturation; linolenic—three degrees; eicosapentaenoic—five degrees; and so on. You can see this increasing complexity as we move up the food chain.

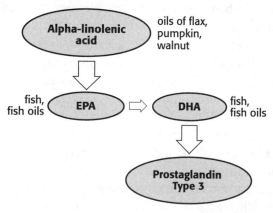

Fig 8   Omega-3 fats

For example, plankton, the staple food of small fish, is rich in alpha-linolenic acid. Carnivorous fish such as mackerel or herring eat the small fish that have converted some of their alpha-linolenic acid to more complex fats. The carnivorous fish continue the conversion. Seals eat them and have the highest EPA and DHA concentration, and then the Inuit people eat the seals and benefit from the ready-made meal of EPA and DHA. That's why the Inuit have the lowest risk of heart disease, despite eating a diet high in cholesterol.

The primary source of EPA and DHA is coldwater fish, especially fish that eat fish, namely herring, mackerel, salmon, and tuna. We normally need 300 –400 mg of both DHA and EPA a day, and perhaps double or triple this to correct a problem, for example, a learning difficulty or heart disease. The conversion in the body of alpha-linolenic acid to DHA is not very efficient. For this reason vegetarians rarely have sufficient EPA and DHA levels, unless they eat significant quantities of flaxseeds (also known as linseeds), which are the richest source of alpha-linolenic acid. So during critical periods of development it may be preferable, or essential, to get a direct source of EPA and DHA from fish or an indirect supply by eating flax seeds or flaxseed oil. This would certainly be recommended in order for a pregnant or breast-feeding woman to pass on sufficient EPA and DHA to her child. The World Health Organization now recommends that formulas include these oils, which can then increase blood levels of these vital brain-friendly nutrients.[12] DHA is especially important in pregnancy and infancy because it is literally used to build the brain. One-quarter of the dry weight of the brain is DHA.

The best diet from the point of view of omega-3 fats is a "fishitarian" diet, where you eat fish three times a week, or a seed-eating vegan diet. Not only is it important to eat a direct source of omega-3 fats such as fish or a rich, indirect source such as flaxseeds, but also to eat less saturated and processed fats. Eggs of chickens fed a high omega-3 diet (usually flaxseeds) can also provide significant quantities of omega-3.

An ongoing research program at Hammersmith Hospital in London has identified that the babies of vegan breast-feeding mothers are brainier, probably because their breast milk, compared to infant formula or the breast milk of dairy-eating vegetarians or omnivores, provides more of the essential fatty acids needed for the development of neural membranes. According to Louise Thomas, a member of the Hammersmith team, the balance of saturated vs. polyunsaturated fat in fat tissue could act as a marker for intelligence.[13] Donald Rudin, a doctor and medical researcher, has shown that flax oil can improve the behavior of schizophrenics and juvenile delinquents who fail to respond to counseling.[14] It can also improve visual function, color perception, and mental acuity.

The Omega-6s

The other essential fat family is omega-6. Of all the tissues of the body, the brain has the highest proportion of omega-6 fats.

The grandmother of the omega-6 fat family is linoleic acid. Linoleic acid is converted by the body into gamma-linolenic acid (GLA). Evening primrose oil and borage oil (also known as starflower oil) are the richest known sources of GLA.

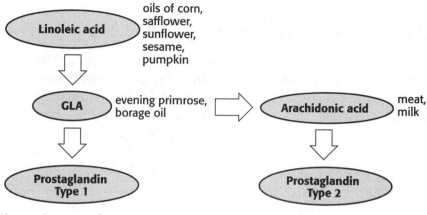

Fig 9   Omega-6 fats

Supplementing GLA, usually from evening primrose oil, has proven effective in a wide variety of mental health problems. Numerous studies have shown that schizophrenics have low levels of omega-6 fats.[15] [16] [17] [18] A large-scale placebo-controlled trial using evening primrose oil showed significant improvement in this debilitating condition.[19] However, results became even more spectacular when vitamins B_6, zinc, niacin, and vitamin C were added, all of which are needed by the body to turn essential fats, both omega-3 *and* 6, into prostaglandins.[20] This produced marked improvements in memory, the symptoms of schizophrenia, and also tardive dyskinesia, a side effect of some medications for psychiatric disorders.

Adding evening primrose oil to the diets of alcoholics going through withdrawal dramatically reduces symptoms, and in the long term improves memory.[21] [22] [23] [24] [25] Due to its reported effects on memory, evening primrose oil was given to Alzheimer's patients in a controlled trial and once again, highly significant improvements in memory and mental function were found.[26] Evening primrose oil has also been well-proven to reduce premenstrual symptoms.

One omega-6 fat has something of a Jekyll and Hyde nature: arachidonic acid. While there is no question that it is essential for brain function, too much is associated with promoting inflammation. It can be derived either directly from meat or animal produce, or indirectly from linoleic acid or GLA. The latter may be preferable because, as well as producing arachidonic acid, they produce anti-inflammatory substances that balance its inflammatory effects.

In other words, let your body make its own arachidonic acid by eating seeds and their oils, rather than lots of meat and dairy produce.

Where to Find Omega-3 and Omega-6 Fats

As we've seen, the seeds with the highest levels of omega-3 fats are flaxseeds. Hemp and pumpkin seeds are rich sources too. Remember, though, that these have to be converted into EPA and DHA by the body and that fish, especially coldwater fish, are the best *direct* source of these brain boosters. This is why fish-eaters like the Japanese have three times the omega-3 fats in their body fat than the average American. Vegans, who eat more seeds and nuts, have twice the omega-3 fat level in their body fat than the average American.

The best seeds for omega-6 fats are hemp, pumpkin, sunflower, safflower, sesame, and corn. Walnuts, soybeans, and wheatgerm are also rich in omega-6 fats.

Best Foods for Brain Fats

Omega 3	Omega 6
Flax (linseed)	Corn
Hemp	Safflower
Pumpkin	Sunflower
Walnut	Sesame

EPA & DHA	GLA
Salmon	Evening primrose
Mackerel	Borage oil
Herring	Blackcurrant seed
Sardines	
Anchovies	**Arachidonic Acid**
Tuna	Meat
Marine algae	Dairy produce
Eggs	Eggs
	Squid

So what should you eat to get an optimal intake of these essential fats? There are three possibilities: eat seeds and fish; eat seed oils, which are more concentrated in essential fats but don't provide other nutrients such as minerals, which are rich in the whole seeds; or supplement concentrated fish oils and seed oils such as flax, evening primrose, or starflower borage oil.

Seeds and Fish

If you want to do it with seeds, put one measure each of sesame, sunflower, and pumpkin seeds, and three measures of flaxseeds, in a sealed jar. Keep it in the fridge, away from light, heat, and oxygen. Simply adding one heaping tablespoon of these seeds, ground in a coffee grinder, to your breakfast each morning guarantees a good daily intake of essential fatty acids. I'd recommend also eating 100 g of oily fish twice a week.

Seed Oils

If you want to do it with oils, the best place to start is an oil blend that offers a 1:1 ratio of omega-3 and omega-6 fats. You want an oil blend that is cold-pressed, preferably organic and kept refrigerated before you buy it. These are now widely available in health food stores. You need about a teaspoon a day of such an oil and can add it to salads and other foods (without heating) or just take it by itself. Hemp-seed oil is the next best thing. It provides 19 percent alpha-linolenic acid (omega-3), 57 percent linoleic acid and 2 percent GLA (both omega-6).

Essential Fat Supplements

As far as supplements are concerned, for omega-6 your best bet is starflower oil (borage oil) or evening primrose oil. Starflower oil provides more GLA, and you need at least 100 mg of GLA a day. Fish oils are best for omega-3, and you need at least 200 mg of EPA and 200 mg of DHA—or 400 mg of these two combined. So, either supplement one GLA capsule and one fish oil capsule rich in EPA and DHA, or find a supplement that combines EPA, DHA, and GLA, and take two a day.

These levels of essential fats promote brain function and health. These quantities should be doubled if you scored high on the Essential Fats Check (see page 25), until your symptoms go away. (If you have a mental health problem that responds well to essential fats, you may even need more, but this is explained in later chapters.)

In summary, here are some general guidelines to ensure you get enough brain fats:

- Eat seeds and nuts—the best seeds are flax, hemp, pumpkin, sunflower, and sesame. You get more goodness out of them by grinding them first and sprinkling on cereal, soups, and salads.

- Eat coldwater carnivorous fish—a serving of herring, mackerel, salmon, or fresh tuna two or three times a week provides a good source of omega-3 fats.

- Use cold-pressed seed oils—either choose an oil blend or hemp oil for salad dressings and other cold uses, such as drizzling on vegetables instead of butter.

- Minimize your intake of fried food, processed food, and saturated fat from meat and dairy.

- Supplement fish oil for omega-3 fats and starflower or evening primrose oil for omega-6 fats.

In practical terms, you may want to pursue a combined strategy to ensure an optimal intake of brain fats. Here's what I recommend:

A tablespoon of ground seeds	— most days (five out of seven)
Cold-pressed seed oil blend	— in salad dressings and on vegetables
Coldwater carnivorous fish	— twice a week
EPA/DHA/GLA supplement	— once a day

Chapter 5

PHOSPHOLIPIDS—YOUR MEMORY'S BEST FRIENDS

Phospholipids are the "intelligent" fats in your brain. They are the insulation experts, helping make up the myelin that sheathes all nerves and so promoting a smooth run for all the signals in the brain. Not only do phospholipids enhance your mood, mind, and mental performance, they also protect against age-related memory decline and Alzheimer's disease.

There are two kinds of phospholipids—phosphatidyl choline and phosphatidyl serine. Supplementing phosphatidyl choline and phosphatidyl serine has some very positive benefits for your brain. Research on rats at Duke University Medical Center in the United States demonstrated that giving choline during pregnancy creates the equivalent of superbrains in the offspring.

The researchers fed pregnant rats choline halfway through their pregnancies. The infant rats whose mothers were given choline had vastly superior brains with more neuronal connections, and consequently, improved learning ability and better memory recall, all of which persisted into old age. This research showed that giving choline helps restructure the brain for improved performance.[27]

The positive effects of supplementing phosphatidyl serine are equally amazing. In one study, supplementing PS improved the subjects' memories to the level of people twelve years younger. Dr. Thomas Crook from the Memory Assessment Clinic in Bethesda, Maryland, gave 149 people with age-associated memory impairment a daily dose of 300 mg of PS or a placebo. When tested after twelve weeks, the ability of those taking PS to match names to faces (a recognized measure of memory and mental function) had vastly improved.[28]

The Lowdown on Phospholipids

Although your body can make phospholipids, getting some extra from your diet is even better. The richest sources of phospholipids in the average diet are egg yolks and organ meats. Nowadays we eat much less of both than we did a few decades ago. Since egg phobia set in, amid the unfounded fears that dietary cholesterol was the major cause of heart disease, our intake of phospholipids has gone down dramatically. Conversely, the number of people suffering from memory and concentration problems has gone up.

Now you can understand why lions and other animals at the top of the food chain eat the organs and brain first. Foxes are one of the most adaptive of all animals in Britain. Their favorite meal is the heads of chickens. They're not stupid.

Why Eggs are Good for You

But we are, or at least are in danger of becoming so, unless we include phospholipids in our diet. One way to do this is to eat more eggs. But aren't they high in fat and cholesterol? As we learned in the last chapter, essential fats are good for you. The kind of fat in an egg depends on what you feed the chicken. If you feed them a diet rich in omega-3 fats, for example flaxseeds or fishmeal, you get an egg high in omega-3. An egg is as healthy as the chicken that laid it. As long as you don't fry them, eggs are a great brain food, and the richest dietary source of choline.

As for cholesterol, we forget that it is essential for good health. Your brain contains vast amounts of it, and it is used to make the sex hormones estrogen, progesterone, and testosterone. It is simply a myth that eating eggs high in cholesterol gives you heart disease.

Here's one of many studies that prove it. Dr. Alfin-Slater from the University of California gave twenty-five healthy people with normal blood cholesterol levels two eggs per day (in addition to the other cholesterol-rich foods they were already eating as part of their normal diet) for eight weeks. A further twenty-five healthy people were given one extra egg per day for four weeks, then two extra eggs per day for the next four weeks. The results showed no change in blood cholesterol.[29] Other studies show the same thing. Eating eggs neither raises blood cholesterol, nor causes heart disease. A free-range, organic, omega-3-rich egg is a superfood, especially if you don't fry it.

Lecithin Is a Direct Source of Phospholipids

Lecithin is the best source of phospholipids and is widely available in health food shops, sold either as lecithin granules or capsules. "Lecithin is practically a wonder drug as far as cognitive impairment is concerned," says Dr. Dharma Singh Khalsa, author of *Brain Longevity* and an expert in nutrition and its role in enhancing memory. The ideal daily intake to keep your brain in top shape is 5 g of lecithin, or half this if you take "high PC" (phosphatidyl choline) lecithin. The easiest and cheapest way to take this is to add a tablespoon of lecithin, or a heaping teaspoon of high-PC lecithin, to your cereal in the morning. Or you can take lecithin supplements. Most capsules provide 1200 mg, so you would need four a day. In case you were wondering, lecithin doesn't make you fat. In fact, quite the opposite: It helps the body digest fat.

While an optimal intake of phospholipids helps your brain sing by improving the insulation around nerves, choline and serine are also brain nutrients in their own right.

Choline: Memories Are Made of This

Acetylcholine, the memory neurotransmitter, is made directly from choline. A deficiency in it is probably the single most common cause for declining memory. Fish, especially sardines, are rich in it, hence the old wives' tale of fish being good for the brain. Eggs are also a major source of choline, followed by liver, soybeans, peanuts, and other nuts.

Supplementing choline not only makes more acetylcholine,[30] the memory neurotransmitter, it is also a vital building material for nerve cells and the receptor sites for neurotransmitters. According to Professor Wurtman from the Massachusetts Institute of Technology, if your choline levels are depleted, your body grabs the choline that you need to build your nerve cells to make more acetylcholine.[31] So Wurtman believes that providing the brain with enough of this smart nutrient is essential. Phosphatidyl choline, nicknamed PC, which is what you get in eggs and lecithin, is the most usable form of this vital brain nutrient. There's a side benefit too—choline improves liver function.[32]

PS: Don't Forget the Phosphatidyl Serine

Nicknamed PS, phosphatidyl serine is equally important for maintaining and promoting your memory. Known as the memory molecule, PS is a smart nutrient that can genuinely boost your brain power. While the body can make its own PS, we rely on receiving some directly from our diet, which makes PS a semiessential nutrient. The trouble is that modern diets are deficient in PS—unless you happen to eat a lot of organ meats, in which case you may take in 50 mg a day. A vegetarian diet is unlikely to achieve even 10 mg a day. Supplementing 100–300 mg a day can make a real difference.

The ability of PS to "roll back the clock" in those with age-related memory decline has also been observed in numerous animal trials.[33] Other studies with humans have found that PS supplementation can also benefit those with only mild memory impairment,[34] and in addition to improving memory can alleviate depressive symptoms and seasonal affective disorder (SAD).[35][36]

The secret to the memory-boosting properties of PS is probably due to its ability to help brain cells communicate, as it is a vital part of the structure of the brain's receptor sites.

In summary, here are some general guidelines to help ensure you have an optimal intake of phospholipids, the memory molecules:

- Add a tablespoon of lecithin granules or a heaping teaspoon of high-PC lecithin to your cereal every day.

- Or eat an egg—preferably free-range, organic, and high in omega-3s.

- Supplement a brain-food formula providing phosphatidyl choline and phosphatidyl serine.

Chapter 6

Amino Acids—The Alphabet of Mind and Mood

Phospholipids improve the brain's hearing, so to speak, by keeping neurons' receptor sites in good health. Amino acids, which are the building blocks of protein, improve the brain's talking. The words the brain uses to send messages from one cell to another are called **neurotransmitters**, and the letters they are built from are amino acids.

Deficiency in amino acids isn't at all uncommon and can give rise to depression, apathy and lack of motivation, an inability to relax, and poor memory and concentration. Supplementing amino acids has been proven to correct all these problems. For example, a form of the amino acid tryptophan has proven more effective in double-blind trials than the best antidepressant drugs.[37] The amino acid tyrosine improves mental and physical performance under stress better than coffee.[38] The amino acid GABA is highly effective against anxiety.[39]

But to understand why amino acids are your brain's best friends, we need to explore what neurotransmitters actually do.

There are hundreds of different kinds of neurotransmitters in the brain and body, but here are the main players:

- **Adrenaline, noradrenaline, and dopamine** make you feel good, stimulating you, motivating you, and helping you deal with stress.

- **GABA** counteracts these stimulating neurotransmitters, relaxing you and calming you down after stress.

- **Serotonin** keeps you happy, improving your mood and banishing the blues.

- **Acetylcholine** keeps your brain sharp, improving memory and mental alertness.

- **Tryptamines** keep you connected. For example, melatonin keeps you in sync with day and night and the seasons.

There are many other substances in the brain that act much like neurotransmitters, such as endorphins, which give you a sense of euphoria. But these are the big five—the key players in the orchestra of your brain. Your mood, your memory and your mental alertness are all affected by the activity of different kinds of neurotransmitters. If serotonin is up, for example, you are likely to be happy; if dopamine and adrenaline are down, you are likely to feel unmotivated and tired. Having the right balance of these key neurotransmitters is a must if you want to be in tip-top mental health.

How Neurotransmitters Work

Neurotransmitters are released from one neuron and sent across the gap, the synapse, to deliver their messages to the next neuron. Each neurotransmitter only fits into certain receptor sites—the "letter boxes" of the receiving cell. When the message is delivered, an electrical signal passes from one neuron to another.

Once a neurotransmitter has delivered its message, it is released from the receptor site and returns to the synapse. It can be reabsorbed or recycled by the neuron that released it, or it might be broken down and destroyed.

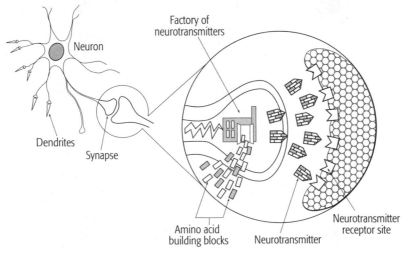

Fig 10   How neurotransmitters work

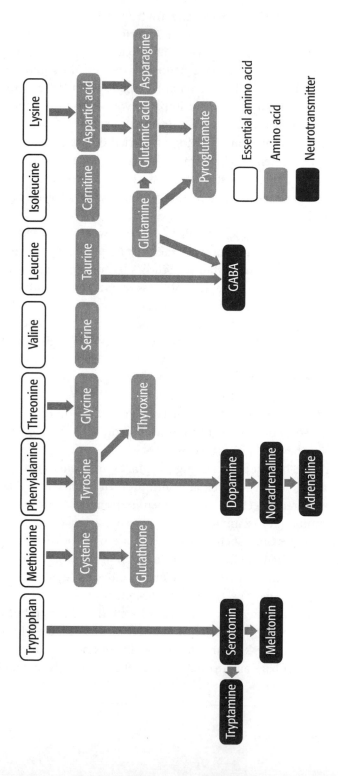

Fig 11 Family tree of key neurotransmitters

These neurotransmitters are made directly from amino acids taken into the body from food. There are eight essential amino acids (see Figure 11). From these eight we can make all the other amino acids our brains and bodies need, and from these we can make neurotransmitters. In Figure 11 you can see how the neurotransmitter *serotonin* is made from the amino acid *tryptophan*. Serotonin is known to help improve your mood, so eating food rich in tryptophan, such as turkey, can improve your mood.

This was shown clearly by an experiment carried out at Oxford University's psychiatry department. Eight women were given a diet devoid of tryptophan. Within eight hours, most of them started to feel more depressed. When tryptophan was added to their diet without their knowledge, their mood improved.[40]

Another example is tyrosine. Tyrosine has been well researched by the military and has been shown to improve mental and physical performance, especially under stressful circumstances. Studies by the United States military found that giving tyrosine to soldiers in stressful conditions of extreme cold, or intense physical activity over prolonged periods of time, shows clear improvements in both mental and physical endurance. More recent research from Holland demonstrates how tyrosine gives you the edge in conditions of stress. Twenty-one cadets were put through a demanding one-week military combat training course. Ten cadets were given a drink containing 2 g of tyrosine a day, while the remaining eleven were given an identical drink without the tyrosine. Those on tyrosine consistently performed better, both in memorizing the task at hand and in tracking the tasks they had performed.[41]

Later on we'll see how supplementing specific amino acids such as these can help solve a wide variety of mental health problems. They work because amino acids have direct effects on neurotransmitters, as do many prescribed drugs. Amphetamines, for example, work by causing an excessive release of adrenaline. Antidepressants such as Prozac work by blocking serotonin reuptake, hence keeping more for a longer duration in the synapse. But these drugs, as we'll see later in Chapter 21, have many undesirable side effects and essentially work against your body's natural design, not with it.

Nutrients such as amino acids work just as well, if not better, but don't have the side effects except in massive doses, because making use of them is part of your brain and body's natural design. So, the best way to tune up your brain is to ensure you have an adequate intake of amino acids in your diet. This means eating protein.

Protein Power

Protein is vital. Since almost all neurotransmitters are made from it, you can influence how you feel by giving yourself the ideal quantity and quality of protein every day. By taking this in an easily absorbed form it can be put to good use by your body and brain. The better the quality and "usability" of the protein you eat, the less you actually need to be optimally nourished.

The quality of a protein is determined by its balance of amino acids. Though there are twenty-three amino acids from which the body can build everything, from a neurotransmitter to a neuron, you actually need to eat only the eight so-called "essential" amino acids because the body can make the rest from these. The better the balance of amino acids—expressed as a unit called an NPU, which stands for "net protein usability"—the more you can make use of the protein.

The chart below shows the top twenty-four individual foods and food combinations in terms of NPUs, or protein quality. Combining legumes with rice, for example, is a great way of increasing protein content. It also shows how much of a food, or food combination, you need to eat to get a 20 g serving of protein. A man needs to eat the equivalent of three to four of these servings, while a woman needs to eat two to three, every day.

A typical day's allotment of protein for a man might therefore include an egg for breakfast (10 g), a 200 g (7 oz) salmon steak for lunch (40 g), and a serving of beans with dinner (20 g).

For a vegetarian, a typical day's worth might be a small tub of yogurt and a heaping tablespoon of seeds on an oat-based cereal for breakfast (20 g), and a 275 g (10 oz) serving of tofu (20 g) and vegetable steam-fry, served with either a cup of quinoa (20 g), or a serving of beans with rice (20 g) as part of dinner. The trick for vegetarians is to eat "seed" foods—that is, foods that would grow if you planted them. These include seeds, nuts, beans, lentils, peas, corn, or the germ of grains such as wheat or oat. "Flower" foods such as broccoli or cauliflower are also relatively rich in protein.

Note that the cup measures indicated are Imperial.

Packed with Protein: The Top 24

Food	Percentage of calories as protein	How much for 20 g (³/₄ oz)	Protein quality (NPU)
Grains/Beans			
Quinoa	16	100 g (3.5 oz)/1 cup dry weight	Excellent
Tofu	40	275 g (10 oz)/1 packet	Reasonable

Food	Percentage of calories as protein	How much for 20 g (¾ oz)	Protein quality (NPU)
Corn	4	500 g (1 lb 2 oz)/3 cups cooked weight	Reasonable
Brown rice	5	400 g (14 oz)/3 cups cooked weight	Excellent
Chickpeas	22	115 g (4 oz)/0.66 cup cooked weight	Reasonable
Lentils	28	85 g (3 oz)/1 cup cooked weight	Reasonable
Fish/meat			
Tuna, canned	61	85 g (3 oz)/1 small tin	Excellent
Cod	60	35 g (1.25 oz)/1 very small piece	Excellent
Salmon	50	100 g (3.5 oz)/1 small piece	Excellent
Sardines	49	100 g (3.5 oz)//1 baked	Excellent
Chicken	63	75 g (2.5 oz)/1 small roasted breast	Excellent
Nuts/seeds			
Sunflower seeds	15	185 g (6.5 oz)/1 cup	Reasonable
Pumpkin seeds	21	75 g (2.5 oz)/ 0.5 cup	Reasonable
Cashew nuts	12	115 g (4 oz)/1 cup	Reasonable
Almonds	13	115 g (4 oz)/1 cup	Reasonable
Eggs/dairy			
Eggs	34	115 g (4 oz)/2 medium	Excellent
Yogurt, natural	22	450 g (1 lb)/3 small pots	Excellent
Cottage cheese	49	125 g (4.5 oz)/1 small pot	Excellent
Vegetables			
Peas, frozen	26	250 g (9 oz)/2 cups	Reasonable
Other beans	20	200 g (7 oz)/2 cups	Reasonable
Broccoli	50	40 g (1.5 oz)/ 0.5 cup	Reasonable
Spinach	49	40 g (1.5 oz)/0.66 cup	Reasonable
Combinations			
Lentils and rice	18	125 g (4.5 oz)/small cup dry weight	Excellent
Beans and rice	15	125 g (4.5 oz)/small cup dry weight	Excellent

Supplementing Amino Acids

While eating protein is the best way to start to get these essential amino acids, supplementing amino acids is the best way to guarantee you are receiving optimal amounts. This is especially relevant to some people who seem to be prone to neurotransmitter deficiencies and more dependent on certain amino acids than others. Some people who are prone to depression, for example, find that supplementing tryptophan or 5-hydroxy-tryptophan (5-HTP) keeps depression at bay.

One of the advantages of supplementing individual amino acids is that they are more easily absorbed this way. The reason for this is that amino acids compete for absorption, so if you supplement one such as tryptophan or 5-HTP, without eating protein-rich food at the same time, you absorb more into the bloodstream. Supplementing with fruit may be even better because the presence of carbohydrates is known to help the absorption of this amino acid.

Supplementing individual amino acids, besides from food or with fruit, is best done as and when you need it. As we investigate nutritional solutions to a variety of mental health problems, I'll be recommending certain individual amino acids to help bring you back into balance.

Another option to ensure a good balance of amino acids is to supplement a powder containing the right balance of "free-form" amino acids. These free- form amino acids don't require digestion in the same way that protein does, so they are easily absorbed. They do, however, compete with each other, so they are not as effective as supplementing an individual amino acid.

A decent protein powder should provide the following key brain-boosting amino acids, and more, in these kinds of amounts in a daily serving:

Glutamine/glutamic acid	2,000 mg
Tyrosine	1,000 mg
GABA/taurine	1,500 mg
Tryptophan	500 mg*
Phenylalanine	1,000 mg

*Please note: in some countries the amount of tryptophan in supplements is restricted; it is banned for sale in the United States.

Note that if you are supplementing free-form amino acids, be careful not to overdo it if you also choose to supplement individual amino acids. Don't exceed my recommendations for each individual amino acid. You'll find these in Part 3.

The protein powder could be added to your breakfast cereal or to a nutritious fruit shake. You can have too much protein, however, so more doesn't always mean better. Once daily protein intake goes above 85 g a day (depending on your exercise level and hence requirement) this can have negative health consequences. Breakdown products of protein, such as ammonia, are toxic to the body and stress the kidneys in their elimination. Too many amino acids means too much acid in the blood. The body neutralizes this by releasing calcium from bone. It is now well established that very high protein diets contribute to osteoporosis. So, make sure you get enough, not too much.

In summary, here are some general guidelines to help ensure you have an optimal intake of amino acids—the alphabet of mind and mood:

- Have three servings of the protein-rich foods shown above a day if you are a man, and two if you are a woman.

- Choose good vegetable protein sources, including beans, lentils, quinoa, tofu (soy), and "seed" vegetables.

- If eating animal protein, choose lean meat or preferably fish, organic whenever possible.

- Consider supplementing some free-form amino acids, or individual amino acids if you have a related mental health problem.

Chapter 7

Intelligent Nutrients— The Brain's Master Tuners

In every great production, there are hundreds of people "behind the scenes" who support the main players. The same is true with your brain. These are the vitamins and minerals. One of their main roles is to help turn glucose into energy, amino acids into neurotransmitters, simple essential fats into more complex fats like GLA or DHA and prostaglandins, and choline and serine into phospholipids. They help build and rebuild the brain and nervous system and keep everything running smoothly. They are your brain's best friends.

Knowing this, we decided to test what would happen to the intelligence of schoolchildren if given an optimal intake of vitamins and minerals. Gwillym Roberts, a schoolteacher and nutritionist from the Institute for Optimum Nutrition, and Professor David Benton, a psychologist from Swansea University, put sixty schoolchildren onto a special multivitamin and mineral supplement designed to ensure an optimal intake of key nutrients.[42] Without their knowledge, half these children were placed on a placebo.

After eight months on the supplements, the nonverbal IQs in those taking the supplements had risen by over 10 points! No changes were seen in those on the placebos. This study, published in the *Lancet* in 1988, has since been proven many times in other studies. Most have used RDA levels of nutrients, much lower than our original study, but still show increases in IQ averaging 4.5 points. But why do vitamins and minerals raise IQ? The answer is that children, and adults, think faster and can concentrate for longer with an optimal intake of vitamins and minerals. (See Chapter 12 for more on this.)

The Ultimate Head Start

The sooner you start optimally nourishing your brain, the better. Of course, that puts the responsibility on the mother while pregnant and breast-feeding. A sixteen-year study by the Medical Research Council shows just how critical optimum nutrition is in the early years. They fed 424 premature babies either a standard or an enriched milk formula containing extra protein, vitamins and minerals. At eighteen months, those fed standard milk "were doing significantly less well" then the others and at eight years old had IQs up to 14 points lower![43]

Every one of the 50 known essential nutrients, with the exception of vitamin D, plays a major role in promoting mental health. Here are some of the key brain nutrients, the symptoms that occur in deficiency, and the best foods to eat to help you get enough.

The B Vitamins

The B-complex group of vitamins are vital for mental health. Deficiency of any one of the eight B vitamins will rapidly affect how you think and feel. This is because they are water soluble and rapidly pass out of the body. So we need a regular intake throughout the day. Also, since the brain uses a very large amount of these nutrients, a short-term deficiency will affect mental abilities. While the deficiency symptoms of B vitamins are well known, we still do not know exactly why many of the symptoms occur. Each B vitamin has so many functions in the brain and nervous system for which there are many logical explanations but few hard proofs. Many people choose to safeguard against deficiency by taking a B-complex supplement or a multivitamin every day.

Vitamin B$_1$ (Thiamine)

Vitamin B$_1$ helps turn glucose, the fuel for the brain, into energy. So, one of the first symptoms of deficiency is mental and physical tiredness. People low in this vitamin have poor attention span and concentration. David Benton, one of the leading experts in nutrition and IQ, has found that low levels of thiamine correlate with poor cognitive function in young adults, and that thiamine supplementation was associated with reports of feeling more clearheaded, composed, and energetic, and having faster reaction times, even in those whose thiamine status, according to the traditional criterion, was adequate.[44][45]

Major Nutrients, Best Foods, and Symptoms of Deficiency

Nutrient	Effects of deficiency	Food sources
Vitamin B_1	Poor concentration and attention	Whole grains, vegetables
Vitamin B_3	Depression, psychosis	Whole grains, vegetables
Vitamin B_5	Poor memory, stress	Whole grains, vegetables
Vitamin B_6	Irritability, poor memory, depression, stress	Whole grains, bananas
Folic Acid	Anxiety, depression, psychosis	Green leafy vegetables
Vitamin B_{12}	Confusion, poor memory, psychosis	Meat, fish, dairy products, eggs
Vitamin C	Depression, psychosis	Vegetables and fresh fruit
Magnesium	Irritability, insomnia, depression	Green vegetables, nuts, seeds
Manganese	Dizziness, convulsions	Nuts, seeds, tropical fruit, tea
Zinc	Confusion, blank mind, depression, loss of appetite, lack of motivation and concentration	Oysters, nuts, seeds, fish

Vitamin B_3 (Niacin)

Of all the nutrients connected with mental health, niacin, or vitamin B_3, is the most famous. Niacin was first discovered because deficiency was identified as the cause for pellagra, a disease in which people developed mental illness, diarrhea, and eczema. Due to the pioneering work of Drs. Abram Hoffer and Humphrey Osmond, niacin has been extensively researched as a treatment for schizophrenia and was found highly effective in acute schizophrenia in doses of several grams (see Chapter 25). The RDA is only 18 mg! Getting enough niacin does more than stop you from developing a psychosis. In one study, 141 mg of niacin every day improved memory by more than 10 percent in both young and old people.[46]

Vitamin B$_5$ (Pantothenic Acid)

Pantothenic acid, also called vitamin B$_5$, is another potent memory booster. It is needed to make both stress hormones and the memory-boosting neurotransmitter, acetylcholine. Supplementing extra B$_5$, particularly with choline, can sharpen your memory (see Chapter 13).

Vitamins B$_6$, B$_{12}$, and Folic Acid

These three, together with niacin, control a critical process in the body called methylation. This is vital in the formation of almost all the neurotransmitters. Methylation abnormalities lie behind many mental health problems, as we'll find out later in this book. A lack of B$_6$, for example, means you won't make serotonin efficiently, which could potentially lead to depression. B$_6$ can help relieve stress too, while stress depletes B$_6$. In one study, the level of psychological distress in HIV-infected people decreased as their B$_6$ status improved through supplementation.[47] So, if you're B$_6$ deficient and stressed, you may be heading for depression.

A lot of us are deficient in B$_6$, as well as in folic acid, also known as folate. In a study at the Kings College Hospital psychiatry department in London, a third of 123 patients were found to have low levels of folic acid. They were given either folic acid or placebos for six months. There was a significant improvement only in the group of patients taking folic acid, which included both depressed and schizophrenic patients.[48]

Folic acid deficiency is very common in patients with mental health conditions. As long ago as 1967 a consultant psychiatrist, Dr. Carney from Lancaster Moor Hospital, recommended that anyone with a mental health problem be checked for folic acid and B$_{12}$ deficiency because they are so often found lacking.[49] Vitamin B$_{12}$ is also vital for a healthy nervous system. Without vitamin B$_{12}$, neither the senses nor the brain can work properly. Deficiency has been shown to be present in as many as half of patients with dementia, with an equivalent number showing an inability to absorb it.[50][51] However, it isn't just older people who need it. Low B$_{12}$ levels cause poor mental performance in adolescents, too.[52]

Getting enough B$_6$, B$_{12}$, and folic acid is absolutely vital in pregnancy, both for protecting against developmental problems such as spina bifida and for general intellectual development. Children born to mothers deficient in folic acid show delayed intellectual development.[53]

These nutrients have so many critical roles to play in the brain and nervous system that ensuring you are getting optimal levels of these nutrients is a prerequisite for mental health.

Best of the Rest

We've seen how vital the Bs are in keeping the brain fit. Let's take a look at the rest of the best brain-boosting nutrients.

Vitamin C

Vitamin C does much more than stop you from getting a cold. It has many roles to play in the brain too, including helping to balance neurotransmitters. While not as spectacular in effect as niacin, vitamin C has been shown to reduce the symptoms of both depression and schizophrenia.[54] A number of studies have shown that people diagnosed with mental illness may have much greater requirements for this vitamin and are frequently deficient.[55] In one study patients only started to excrete the same amount of vitamin C as the control group when given 1 g a day—more than ten times the RDA. Dr. Vandercamp, from the VA Hospital in Michigan, found that schizophrenic patients could metabolize ten times more vitamin C than normal people.[56]

These studies show how unique we all are. Some people need ten times more of a nutrient to stay healthy. Even a so-called well-balanced diet isn't enough for many people. That's why it's well worth supplementing your diet to enhance your mind and body.

Calcium and Magnesium—Nature's Tranquilizers

Popping a mineral may be the last thing you'd think of doing when you're feeling anxious, edgy, and unable to relax. Calcium and magnesium will do the trick, though, by helping to relax nerve and muscle cells.

Muscle cramps are an obvious sign of magnesium deficiency. A lack of either calcium or magnesium can also make you more nervous, irritable, and aggressive. Magnesium has been used successfully to treat autistic and hyperactive children, together with other nutrients. Most of all, it helps you to sleep.

Magnesium has many roles to play in the nervous system, and researchers are starting to look more closely at the possibility that magnesium deficiency may be a cause of mental illness. Ironically, when patients are put on psychotropic drugs, both calcium and magnesium levels tend to decline, which just makes matters worse.[57] Supplementing them helps to reduce the unpleasant side effects of these drugs.

Magnesium is perhaps the second most commonly deficient mineral after zinc (see below). Green, leafy vegetables are rich in it because it is part of the chlorophyll molecule, which makes plants green. So are nuts and seeds, particularly sesame, sunflower, and pumpkin seeds. An ideal intake is probably 500 mg a day, which is almost double what most people achieve. A tablespoon of seeds a day, plus 200 mg in a multimineral, is a good way to ensure you're getting enough.

Manganese—The Forgotten Mineral

With manganese, balance is everything. Both too much and too little of this mineral affect the way our brain functions. Excess, found occasionally in miners inhaling dust from manganese ore, results in psychosis and nervous disorders similar to Parkinson's disease. However, this is rare because manganese is both hard to absorb and readily excreted.

Too little manganese may be a factor in schizophrenia and other psychotic problems. Even as early as 1917, manganese chloride was found to be effective for the treatment of schizophrenia. At Princeton's Brain Bio Center, Dr. Carl Pfeiffer revived the interest in these trace metal and found that almost all patients can benefit from extra manganese and zinc.[58 59] He found that high levels of copper displace manganese and help to produce the continuous and excessive overstimulation that characterizes so many psychotic states. He also found that slight manganese deficiency is associated with insomnia, restlessness, nonproductive activity, and elevated blood pressure. Clearly, one doesn't have to be psychotic to experience these common signs of deficiency. Manganese deficiency can also cause fits and convulsions (see Chapter 33).

As with many trace minerals, the difference between the amount required to prevent deficiency (defined for animals as the level at which growth and reproduction are affected) and the amount needed for optimum health vary considerably. There is no RDA for this essential mineral, although most recommend a daily intake of 2.5–5 mg. Some people need ten times this amount![60]

Manganese is found mainly in seeds, nuts and grains, and tropical fruit, such as bananas and pineapples. Tea is very rich in it. Because it's extremely poorly absorbed and easily excreted from the body, however, it's well worth supplementing 5 mg a day, and 20 mg if you have a mental health problem.

Think Zinc

Zinc is the most commonly deficient mineral, and the most critical nutrient for mental health. The average intake in Britain is 7.5 mg, which is half the RDA of 15 mg. This means that half the British population gets less than half the level of zinc thought to protect against deficiency. Zinc deficiency is associated with schizophrenia, depression, anxiety, anorexia, delinquency, hyperactivity, autism—in short, it's implicated in a huge range of mental health problems.

There are also many circumstances that increase one's need for zinc, quite apart from not getting enough from the diet. These include stress, infections, PMS and other hormone imbalances, using the contraceptive pill, excess copper, frequent alcohol consumption, blood sugar problems, and an inherited extra need for zinc. In the body, it is concentrated in sperm and rapidly lost with excessive ejaculation. Zinc is found in any "seed" food such as nuts and seeds and the germ of grains. Meat and fish are rich sources, but none is richer than oysters: A single oyster can provide as much as 15 mg of zinc! And this is why they're recommended as an aphrodisiac—at least for men.

In summary, here are some general guidelines to help ensure you have an optimal intake of vitamins and minerals to keep your brain in tune:

- Eat at least five, and ideally seven, servings of fresh fruit and vegetables a day.

- Eat nuts and seeds regularly, and choose whole foods, such as whole grains, lentils, beans, and brown rice, rather than refined food.

- Supplement a multivitamin and mineral that gives you at least 25 mg of all the B vitamins, 10 mcg of B_{12}, 100 mcg of folic acid, 200 mg of magnesium, 3 mg of manganese, and 10 mg of zinc.

PART 2

PROTECTING YOUR BRAIN

Optimum brain nutrition isn't just about getting the
right nutrients. It's also about minimizing the
"anti-nutrients." These include oxidants, alcohol,
sugar, stimulants, stress, toxic minerals, and
allergy-provoking foods: the Seven Brain Drainers.

Chapter 8

THE BRAIN AGERS—
OXIDANTS, ALCOHOL, AND STRESS

Maximizing your mental powers isn't just about what you eat. It's also about what you don't eat (and what you do drink and smoke). Your brain and nervous system are made out of essential fat, protein, and phospholipids, all of which can be damaged by oxidants—the body's own nuclear waste—as well as by alcohol and too much stress.

Oxidants: Up in Smoke

First we'll look at one of today's burning issues: oxidants. They're a real hazard in our fume-filled, polluted, fast-food century.

Don't Fry Your Brain

As we saw earlier, the dry matter of the brain is 60 percent fat, and the kind of fat you eat alters the kind of fat in your brain. The worst fats you can eat are called "trans" fats. These damaged fats are found in deep-fried food and foods containing hydrogenated vegetable oils. So, if you want to minimize your exposure to trans fats, limit your intake of fried and especially deep-fried food, and don't buy foods containing hydrogenated fats. Check the list of ingredients in processed foods: If a food has the "H" word in the ingredients, don't put it in your basket!

Why are trans fats so bad for you? After you eat them, they can be taken directly into the brain and appear in the same position as DHA in brain cells, where they mess up thinking processes. They also block the conversion of essential fats into vital brain fats such as GLA, DHA, and prostaglandins. Twice as many trans fats appear in the brains of people deficient in omega-3 fats. So a combined deficiency in omega-3 fats and an excess of trans fats—the hallmark of the French-fry generation—is a bad scenario.

According to recent estimates, the total fat intake of an American man may be 150–250 g a day (70–100 g is the recommended amount), up to a quarter of which comes from trans fats. A serving of French fries or fried fish can each deliver 8 g, a doughnut 12 g, and a bag of chips more than 4 g. All these spell trouble.

As the brain is more than half fat, there is a real danger of these becoming oxidized, or going rancid. Fried food, smoking, and pollution are three main factors that introduce oxidants into the body, which cause a chain reaction of damage to the essential fats attached to phospholipids (see Figure 12) in nerve cell membranes. As you can see in the figure below, vitamin E helps protect your brain from these damaging effects.

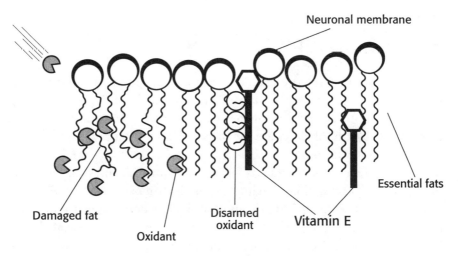

Fig 12   How oxidants damage your brain

Smoking Like Crazy

A single puff of a cigarette contains a trillion oxidants, which rapidly travel into your brain. It also carries high levels of the heavy metal cadmium, the gradual accumulation of which depletes zinc. As discussed in the last chapter, zinc has several crucial roles to play in brain development and maintenance, not least of which are the prevention of oxidation and the synthesis of serotonin and melatonin.[1] Low zinc is implicated in schizophrenia, and the frequency of smoking among schizophrenic patients has been observed to be significantly greater than in the general population.[2]

Researchers at Duke University in the United States have shown how nicotine withdrawal can interfere with serotonin activity and development of the brain, leading to depression in the children of women who smoke during pregnancy or in adolescent smokers.[3] Meanwhile, a study by Dr. Corvin of St. James's Hospital in Dublin found that smoking doubled the incidence of psychotic symptoms among patients with manic depression.[4]

One more thing. Smoking is a known risk factor leading to strokes—the third most common cause of death—where the brain is starved of blood because of damage to the arteries supplying it.[5]

Less avoidable are the oxidants from exhaust fumes, particularly diesel. These have an insidious effect on your body and brain. They also explain why lung cancer incidence among nonsmokers is going up in cities.

It's no surprise to find that the risk for Alzheimer's disease is much higher in smokers and people who eat lots of fried and processed fats. More on this in Chapter 36.

Antioxidants Protect Your Brain

There may not be a lot you can do to avoid many pollutants, but you can protect your brain from the inside. Antioxidants are the antidote to oxidants. If oxidants are the sparks from the fire of anything burnt, be it food, a cigarette, or gas, antioxidants are like fireproof gloves that prevent the sparks from damaging your brain.

Most important for the brain is the fat-based antioxidant, vitamin E. This prevents the chain reactions of damage caused when oxidants enter the brain (see Figure 12). A United States study of 4,809 elderly people found that decreasing serum levels of vitamin E were consistently associated with increasing levels of poor memory.[6] Vitamin E is properly called "d-alpha tocopherol," and its relatives gamma-tocopherol and tocotrienols are also important for the brain. These are only found in the better quality supplements that contain vitamin E together with "mixed tocopherol." They are also present in vitamin E-rich foods, such as seeds, cold-pressed seed oils, and fish.

There are other vital antioxidants. Vitamin C, for example, helps "recycle" vitamin E once it has grabbed hold of an oxidant. A twenty-two-year Swiss study has confirmed that for people aged sixty-five and older, higher ascorbic acid levels are associated with better memory performance.[7] Russell Matthews and colleagues of the Harvard Medical School Neurochemistry

Laboratory in Boston have shown how supplementing coenzyme Q_{10} can increase energy production in the brain and protect it from neurotoxins.[8] Levels of coenzyme Q_{10} are up to 35 percent lower in the brains of schizophrenics than in the rest of the population.[9]

In fact, there are many members of the fire-fighting team. The main players are shown below, in Figure 13, which shows how the body detoxifies an oxidant from fried food.

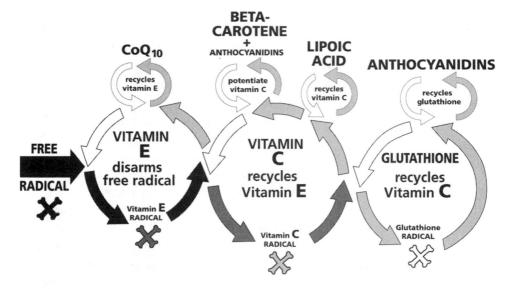

Fig 13 How antioxidants disarm an oxidant or "free radical"

To give yourself maximum protection, it's worth both eating foods high in these antioxidants and supplementing a good all-around antioxidant supplement. These are the best foods for each anti-aging antioxidant:

- **Beta-carotene**—carrots, sweet potatoes, dried apricots, squash, watercress
- **Vitamin C**—broccoli, peppers, kiwifruit, berries, tomatoes, citrus fruit
- **Vitamin E**—seeds and their cold-pressed oils, wheat germ, nuts, beans, fish
- **Selenium**—oysters, Brazil nuts, seeds, molasses, tuna, mushrooms
- **Glutathione**—tuna, beans, nuts, seeds, garlic, onions
- **Anthocyanidins**—berries, cherries, red grapes, beetroot, prunes
- **Lipoic acid**—red meat, potatoes, carrots, yams, beets, spinach
- **Coenzyme Q_{10}**—sardines, mackerel, nuts, seeds, soy oil.

Make sure you also supplement an antioxidant formula containing all these. Eating these antioxidant-rich foods and supplementing antioxidant nutrients is your best protection against Alzheimer's disease and memory decline in old age. Supplementing vitamin E, for example, has been proven to prevent Alzheimer's disease and slow down its progression.

Alcohol Pickles Your Brain

Alcohol is the brain's worst enemy. As soon as you start getting drunk you're damaging your brain. The brain is incapable of detoxifying alcohol, so once the liver's capacity is exceeded, alcohol starts to loosen up and disrupt normal communication signals in the brain, worsening memory. That's one of the reasons we like it—to forget about our worries.

Alcohol worsens your memory by dissolving fatty acids within brain cells and replacing DHA with a poor substitute, DPA. It also blocks the conversion of fats into DHA and prostaglandins. These are the main reasons why alcohol consumption is associated with mental impairment. It also knocks out vitamins, so the more you drink the more nutrients you need.

While alcohol is without question a neurotoxin, evidence of lowered intelligence with moderate alcohol use, meaning one or two drinks a day, is lacking. A study by the National Institute of Public Health in the Netherlands actually found less risk of poor cognitive function among those who had one or two drinks a day, compared to abstainers. The same is not true for high alcohol consumers whose intellectual performance is definitely impaired.

All this begs the question of how much is too much, and why might small amounts of alcohol not affect mental performance? There are two theories. One is that smaller amounts of alcohol, which temporarily promote GABA, the brain's relaxing neurotransmitter, may keep you "chilled." As you'll see later, lower stress levels are good for the brain. The other is that, if you're not getting drunk, the liver is effectively detoxifying alcohol.

Alcohol and Pregnancy: A Bad Mix

Alcohol can cause the most damage in women who have just become pregnant. The time of greatest risk is two days before or after the moment of conception. This is because it can cause gene damage that results in the baby being born with "fetal alcohol syndrome," a condition that affects growth, the nervous system, and intellectual development.

The first caution against alcohol during pregnancy comes in the Bible. In the *Book of Judges* in the Old Testament, the Lord advises Manoah's wife, who had become pregnant, not to "eat of anything that cometh of the vine, neither let her drink strong wine or strong drink." The Royal College of Obstetricians and Gynaecologists are less strict. They say that there is little danger below two units of alcohol a day (two small glasses of wine or one pint of beer), or ten units a week. Not all agree. Professor Derek Bryce-Smith, whose research helped identify the dangers of toxic metal excess and mineral deficiency in relation to miscarriage and birth defect risk, believes "it is absurd to think there is a safe cut-off level." Researchers at San Diego State University, California, have recently confirmed that children prenatally exposed to alcohol can suffer from serious cognitive deficits including learning, memory, and behavioral problems, as well as alcohol-related changes in brain structure.[10]

Personally, I think it is not worth taking the risk. Alcohol is potentially damaging at any time of life, but particularly damaging at the beginning and end.

Why Stress Makes You Forgetful

Have you ever noticed that you forget things when you're stressed? That's because stress increases levels of the hormone cortisol, and cortisol damages your brain. According to research by Professor Robert Sapolsky of Stanford University, two weeks of raised cortisol levels caused by stress leaves dendrites, those connections between brain cells, shriveled up[11]. Using a brain imaging technique, Douglas Bremner of Yale University, Connecticut, has shown that the part of the brain responsible for learning and memory is smaller in patients with post-traumatic stress disorder, and that this correlates with poorer memory.[12] So, if your game plan in life is to work your butt off, make a million, and retire, you may retire with half a brain! That's the bad news.

The good news is that Professor Sapolsky's research showed that dendrites do grow back once cortisol levels decline. In other words, stay cool. Chapter 16 explains how to do that.

The danger of stress-triggered raised cortisol levels over long periods of time should not be underestimated. Numerous studies have linked elevated cortisol levels with impaired memory function.[13] [14] It is almost certainly a major contributor to the increased incidence of memory decline in later years and Alzheimer's disease. Researchers at the La Sapienza University in Rome have shown that cortisol levels are significantly higher in Alzheimer's patients than in controls and correlate with the severity of the disease.[15] Linda Carlson and colleagues at McGill University in Montreal have confirmed that in Alzheimer's patients, the higher the cortisol, the worse their memory.[16] They also found that the higher the levels of another stress hormone, DHEA, the better their memory.

DHEA: The Anti-Aging Adrenal Hormone

One of the more reliable indicators of adrenal exhaustion is a person's level of an adrenal hormone called DHEA, an abbreviation for "dehydro-epiandrosterone." DHEA not only helps control stress, it also maintains proper mineral balance, helps control the production of sex hormones, and builds lean body mass while reducing fat tissue. Increased levels of DHEA, nicknamed the anti-aging hormone, have many benefits associated with youth. Levels start to decline after the age of twenty, especially in people who live in a state of prolonged stress. DHEA levels can be measured in blood and saliva, and low levels can be boosted by DHEA supplementation, together with stress management through diet, exercise, and lifestyle changes. Owen Wolkowitz and colleagues from the University of California, San Francisco, have shown how DHEA supplementation can dramatically improve memory and depression.[17]

Prolonged stress also disturbs blood sugar balance, and as you'll see in the next chapter, this blunts memory and alertness, as well as potentially damaging the brain.

In summary, here are a few simple steps you can take to avoid the brain agers:

- Avoid foods containing hydrogenated fats.

- Limit your intake of fried foods and processed foods.

- Eat foods rich in antioxidants—fruits, vegetables, seeds, and fish.

- Supplement an antioxidant formula containing beta-carotene, vitamin C, vitamin E, selenium, glutathione, anthocyanidins, lipoic acid, and coenzyme Q_{10}.

- Stop smoking.

- Avoid or limit alcohol. If you don't get drunk, you're not damaging your brain.

- Do all you can to reduce your stress level (see Chapter 16).

Chapter 9

SUGAR AND STIMULANTS MAKE YOU STUPID

A s we learned in Chapter 3, complex carbohydrates are the best fuel for the brain, and sugar the worst. There are many reasons for this.

Not So Sweet

First, the more sugar and refined carbohydrates—such as commercial cereals, biscuits, buns, cakes, and sweets—that you eat, the more you become unable to maintain even blood sugar levels. The symptoms of blood sugar problems, technically called disglycemia, are many, and include fatigue, irritability, dizziness, insomnia, excessive sweating (especially at night), poor concentration and forgetfulness, excessive thirst, depression and crying spells, digestive disturbances, and blurred vision. One of the world's experts on blood sugar problems, Professor Gerald Reaven from Stanford University in California, estimates that 25 percent of normal, non-obese people have "insulin resistance." This means their bodies don't respond properly to their own insulin, whose job is to keep the blood sugar level even. In my experience, I would guess that well over 50 percent of people with mental health problems, from depression to schizophrenia, have blood sugar problems as a major underlying cause.

The second reason sugar is so bad for you is that it uses up your body's stores of vitamins and minerals and provides next to none. Every teaspoon of sugar uses up B vitamins, for example, which therefore makes you more deficient. B vitamins are vital for maximizing your mental performance. About

98 percent of the chromium present in sugarcane is lost in turning it into sugar. This mineral is vital for keeping your blood sugar level stable.

The third reason is conclusive evidence that high sugar consumption is linked to poor mental health. Researchers at the Massachusetts Institute of Technology found that the higher the intake of refined carbohydrates, the lower the IQ. In fact, the difference between the high sugar consumers and the low sugar consumers was a staggering twenty-five points![18] Sugar has been implicated in aggressive behavior,[19 20 21 22 23 24] anxiety,[25 26] hyperactivity and attention deficit,[27] depression,[28] eating disorders,[29] fatigue,[30] learning difficulties,[31 32 33 34] and PMS.

Dr. Carl Pfeiffer, founder of Princeton's Brain Bio Center, classified blood sugar problems as one of the five main underlying factors in schizophrenia. You can become antisocial, aggressive, fearful, phobic, psychotic, and suicidal, all by having a simple blood sugar problem. So rule number one if you want to optimize your mental performance or have a mental health problem is: Quit sugar and cut back on refined carbohydrates.

Glucose Damages the Brain

Glucose itself is not toxic, provided you can keep your blood sugar level even. But the minute your blood sugar level goes above the maximum threshold, which is what happens in the severest level of dysglycemia, called diabetes, glucose becomes toxic to the brain. This is why diabetics develop nerve, eye, and brain damage.

The reason this happens is that an excess of glucose, much like oxidants, damages nerve cells and stops them from working properly. This happens because glucose reacts with proteins in the brain and nervous system. This reaction, called glycation, stops the protein from moving freely, and membranes start to get thicker and "gunked up," slowing down brain communication. Excesses of glucose also cause inflammation in the brain, which is the body's way of saying something's wrong.[35] The hallmark of Alzheimer's disease is the presence of inflamed and damaged tissue in the brain, caused, in part, by this process. (More on this in Chapter 36.)

As more and more people are becoming disglycemic, the incidence of related conditions—obesity, age-related memory loss, Alzheimer's disease, heart disease, and diabetes—are also on the increase.

Are You a Stimulant Addict?

Sugar is only one side of the coin, as far as blood sugar problems are concerned. Stimulants and stress are the other. As you can see from the figure below, if your blood sugar level dips, there are two ways to raise it. One is to eat more glucose, and the other is to increase your level of the stress hormones adrenaline and cortisol. There are two ways you can raise adrenaline and cortisol. Consume a stimulant—tea, coffee, chocolate, or cigarettes. Or react stressfully, causing an increase in your own production of adrenaline.

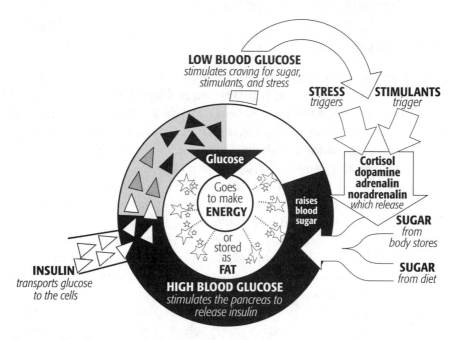

Fig 14   Blood sugar imbalance

Knowing this, you can see how easy it is to get caught up in the vicious cycle of stress, sugar, and stimulants. It will leave you feeling tired, depressed, and stressed much of the time.

Here's how it works. Through excess sugar, stress, and stimulants you lose your blood sugar control and wake up each morning with low blood sugar levels and not enough adrenaline to kickstart your day. So you adopt one of two strategies:

- Either you reluctantly crawl out of bed on remote control and head for the kettle, make yourself a strong cup of tea or coffee, light up a cigarette, or have some fast-releasing sugar in the form of toast, with some sugar on it called jam. Up goes your blood sugar and adrenaline levels, and you start to feel normal.

- Or you lie in bed and start to think about all the things that have gone wrong, could go wrong, will go wrong. You start to worry about everything you've got to do, haven't done, and should have done. About ten minutes of this gets enough adrenaline pumping to get you out of bed.

If this sounds like you, you're caught in that vicious circle, with all its negative effects on your mind and mood.

Caffeine Blunts the Mind

Here's the irony. The reason people get hooked on drinking coffee, particularly in the morning, is that it makes you feel better, more energized, and alert. But, wondered Dr. Peter Rogers, a psychologist at Bristol University, does coffee actually increase your energy and mental performance, or just relieve the symptoms of withdrawal? When he researched this, he found that, after that sacred cup of coffee, coffee drinkers don't feel any better than people who never drink coffee. Coffee drinkers just feel better than they did when they woke up.[36] In other words, drinking coffee relieves the symptoms of withdrawal from coffee. It's addictive.

Coffee is not only addictive, it worsens mental performance. A study published in the *American Journal of Psychiatry* studied 1,500 psychology students and divided them into four categories depending on their coffee intake: abstainers, low consumers (1 cup or equivalent a day), moderate (1–5 cups a day), and high (5 or more cups a day). The moderate and high consumers were found to have higher levels of anxiety and depression than the abstainers, and the high consumers had the greatest incidence of stress-related medical problems, as well as lower academic performance.[37] A number of studies have shown that the ability to remember lists of words is made worse by caffeine. According to one researcher, "Caffeine may have a deleterious effect on the rapid processing of ambiguous or confusing stimuli...." That sounds like a description of modern living!

Exhaustion in a Cup

Caffeine blocks the receptors for a brain chemical called "adenosine," whose function is to stop the release of the motivating neurotransmitters dopamine and adrenaline. With less adenosine activity, levels of dopamine and adrenaline increase, as does alertness and motivation. Peak concentration occurs thirty to sixty minutes after consumption.

The more caffeine you consume, the more your body and brain become insensitive to their own natural stimulants, dopamine and adrenaline. You then need more stimulants to feel normal, and keep pushing the body to produce more dopamine and adrenaline. The net result is adrenal exhaustion— an inability to produce these important chemicals of motivation and communication. Apathy, depression, exhaustion, and an inability to cope set in.

Coffee isn't the only source of caffeine. There's as much in a strong cup of tea as a regular cup of coffee. Caffeine is also the active ingredient in most cola and other energy drinks such as Red Bull, which sold over 100 million cans last year. Chocolate and green tea also contain caffeine, but much less than these drinks.

Caffeine Buzzometer

Here are the caffeine levels in a number of popular products:

Product	Caffeine content
Coca-Cola Classic 350 ml (12 fl oz)	46 mg
Diet Coke 350 ml (12 fl oz)	46 mg
Red Bull	80 mg
Hot cocoa 150 ml (5 fl oz)	10 mg
Coffee, instant 150 ml (5 fl oz)	40–105 mg
Coffee, espresso, cappuccino, latte	30–50 mg
Coffee, filter 150 ml (5 fl oz)	110–150 mg
Coffee, Starbucks (grande)	500 mg
Decaffeinated coffee 150 ml (5 fl oz)	0.3 mg
Tea 150 ml (5 fl oz)	20–100 mg
Green tea (5 fl oz)	20-30 mg
Chocolate cake (1 slice)	20–30 mg
Bittersweet chocolate 28 g (1 oz)	5–35 mg
Pro Plus	50 mg
PEP	30 mg

Kicking the Habit

If you want to be in tip-top mental health, stay away from stimulants. This is doubly important for those with mental health problems because too much caffeine can, in some, produce symptoms that lead to a diagnosis of schizophrenia or mania. This may happen because high caffeine consumers can both become allergic to coffee and unable to detoxify caffeine. The net effect is serious disruption of both mind and mood.[38]

Here's how you can give up caffeine:

Coffee contains three stimulants—caffeine, theobromine and theophylline. Although caffeine is the strongest, theophylline is known to disturb normal sleep patterns, and theobromine has a similar effect to caffeine, although it is present in much smaller amounts in coffee. So decaffeinated coffee isn't exactly stimulant-free. As a nutritionist, I have seen many people cleared of minor health problems such as tiredness and headaches just from cutting out their two or three coffees a day. The best way to find out what effect it has on you is to quit for a trial period of two weeks. You may get withdrawal symptoms for up to three days. These reflect how addicted you've become. After that, if you begin to feel perky and your health improves, that's a good indication that you're better off without coffee. The most popular alternatives are Caro Extra or Bambu (made with roasted chicory and malted barley), dandelion coffee (Symingtons or Lanes), or herb teas.

Tea is the great British addiction. A strong cup of tea contains as much caffeine as a weak cup of coffee and is certainly addictive. Tea also contains tannin, which interferes with the absorption of vital minerals such as iron and zinc. Particularly addictive is Earl Grey tea containing bergamot, itself a stimulant. If you're addicted to tea and can't get going without a "cuppa," it may be time to stop for two weeks and see how you feel. The best-tasting alternatives are Rooibos tea (red bush tea) with milk, and herbal or fruit teas. Drinking very weak tea from time to time is unlikely to be a problem.

Chocolate bars are usually full of sugar. Cocoa, the active ingredient in chocolate, provides significant quantities of the stimulant theobromine, whose action is similar to caffeine's, though not as strong. It also contains small amounts of caffeine. Theobromine is also obtained in cocoa drinks like hot chocolate. As chocolate is high in sugar and stimulants, and delicious as well, it's all too easy to become a chocoholic. The best way to quit the habit is to have one month with NO chocolate. Instead, eat healthy "sweets" from health food shops that are sugar-free and don't contain chocolate. After a month you will have lost the craving.

Cola and "energy" drinks contain anything from 46 to 80 mg of caffeine per can, which is as much as a cup of coffee. In addition, these drinks are often high in sugar and colorings, and their net stimulant effect can be considerable. Check the ingredients list, and stay away from drinks containing caffeine and chemical additives or colorings.

Changing any food habit can be stressful in itself, so it is best not to quit everything in one shot. A good strategy is to avoid something for a month and then see how you feel. One way to greatly reduce the cravings for foods you've got hooked on is by having an excellent diet. Since all stimulants affect blood sugar levels, you can keep yours even by always having something substantial for breakfast, such as an oat-based, not too refined cereal; unsweetened live yogurt with banana, ground sesame seeds and wheatgerm; or an egg. You can snack frequently on fresh fruit. The worst thing you can do is go for hours without eating. Eating a highly alkaline-forming diet can reduce cravings for cigarettes and alcohol. This means eating lots of fresh vegetables and fruit. These high-fiber foods also help to keep your blood sugar levels even.

As we saw in Chapter 7, vitamins and minerals are important too because they help to regulate your blood sugar level, and hence your appetite. They also minimize the withdrawal effects of stimulants and the symptoms of food allergy. The key nutrients are vitamin C, the B complex vitamins, especially vitamin B_6, and the minerals calcium and magnesium. Fresh fruit and vegetables provide significant amounts of vitamin C and B vitamins, while vegetables and seeds, such as sunflower and sesame, are good sources of calcium and magnesium. For maximum effect, however, it is best to supplement these nutrients as well as eating foods rich in them. I recommend a high-strength multivitamin, plus 2,000 mg per day of vitamin C and 200 mcg of chromium.

In summary, here are a few simple steps you can take to balance your blood sugar, as well as following the advice in Chapter 3:

- Avoid sugar and foods containing sugar. This means anything with added glucose, sucrose, and dextrose. Fructose is not so bad, but still best reduced.

- Break your addiction to caffeine by avoiding coffee, tea, and caffeinated drinks for a month, while improving your diet. Once you are no longer craving caffeine, the occasional weak cup of tea or very occasional coffee is not a big deal.

- Break your addiction to chocolate. Once you are no longer craving it, the occasional piece of chocolate is not a problem, but choose the dark, low-sugar kind.

Chapter 10

AVOIDING BRAIN POLLUTION

In the last fifty years alone, 3,500 new chemicals have been added to food. A further 3,000 have been introduced into our homes.[39] Heavy metals like lead and cadmium are so commonplace in our twenty-first century environment that the average person has body levels 700 times higher than those of our ancestors.[40] Most of our food is sprayed with pesticides and herbicides. In fact, up to a gallon of them may have been sprayed on the fruit and vegetables consumed by the average person in a year.

All of these are classified as antinutrients—substances that interfere either with our ability to absorb or to use essential nutrients, or in some cases, promote the loss of essential nutrients from the body.

Nobody really knows how much this modern cocktail of antinutrients messes up our mental health. But we do know that high intakes of lead, cadmium, certain food colorings, and other chemicals can have a disastrous effect on intellectual performance and behavior.

A high intake of antinutrients has been associated with mood swings, poor impulse control and aggressive behavior, poor attention span, depression and apathy, disturbed sleep patterns, and impaired memory and intellectual performance. If these symptoms are present, the nutritional approach to promoting mental health includes testing for high levels of antinutrients and, if found, removing the source and detoxifying the body. Here are some examples of antinutrients, their sources, effects in excess on mental health, and nutritional protectors that help to lower body levels of these unwanted substances.

Antinutrient	Effect	Source	Protector
Lead	Hyperactivity, aggression	Exhaust fumes	Vitamin C, Zinc
Cadmium	Aggression, confusion	Cigarettes	Vitamin C, Zinc
Mercury	Headaches, memory loss	Pesticides, fillings	Selenium
Aluminum	Associated with senility	Cookware, water	Zinc, Magnesium
Copper	Anxiety and phobia	Water	Zinc
Tartrazine	Hyperactivity	Food colorings	Zinc

Anatomy of the Antinutrients

Now let's take a closer look at just what these culprits can do to our mental health.

Lead: One Big Headache

Researchers at the California Institute of Technology have been studying changes in lead concentrations throughout the world—in ocean beds, soil samples, and even snow. Their work shows that lead concentration, even in unpolluted Greenland, has risen between 500 and 1,000 times since prehistoric ages. Comparisons of lead found in humans showed a similar increase. The question we must ask is, what effect is this having on us?

Children are most at risk of lead toxicity. This is especially so up to age twelve, when lead can create irreversible brain damage. The most common symptoms in children are an inability to concentrate, disturbed sleep patterns, uncharacteristic aggressive outbursts, fussiness about food, sinus conditions, and headaches. Adults are more likely to experience a chronic lack of physical and mental energy, together with restlessness, insomnia, irritability, confusion, anxiety, delusions, depression, disturbing dreams, neurological problems, headaches, and convulsions.

Lowering IQ

The first study to shake the status quo on lead toxicity was the Needleman study. Herbert Needleman, an associate professor of child psychiatry, looked at a group of 2,146 children in first and second grade schools in Birmingham, Alabama. He examined lead concentrations in shed baby teeth to obtain more long-term levels than shown by a simple blood test. He then asked the school teachers to rate the behavior of children they had taught for at least two months. This was done using a questionnaire designed to measure the teacher's rating of children for a number of characteristics. He also ran a series of behavioral, intellectual, and physiological tests on each child before dividing the children into six groups according to their lead concentration in teeth.

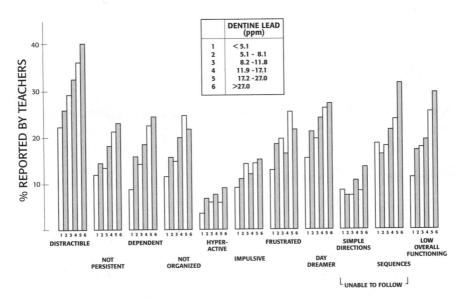

Fig 15   Classroom behavior in relation to dentine lead concentration

As you can see, his results showed a clear relationship between lead concentrations and bad school behavior, as rated by the teachers without any knowledge of the children's lead levels. Needleman also found the average IQ for the high-lead children was 4.5 points below that of the low-lead group. Reaction time (a measure of attention capability) was also consistently worse in those with higher lead levels. EEG readings (which measure brain wave patterns) also showed clear differences based on lead concentration. Perhaps the most interesting result was that none of the high-lead children had an IQ above 125 points (100 is average), compared to 5 percent in the low-lead group.[41]

Richard Lansdown, principal psychologist at the London Hospital for Sick Children, and William Yule, psychologist at the University of London, decided to replicate the essentials of Needleman's study on London children using lead levels in the blood instead of teeth. The 160 children involved had blood lead levels from 7 to 33 micrograms per deciliter, averaging 13.5

mcg/dl (35 mcg/dl is the "safe" level recommended by the Lawther Report *Lead and Health*, 1980). This is similar to other national studies of mean lead levels. Again, the teachers rated the children's behavior, and IQ and other tests were made. Lansdown's results were even more striking than Needleman's. The difference in IQ score between high- and low-lead children was seven IQ points. Once again, none of the high-lead group children had IQs above 125, while in the low-lead group, 5 percent did.[42]

A further study by Gerhard Winneke Ph.D., Director of the Medical Institute of Environmental Hygiene in Düsseldorf, found essentially the same results. He studied 458 children with an average blood level of 14.2 mcg/dl and found an IQ deficit of five to seven points between those with high and low lead levels.[43]

In Britain the blood levels allowed in industrial workers are 80 mcg/dl for men and 40 kmcg/dl for women. In the United States the level is 40 mcg/dl regardless of sex. Yet these landmark studies from the 1980s have shown conclusively that levels of lead as low as 13 mcg/dl can affect behavior and lower intelligence in children. When we consider that the average EEC lead level in the 1980s was 13 mcg/dl, we must come to the appalling conclusion that lead was then damaging the minds of one in two children in the EEC. With lead-free gas now common, the situation is improving. However, this is not the end of the story.

A follow-up study of children with elevated lead levels found, eleven years later, a sevenfold increase in the odds of failure to graduate from high school, lower class standing, greater absenteeism, more reading disabilities, and deficits in vocabulary, fine motor skills, reaction time, and hand-eye coordination.[44] The toxic effects of lead on the brain will be with us for some time yet.

The important lesson from lead is that tiny changes in what we ingest can have vast consequences for our health, which, although invisible to the eye, can and has been proven by research. Banning lead in gas was the first campaign of the Institute for Optimum Nutrition. There are many others yet to be won.

Cadmium: Peril as You Puff

Cadmium is another heavy metal that is associated with disturbed mental performance and increased aggression. The most common source is in cigarettes. Cadmium levels in the blood correlate well to the number of cigarettes smoked. There is also cadmium in car exhaust fumes and small amounts in food, especially if it's refined, since beneficial minerals that act as cadmium protectors are taken out in the refining process.

Aluminum: Toxic Intruder

Aluminum is in widespread use in food packaging and turns up in many common household products. It's in antacids, toothpaste tubes, aluminum foil, pots and pans, and water. There is an association between aluminum and Alzheimer's disease, discussed in Chapter 36. Not all aluminum will enter the body. Only under certain circumstances will aluminum leach, for example, from a pan. Old-fashioned aluminum cookware, if used to heat something acidic like tea, tomatoes, or rhubarb, will leach particles of aluminum into the water. Also, the more zinc deficient you are, the more you absorb.

Mercury: Why Hatters Were Mad

Mercury is the reason nineteenth century hatters went mad. By polishing top hats with mercury, they became overloaded with this toxic element, which disturbs brain function and makes you crazy. Mercury is very toxic indeed, and small amounts reach us from contaminated foods and from tooth fillings. Of particular concern is fish caught in polluted waters. Mercury is used in a number of chemical processes, and accidents and illegal dumping have led to increased mercury levels in some areas, including the English Channel. Fish, especially larger fish like tuna, store the mercury that we then ingest. Fortunately, tuna is also high in selenium, a mercury protector. Mercury has also been used as a constituent of thimerosal, found in diptheria and hepatitis vaccines. This has recently been stopped.

The Copper Controversy

Copper is both an essential mineral and a toxic one. It's rare to be deficient in copper, except in people with diets very high in refined foods, largely because of copper pipes. These leach small amounts of copper into water. However, if you live in a soft-water area or in a house with new copper piping that hasn't yet calcified, you can be exposed to toxic levels of copper. Copper and zinc are enemies. So, if you are zinc deficient, you may not be able to get rid of excess. The birth control pill also raises copper levels.

So it's not so hard to get too much copper, which is associated with anxiety, paranoia, and schizophrenia. Consider this story. I met a principal of a school for "problem" children. We got to talking about the effects of lead and other toxic metals on behavior. We decided to set up a challenge. On return, he'd send me a dozen hair samples from different students, which I would analyze and use to predict their behavior. I ran the hair mineral analyses and found three abnormal results. One had a very high lead level. I predicted aggressive behavior, hyperactivity, and poor attention span. I was right. The child in question was the worst behaved in the school! Two others had high copper levels. I predicted anxiety. They turned out to be a schoolteacher and his wife. They had recently moved into a new house, built on the grounds of the school, with new copper pipes in a soft-water area. The wife had started to become more and more anxious and had been prescribed medication. The husband was apparently free of symptoms.

This story illustrates how easy it is to be copper toxic without knowing it. Copper excess, which can cause extreme fears, paranoia, and hallucinations, is rarely checked or tested in those with mental health problems, despite the fact that is has been often reported in people with schizophrenia.[45] The copper may be the result of drinking water passing through copper pipes, copper pots and pans, the contraceptive pill, and even copper IUDs. Or it can be the result of vitamin C, B$_3$, or zinc deficiency, all of which are zinc antagonists. It also highlights the importance of drinking filtered or bottled water.

How to Handle the Heavies

We've seen the problem. Now, how to fix it? First you need to discover which, if any, toxic minerals are affecting you.

Hair Mineral Analysis: Your Heavy Metal MOT

There's a simple way to find out if these heavy and toxic minerals are affecting you— a hair mineral analysis. By analyzing a small amount of hair, you can be effectively screened, not only for the bad guys such as lead, cadmium, mercury, and aluminum, but also for the good guys such as magnesium, zinc, chromium, manganese, and so on. For around $50 it's well worth it.

One of the leading labs in London is Biolab. Having analyzed some 50,000 samples of hair, blood, and sweat (collected by placing a patch on the back), they found something disturbing.[46] Every one of these toxic minerals accumulates with age, while levels of essential minerals decline. Dr. Stephen Davies, who led this study, concludes that our overexposure to toxic elements and lack of essential elements from poor diets have exceeded the human body's capacity to adapt and successfully detoxify. The lack of sufficient essential elements makes lead, cadmium, mercury, and aluminum even more toxic.[47] The combination of these factors is no doubt lowering our overall intellectual performance and emotional stability.

Detoxifying Your Brain

You can easily test your own mineral levels with a Hair Mineral Analysis. Look in the Resources section on page 364 under "Laboratory Testing." But what do you do if you have raised levels of toxic minerals?

Once we've ingested toxic minerals, they must compete with other minerals for absorption. These minerals are called antagonists and form our first line of defense. Once the mineral has been absorbed, some natural body substances latch on to it and try to take it out of the body. These are called chelators (pronounced key-lay-tors).

It is the latter principle which lies behind the administration of two drugs, penicillamine and EDTA.

Vitamin C vs. Lead

One of the problems with lead poisoning is that once it is in the brain, where most damage is done, it is very difficult to remove. Neither penicillamine nor the more potent EDTA chelating drugs have much effect because neither can readily cross the blood-brain barrier. But vitamin C can. In a study on rats with high concentrations of lead in their brains, administering EDTA resulted in an 8 percent lowering of lead, while vitamin C decreased levels by 22 percent.[48]

Vitamin C is an all-arounder with the ability to latch on to most heavy metals in the blood and escort them out, sacrificing itself in the process. So high metal burdens call for more vitamin C. It is effective for removing lead, arsenic, and cadmium and is a most important part of any detoxification program.

Zinc vs. Lead and Cadmium

Another substance known to lower lead is zinc, which acts as an antagonist to lead by preventing its absorption in the gut. One study by Dr. Carl Pfeiffer at Princeton's Brain Bio Center administered 2,000 mg of vitamin C and 60 mg of zinc (as zinc gluconate) to twenty-two workers at a lead battery plant, all of whom had elevated lead levels. Complete blood tests were taken at the start of the study and after six, twelve, and twenty-four weeks. The average blood lead level at the start was 62.1 mcg/dl. The results showed the steady decrease of lead levels over the twenty-four week period, although the workers were still receiving similar exposure at work. Zinc also lowers body and brain levels of cadmium. Indeed, most of us could benefit from extra zinc.

Calcium vs. Heavy Metals

Calcium is also effective at keeping down lead levels since lead otherwise stores more easily in our bones. Keeping calcium levels topped up pushes lead out and prevents the rapid rise in toxic minerals which, according to research by Dr. Ellen O'Flaherty at the University of Cincinnati College of Medicine, goes up by 15 percent following menopause.[49] Calcium is particularly effective at keeping down cadmium and aluminum levels. Toxic elements such as lead and uranium accumulate in bone tissue over a lifetime of repeated exposure and are released into the bloodstream as bone tissue breaks down. Bone loss can increase dramatically following menopause, which explains the rise in blood lead levels found in O'Flaherty's research.

Selenium vs. Mercury

Selenium is a mercury antagonist and normally protects us from the mercury present in most seafood. Supplementing an extra dose is always a good idea if there are signs of excess mercury. It also has a similar protective effect with arsenic and cadmium, although it is not so pronounced.

Foods that Fight Heavy Metals

In terms of specific foods, there are a few that can help keep your brain clean. Sulphur-containing amino acids are found as the proteins in garlic, onions, and eggs. The specific amino acids are called methionine and cystine and protect against mercury, cadmium, and lead toxicity. Alginic acid in seaweed, and pectin in apples, carrots, and citrus fruits also help chelate and remove heavy metals, thereby promoting your health. One more reason for an apple a day.

Avoid Food Additives

Over 200,000 tons of chemical additives are added to food each year, or approximately ten pounds per person. Some of us, perhaps all of us, aren't coping well with this level of chemical onslaught.

One of these, tartrazine (E102) has been consistently linked to hyperactivity in children, yet it is still added into many popular soft drinks for children in order to color the drink yellow/orange. A closer look at this food chemical reveals something rather sinister.

Dr. Neil Ward from the University of Surrey decided to test what happens to minerals when drinks containing tartrazine were consumed. He gave children either a drink with tartrazine or an identical one without. He found that adding tartrazine to drinks increased the amount of zinc excreted in the urine, perhaps by binding to zinc in the blood and preventing it from being used by the body.[50] In this study, like many others, he also found emotional and behavioral changes in every child who drank the drink containing tartrazine. Four out of the ten children in the study had severe reactions, three developing eczema or asthma within forty-five minutes of ingestion.

Tartrazine is one of the first of over 1,000 chemical food additives to be proven to be an antinutrient. At this point in time we really have no idea what the combined effect of the literally hundreds of man-made chemicals have on health. My advice is to avoid foods with long lists of additives. There are a few, however, that are good for you. These are the colors E101 (vitamin B$_2$), E160 (carotene, vitamin A); the antioxidants E300-304 (vitamin C), E306-309 (tocopherols, like vitamin E); the emulsifier E322 (lecithin); and stabilizers E375 (niacin) and E440 (pectin). Stay away from the rest.

A clinical nutritionist can check for the presence of many of these antinutrients and devise a lifestyle, diet, and supplement program to eliminate this potential contributor to mental instability. The consequence of decreasing the burden of these antinutrients is a greater ability to cope with the unavoidable stresses life gives us to deal with and improve mental performance.

In summary, here are a few simple steps you can take to avoid antinutrients that pollute your brain:

- Avoid foods containing chemical food additives.

- Don't smoke, and stay away from smoky places.

- Eat mineral-rich foods such as seeds and nuts.

- Supplement vitamin C every day, which protects you from toxic minerals.

- If you have a mental health problem, have a Hair Mineral Analysis done, available through clinical nutritionists (see Resources).

Chapter 11

Brain Allergies

"One man's meat is another man's poison." This is many people's experience. Some foods are suitable, some aren't. Some days you feel good, some days you don't. Often, there is the awareness that it may be connected to what you eat, but the riddle isn't always easy to decipher.

The knowledge that allergies to foods and chemicals can adversely affect moods and behavior in susceptible individuals has been known for a very long time. Early reports, as well as the current research, have found that allergies can affect any system of the body, including the central nervous system. They can cause a diverse range of symptoms including fatigue, slowed thought processes, irritability, agitation, aggressive behavior, nervousness, anxiety, depression, schizophrenia, hyperactivity, and varied learning disabilities.[51] [52] [53] [54] [55] [56] [57] [58] Allergic intolerance in susceptible individuals can be caused by a variety of substances, though many people have reactions to common foods and chemicals.

The most convincing evidence for this comes from a well-conducted double-blind, placebo-controlled crossover trial by Dr. Joseph Egger and his team, who studied seventy-six hyperactive children to find out whether diet can contribute to behavioral disorders. The results showed that 79 percent of the children tested reacted adversely to artificial food colorings and preservatives, primarily tartrazine and benzoic acid, which produced a marked deterioration in behavior. However, no child reacted to these alone. In fact, forty-eight different foods were found to produce symptoms among the children tested. For example, 64 percent reacted to cow's milk, 59 percent to chocolate, 49 percent to wheat, 45 percent to oranges, 39 percent to eggs,

32 percent to peanuts, and 16 percent to sugar. Interestingly enough, it was not only the children's behavior that improved after the individual dietary modifications. Most of the associated symptoms also improved considerably, such as headaches, fits, abdominal discomfort, chronic rhinitis, aches in limbs, skin rashes, and mouth ulcers.[59]

Another similar double-blind controlled food trial by Dr. Egger and his team was conducted with eighty-eight children suffering from frequent migraines. As before, most children reacted to several foods and chemicals. However, the following foods and chemicals were found to be most prevalent: cow's milk provoked symptoms in twenty-seven children, egg in twenty-four, chocolate in twenty-two, both oranges and wheat in twenty-one, benzoic acid in fourteen, and tartrazine in twelve. Yet again, after dietary modification, not only did their migraines improve, but also associated physical disorders such as abdominal pain, muscle aches, fits, rhinitis, recurrent mouth ulcers, asthma, eczema, and a variety of behavioral disorders.[60]

Adults are also affected by food and chemical allergies. When Dr. William Philpott, an American allergy expert, examined 250 emotionally disturbed patients for a possible presence of food or chemical allergies, he found that the highest percentage of symptoms occurred in patients diagnosed as psychotic. For example, out of fifty-three patients diagnosed as schizophrenic, 64 percent reacted adversely to wheat, 50 percent to cow's milk, 75 percent to tobacco, and 30 percent to petrochemical hydrocarbons. The emotional symptoms caused by allergic intolerance ranged from mild symptoms such as dizziness, blurred vision, anxiety, depression, tension, hyperactivity, and speech difficulties to severe psychotic symptoms.[61]

These studies are prime examples of how problems created by allergies often produce a multitude of physical and mental symptoms and affect many body systems. They affect not just the central nervous system and brain, but also, usually, the whole body in various ways. Furthermore, these allergies are very specific to the individual, as are the symptoms they create. Therefore, any diagnosis can only be made individually by using an elimination and challenge diet.

Two recent reports estimate that two in every ten people now suffer from allergies.[65] [66] The young developing nervous system is particularly vulnerable to any allergenic or toxic overload, leading frequently to various behavioral disorders such as hyperactivity and learning disabilities. A further survey estimates that at least one child in ten may react adversely to common foods and food additives.[67]

Pinpointing the Troublemakers

Here are a few examples of how an elimination and challenge diet have been used safely and effectively in treating people suffering from various mental health problems.

Study 1

Thirty patients suffering from anxiety, depression, confusion, or difficulty in concentration were tested, using a placebo-controlled trial, to discover whether individual food allergies could really produce mental symptoms in these individuals. The results showed that allergies alone, not placebos, were able to produce the following symptoms: severe depression, nervousness, feeling of anger without a particular cause, loss of motivation, and severe mental blankness. The foods/chemicals that produced the most severe mental reactions were wheat, milk, cane sugar, tobacco smoke, and eggs.[62]

Study 2

Ninety-six patients diagnosed as suffering from alcohol dependence, major depressive disorders, and schizophrenia were compared to sixty-two control sub-jects selected from adult hospital staff members for a possible food or chemical intolerance. The results showed that the group of patients diagnosed as depressives had the highest number of allergies: 80 percent were found to be allergic to barley and 100 percent were allergic to egg white. Over 50 percent of alcoholics tested were found to be allergic to egg white, milk, rye, and barley. Out of the group of people diagnosed as schizophrenics, 80 percent were found to be allergic to both milk and eggs. Only 9 percent of the control group were found to suffer from any allergies.[63]

Study 3

Routinely treated schizophrenics, who on admission were randomly assigned to a diet free of cereal grain and milk while on the locked ward, were discharged from the hospital in about half the time control patients assigned to a high-cereal diet were. Wheat gluten secretly added to the cereal-free diet abolished this effect, suggesting that wheat gluten may be a cause of schizophrenic symptoms in susceptible individuals.[64]

All About Allergies

If allergies are this common, it's vital that we take a closer look at them.

How Food Allergies Affect Your Mind

Most food allergies provoke mental and emotional changes. This is an idea that has been resisted by conventional allergists, but it has been well proven by clinical tests, scientific analysis, and people's experiences.

We've learned that brain cells "communicate" through the action of neurotransmitters. This is the whole foundation of a chemical model of mental health. Yet brain cells are not unique in being able to communicate in this way. Immune cells in the digestive tract, blood, and body tissues also have receptors to many neurotransmitters. Scientists are beginning to discover there's a lot of "talking" going on between the brain and the nervous system, immune system, and endocrine system. In fact, there's a whole new speciality emerging in medicine called "psycho-neuro-immuno-endocrinology," or PNEI for short! One of the most established links is the "talking" between the gut and the brain, via gut hormones and neurotransmitters. In truth, this is a highly fertile ground in medical science today as we gradually learn that the boundaries between mind and body are extremely fuzzy. Simultaneously, we are discovering a much closer connection between allergies and mental health.

To understand this connection, it's necessary to understand what an allergy is in the first place.

What Is an Allergy?

The classic definition of an allergy is "any idiosyncratic reaction where the immune system is clearly involved." The immune system, which is the body's defense system, has the ability to produce "markers" for substances it doesn't like. The classic marker is an antibody called IgE (immunoglobulin type E). These attach themselves to "mast cells" in the body. When the offending food, called an allergen, latches onto its specific IgE antibody, the IgE molecule triggers the mast cell to release granules containing histamine and other chemicals that cause the classic symptoms of allergy—skin rashes, hayfever, rhinitis, sinusitis, asthma, eczema, and severe reactions to, for example, shellfish or peanuts, causing immediate gastrointestinal upsets or swelling in the face or throat. All these reactions are immediate, severe inflammatory reactions.

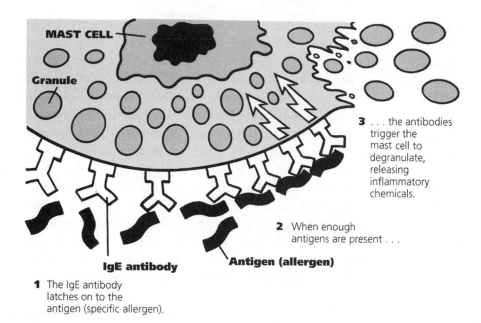

3 . . . the antibodies trigger the mast cell to degranulate, releasing inflammatory chemicals.

2 When enough antigens are present . . .

1 The IgE antibody latches on to the antigen (specific allergen).

Fig 16 How IgE antibodies cause allergic reactions

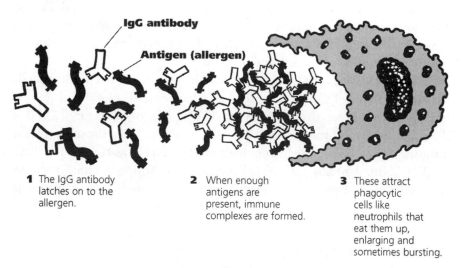

1 The IgG antibody latches on to the allergen.

2 When enough antigens are present, immune complexes are formed.

3 These attract phagocytic cells like neutrophils that eat them up, enlarging and sometimes bursting.

Fig 17 How IgG antibodies cause allergic reactions

The emerging view now is that most allergies and intolerances are not IgE based, but involve another marker, known as IgG. According to Dr. James Braly, medical consultant for York Nutritional Laboratories, which specializes in the IgG ELISA test (see page 361), "Food allergy is not rare, nor are the effects limited to the air passages, the skin, and digestive tract. Most food allergies are delayed reactions, taking anywhere from an hour to three days to show themselves, and are therefore much harder to detect. Delayed food allergy appears to be simply the inability of your digestive tract to prevent large quantities of partially digested and undigested food from entering the bloodstream." This is not a new idea. Since the 1950s, pioneering allergists such as Dr. Theron Randolph, Herbert Rinkel, Dr. Arthur Coca, and, more recently, Dr. William Philpott and Dr. Marshall Mandel, have written about delayed sensitivities causing far-reaching effects on all systems of the body, including the mind.

It is now well established that many, if not the majority, of food intolerances do not produce immediate symptoms, but have a delayed, accumulative effect. This, of course, makes these food intolerances hard to detect by observation alone. I find that the majority of food-sensitive children react to foods after two or more hours. In contrast, IgE reactions are immediate, suggesting that a buildup of IgG antibodies may be a primary factor in food sensitivity.

According to Dr. Jonathan Brostoff, consultant in medical immunology at the Middlesex Hospital Medical School, certain ingested substances can cause the release of histamine, another neurotransmitter now known to have profound effects on mental health, and can also invoke classical allergic symptoms without involving IgE. These substances include lectins (in peanuts), shellfish, tomatoes, pork, alcohol, chocolate, pineapple, papaya, buckwheat, sunflower, mango, and mustard.

Allergic reactions can also occur when there is a substantial production of antibodies (mainly IgG) in response to an allergen in the blood. This results in immune complexes that the body and brain react to (see Figure 17). "It is the sheer weight of numbers that causes a problem," says Brostoff. "These immune complexes are like litter going round in the bloodstream." The litter is cleaned up by cells, principally neutrophils, which act like vacuum cleaners. But if there are too many immune complexes, the neutrophils simply can't keep up.

The Top Ten Allergies

Most food allergies develop in reaction to the protein in food, and particularly foods we eat most frequently. Top of the list is wheat, probably because it contains a substance called gliadin, which irritates the gut wall. Gliadin is allied to gluten, a sticky protein that allows pockets to form when combined with yeast, which is how bread is made. Eating a lot of wheat products isn't good for anyone, especially if you've developed an allergy. The connections between wheat allergy, autism, and schizophrenia are well established (see

Chapters 25 and 28). However, gluten sensitivity can also produce headaches and unsteadiness that go away upon stopping wheat.[68]

Oats contain much less and a different kind of gluten. For this reason, some people who are wheat intolerant are not intolerant to oats.

Dairy produce causes allergic reactions in many people. This includes cheese and yogurt. Some people can tolerate goat's or sheep's milk but not cow's milk. The symptoms are very varied but often include a stuffed nose, frequent colds, bloating and indigestion, "thick" head, fatigue, and headaches. Other foods that can cause allergic reactions include oranges, eggs, other grains apart from wheat, yeast-containing foods, shellfish, nuts, soy, and members of the nightshade family—tomatoes, peppers, potatoes, and aubergine. Some people also develop allergies to tea and coffee, while alcohol, which irritates the gut wall and makes it more leaky, often increases allergic sensitivity to anything eaten.

Testing for Allergies

If you have a history of infantile colic, eczema, asthma, ear infections, hayfever, seasonal allergies, digestive problems (especially bloating), frequent colds, or daily mood swings, or you function better when you don't eat certain foods, you may have a food intolerance.

If you suspect you might have an allergy, there are two courses of action. One is to avoid the suspected substances strictly for two weeks, then reintroduce them in a controlled way, recording your symptoms. This is best done under the guidance of a clinical nutritionist, which is doubly important if you've ever had a severe reaction to food, such as asthma.

The other involves a relatively new blood test, developed over the last eight years, involving a method known as ELISA. This state-of-the-art method of measuring IgG sensitivity will tell you the foods you are currently eating that cause an IgG reaction and how severe that reaction is. Ideally, it is best to also have an IgE ELISA test too. This information can help a clinical nutritionist devise a diet for you that avoids these allergy-provoking foods and replaces them with suitable alternatives. But then what?

Foods that invoke an immediate and pronounced IgE-type reaction may need to be avoided for life. The "memory" of IgE antibodies is certainly long-term, if not forever. In contrast, the cells that produce IgG antibodies have a half-life of six weeks. That means that there are half as many six weeks later. The "memory" of these antibodies is short-term, and within three months there is unlikely to be any residual "memory" of reaction to a food that's been avoided.

Another softer option, after a strict one-month avoidance, is to "rotate" foods so that an IgG-sensitive food is only eaten every four days. This reduces the buildup of allergen-antibody complexes and reduces the chances of symptoms of intolerance. Foods such as wheat and milk that are, by their nature, difficult to digest, are probably best avoided as much as possible for those who show allergic tendencies. This is especially true for wheat, since even IgG sensitivity to wheat appears to be a life-long condition and is possibly genetically predetermined.

Allergy or Indigestion?

Digestive problems are often the underlying factor that leads someone to develop allergies. As you'll see in Chapter 28, most autistic children have digestive problems that cause allergic reactions, which in turn disturb how the brain works. Many allergy sufferers have been found to have low stomach acid, which is essential for digesting food proteins. Dr. James Braly has found zinc deficiency to be extremely common among allergy sufferers. Zinc is not only needed to digest all protein, it's also essential for the production of hydrochloric acid in the stomach. Certain foods, he says, are inherently difficult to digest, the worst being gluten in wheat and casein in dairy products. Wheat and dairy are Britain's top two allergy-provoking foods. He also suspects that many allergy sufferers may have excessively "leaky" digestive tracts, allowing undigested proteins to enter the bloodstream through the gut wall and cause reactions.

So, identifying and avoiding what you react to is one half of the equation. Consumption of alcohol, frequent use of aspirin, deficiency in essential fatty acids, or a gastrointestinal infection or infestation such as candidiasis are all possible contributors to leaky gut syndrome that need to be corrected to reduce intolerance to foods. Frequent use of antibiotics, which wipe out gut bacteria, paving the way for candidiasis, therefore also increases the risk of developing food intolerances.

The emerging view, shared by an increasing number of allergy specialists, is that food sensitivity is a multifactorial phenomenon possibly involving poor nutrition, pollution, digestive problems, and overexposure to certain foods. Removing the foods may help the sufferer recover, but other factors need to be dealt with in order to have a major impact on long-term food intolerance. Due to the complex factors involved in food allergies and intolerance, it is often best to see a clinical nutritionist who can pinpoint the likely culprits from your symptoms and eating patterns, advise you on tests should they prove necessary, and help you correct digestive problems that increase your allergic potential.

In summary, here's how to test for, and reduce, your allergic potential:

- Avoid wheat and dairy products strictly for two weeks and see how you feel. In any case these food groups are best not eaten frequently.

- Improve your digestion by eating plenty of fresh fruit, vegetables, seeds, and fish, which contain essential fats and zinc.

- Keep alcohol, painkillers, and antibiotics to a minimum. These damage the digestive tract.

- If you suspect you've got a food allergy, get yourself tested (see p. 361). A clinical nutritionist can both test what you are allergic to and devise a course of action to reduce your allergic potential.

PART 3

IMPROVING YOUR IQ, MEMORY, AND MOOD

Contrary to popular belief, you can improve your IQ, boost your memory, and enhance your mood at any time of your life. In this part you will find out exactly what you need to do to maximize your mental health and performance throughout your life, stay relaxed, and get a good night's sleep.

Chapter 12

How to Boost
Your Intelligence

It may surprise you to know that you can boost your intelligence, and IQ score, at any age. Some people argue that your real "intelligence"—how smart you are—is innate, something you're born with. But the truth is that your ability to make intelligent decisions depends not only on this aspect of intelligence, but also on the clarity of your mind, how quickly you can think, your attention, how long you can concentrate, and your memory. All of these can be improved with optimum nutrition.

This should not be surprising since the brain, composed of a highly complex network of neurons, is made from what we eat. Thinking is a pattern of activity across this network. The activity, or messengers, are neurotransmitters, which are made from and directly affected by what you eat. When we learn, we actually change the wiring of the brain. When we think, we change the activity of neurotransmitters. This was the logic that made us investigate, in 1986, whether giving a person an optimal intake of nutrients used by the brain and nervous system would improve intellectual performance.

We knew already that a person's nutrient status was associated with intelligence. For instance, in 1960 a study by Dr. A. L. Kubala and colleagues had shown that increased vitamin C status was associated with increased intelligence. Dr. Kubala used IQ as a measure. IQ stands for Intelligence Quotient and is an accepted measure of intelligence, with a score of 100, originally by definition, being average. About 5 percent of people score above 125, and less than 10 percent score below 80, which is considered to be educationally subnormal.

Dr. Kubala divided 351 students into high and low vitamin C groups, depending on the levels in their blood. The students' IQ scores were then measured and found to average 113 and 109, respectively: Those with higher levels of vitamin C in their blood had an average of 4.5 IQ points more.[1]

Gwillym Roberts, a headmaster and researcher at the Institute for Optimum Nutrition, worked out what combination of nutrients would optimally nourish the brain. He then gave these to a pilot group of students, measuring their IQ before and after. Up went their IQ by 10 points.

To test whether these results were valid, Roberts devised a proper "randomized, double-blind, placebo-controlled trial," and, together with David Benton, a psychologist from Swansea University who thought our theory was unlikely but worth testing, ran the trial. We tested a group of sixty children. Without their or our knowledge and at random, we put thirty of them on a special multivitamin and mineral supplement designed to ensure an optimal intake of key nutrients, and the other thirty on an identical placebo. This "double-blind" design meant that neither we nor they could bias the results through our expectations. All children had their IQ scores measured at the start of the trial and then again after eight months.[2]

After eight months on the supplements, the nonverbal IQs in those taking the supplements had risen by an average of over 10 points! Some children were getting more than 20-point improvements in IQ. No changes were seen in those on the placebos, or a control group of students who had not taken any supplements or placebos. The study was published in the *Lancet* medical journal and was the subject of a BBC *Horizon* TV documentary, the day after which every single children's multivitamin in Britain sold out.

This now famous IQ study spawned a dozen similar studies to test if the results were real. The next big study, conducted by Professors Stephen Schoenthaler, John Yudkin, world-famous psychologist Hans Eysenck and Dr. Linus Pauling, involved 615 children given much lower levels of nutrients, at RDA levels. Once again, the results showed that the simple addition of a vitamin and mineral supplement could increase IQ scores by as much as 20 points, with an average increase of at least 4.5 points, this time over three months.[3]

During the press conference revealing the results of this trial, one journalist, referring to those children who had had a 20-point shift in IQ, asked if this could turn a bricklayer into a brain surgeon. The chairman said this was entirely possible. An antagonistic journalist pointed out that the average increase was only 4.5 IQ points and asked what this would do. The spokesman said this would turn them into a journalist!

The truth is that a 4.5 IQ point shift would get many thousands of educationally subnormal children reclassified and returned to "normal" schools. More comprehensive nutritional program have brought several children with IQs in the 40s back into the normal range (see Chapter 26).

But you don't have to be educationally subnormal, nor a child, to benefit. These results have been replicated more than a dozen times (a one-month study at Kings College London,[4] which is too short, showed no effect) and have also been shown in high-IQ kids and in adults,[5] although for reasons yet unknown, more spectacularly in women than men. You do, however, need to be sub-optimally nourished. In other words, once you're getting your ideal intake of nutrients, more won't make you even brighter.

How Do Nutrients Boost IQ?

But how exactly do nutrients increase IQ scores? Wendy Snowden, a researcher from Reading University's psychology department, decided to investigate. Once again, schoolchildren were given supplements or a placebo.[6] The supplemented children showed significant increases in nonverbal IQ scores, but not verbal IQ scores, after ten weeks. A close analysis of performances in the IQ tests showed the same error rate, but the children were able to work faster and attempt more questions after the ten weeks of supplementation. For the verbal IQ test all children completed all questions so there was no room for improvement in work rate. This suggests that the effect of the vitamin and mineral supplements is to increase the speed of processing, which is clearly a significant factor in IQ and presumably in intelligence, as well as attention span. In other words, you think faster and can concentrate for longer.

Brain Fats

As we learned in Chapter 4, eating the right essential brain fats speeds up thinking processes in the brain. While these earlier studies didn't supplement omega-3 fats, there's plenty of evidence that they should have. The levels of omega-3 fats at birth, especially DHA, which is the "brain building" fat, predict intellectual development later in life.[7 8] Children with optimal intakes of omega-3s have the minimum risk of behavioral and learning problems later in life.

Best Fish for Brain Fats

Amount of DHA in 100 g (3½ oz)

Mackerel	1,400 mg
Herring	1,000 mg
Sardines	1,000 mg
Tuna	900 mg
Anchovy	900 mg
Salmon	800 mg
Trout	500 mg

An ideal intake of DHA a day is in the order of 250–500 mg, or double if you have a related mental health problem. This is equivalent to eating 100g of fish, preferably salmon, mackerel, tuna, or herring, three or four times a week. Alternatively, you can take a supplement of fish oils containing DHA. A good-quality cod liver oil supplement can provide up to 200 mg.

The best source of all, at least for babies, is breast milk. Breast milk is naturally rich in DHA, and especially so if the mother eats fish or flaxseeds. Breast-fed babies not only have higher IQs ten years down the track,[9] and better results in examinations, they also have fewer mental health problems.[10]

Balancing Blood Sugar

Keeping an even blood sugar level is critical to intelligence because this affects your ability to concentrate over long periods of time more than anything else. Blood sugar dips not only lower intelligence and concentration, they can also increase aggressive behavior.[11] [12] [13] [14] [15] Eating "slow-releasing" carbohydrates and "grazing, not gorging" is the best way to avoid blood sugar dips. If, on the other hand, you refuel on the move, going from one sugary snack or drink to another, then your blood sugar level is likely to rise and fall like a roller coaster. So, too, will your concentration and mood. See Chapter 3 for the lowdown on what to eat to keep your blood sugar level even.

In summary, the first steps to maximizing your IQ are:

- Ensure an optimum intake of vitamins and minerals, both from diet and supplements.

- Optimize your intake of essential fats, especially omega-3 fats, by eating flaxseeds, oily fish, and/or taking fish oil supplements.

■ **Achieve stable and sustained blood sugar levels.**

These are the basics. But there's still plenty more that you can do to enhance your intelligence and memory (see the next chapter).

Chapter 13

Enhancing Your Memory

If your memory isn't as good as it used to be, your concentration is flagging, and your mind simply isn't as sharp, you may be another victim of a widespread epidemic of brain drain. At best, you may be failing to reach your full potential for mental health. At worst, you may be one of 4 million people now thought to be suffering from age-related memory decline. This reduces your cognitive function too young and leaves you open to an increased risk of developing Alzheimer's disease later in life.

The good news is that mental decline is not inevitable, and you can boost your memory and mental alertness at any age. Research shows clearly that healthy, well-nourished and well-educated people show no signs of declining mental function with age. What's more, while it is true that brain cells die with age, you can also build new brain cells at any age. How? By feeding your brain, both with the right nutrients and the right information. Check yourself out on the questionnaire below to see if there's room for improvement.

Memory Check

Score 1 for each "yes" answer.

- [ ] Is your memory deteriorating?
- [ ] Do you find it hard to concentrate and often get confused?
- [ ] Do you sometimes forget the point you're trying to make?
- [ ] Does it take you longer to learn things than it used to?

☐ Do you find it hard to add up numbers without writing them down?

☐ Do you often experience mental tiredness?

☐ Do you find it hard to concentrate for more than one hour?

☐ Do you sometimes meet someone you know quite well but can't remember his or her name?

☐ Do you often find you can remember things from the past but forget what you did yesterday?

☐ Do you ever forget what day of the week it is?

☐ Do you often misplace your keys?

☐ Do you ever go looking for something and forget what you are looking for?

☐ Do your friends and family think you're getting more forgetful now than you used to be?

☐ Do you frequently repeat yourself?

If your score is:

4 or less: Your memory and concentration are good. The advice in this chapter will help keep you mentally sharp throughout your life.

5 to 10: You are starting to suffer from brain drain. Following all the diet and supplement recommendations in this chapter will help give your memory and concentration a boost.

More than 10: You are experiencing significant memory and concentration impairment and need to do something about it. As well as following all the diet and supplement recommendations in this chapter, read Chapter 35 and see a nutritionist who can assess and help you correct the biochemical imbalances that contribute to memory decline.

How Your Memory Works

Memories are not held in one, but several networked brain cells. These links between brain cells, hardwired by a network of interconnecting neuronal dendrites (see Figure 1b on page 9), are stimulated by learning new information. Rats put into a highly stimulating "Disneyland for rats" rapidly grew new dendrites within four days, according to research by Dr. William Greenough at the University of Illinois.[16] Stress does the opposite. High levels of the stress hormone cortisol makes dendrites shrivel up, according to Professor Sapolsky of Stanford University, whose research found this effect became noticeable after as little as two weeks of stress.[17] Fortunately, dendrites do grow back once cortisol levels decline. In other words, use it or lose it—and stay cool.

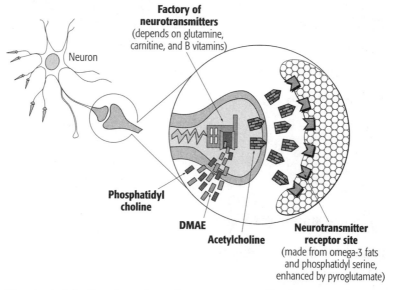

Fig 18   **Acetylcholine in action: the memory molecule**

Memories themselves are thought to be stored by altering the structure of a molecule called RNA within brain cells. For a memory to be made, it must enter the cell by seeing, hearing, or doing something, which accounts for the three kinds of memory—visual, auditory, or kinesthetic. If a memory involves all three, it will exist in a maximum number of brain cells. That's why if you see a telephone number, repeat it to yourself aloud, and punch the numbers on the phone several times, you are more likely to remember it. The brain, particularly the hippocampus region, then decides whether it's worth storing. In Alzheimer's patients, the hippocampus loses its ability to file memories, resulting in an inability to store new memories.

A critical question is how memories are put into storage, retrieved, and connected. The key memory molecule is the neurotransmitter acetylcholine, highly concentrated in the hippocampus. People with Alzheimer's disease, for example, show a marked deficiency of acetylcholine. Even if a memory is intact, if you don't have enough acetylcholine, you can't connect one part of the memory with other parts. For example, you know the face but can't remember the name.

Natural Mind and Memory Enhancers

The best way to enhance your memory and mind, and protect yourself from memory decline, is to ensure an optimal intake of not only essential vitamins, minerals, and fats, but also five nutrients from which your body can make key brain chemicals, plus two herbs. These seven natural mind and memory enhancers are:

- Phosphatidyl choline and DMAE—acetylcholine precursors

- Phosphatidyl serine and pyroglutamate—receptor enhancers

- Glutamine—fuel for brain cells

- Ginkgo biloba and vinpocetine—herbal circulation improvers.

These are becoming widely available and can be found in combination in state-of-the-art brain-boosting supplements, as well as in certain foods.

The Big Five Nutrients

Phosphatidyl Choline: Superbrain Food

The key brain chemical for memory is acetylcholine. A deficiency in it is probably the single most common cause for declining memory. As we saw in Chapter 2, it is derived from phosphatidyl choline, a nutrient in foods.

The richest dietary sources of phosphatidyl choline are egg yolks and fish, especially sardines. Since egg phobia set in, on the false basis that dietary cholesterol was a major cause of heart disease, the average intake of choline from diet has dropped dramatically. The American Medical Association says that up to seven eggs a week is fine. Phosphatidyl choline is also found in lecithin, a supplement that comes in granules and capsules. You need about 1–2 g of phosphatidyl choline a day for maximizing mental function. Most lecithin contains about 20 percent phosphatidyl choline, so you would need 5–10 g of lecithin a day. You can also buy "HiPC lecithin," which is twice as rich in phosphatidyl choline, so you would only need 2.5–5 g a day, or a heaping teaspoon. However, you don't simply make more acetylcholine by eating choline. Vitamin B_5 (pantothenic acid) is essential for the formation of acetylcholine in the body, as are vitamins B_1, B_{12}, and also vitamin C. As always, nutrients work together.

Recent research has shown that taking choline during pregnancy can result in offspring with "superbrains." This research, carried out at Duke University Medical Center in the United States, fed pregnant rats choline halfway through their pregnancies. The infant rats whose mothers were given choline had vastly superior brains, improved learning ability, and better memory recall, all of which persisted into old age. This research showed that giving choline helps restructure the brain for improved performance[18]. Supplementing high doses of choline has also been proven to boost memory in adults. For example, Florence Safford of Florida International University gave forty-one people aged fifty to eighty choline supplements of 500 mg every day for five weeks. They reported having half as many memory lapses, such as forgetting names or losing things.[19]

Supplementing choline can help the young as well as the old. Dr. Ladd and colleagues at the West Valley College in Saratoga, California, gave eighty college students a single 25 g dose of phosphatidyl choline (3.75 g of choline) and found a significant improvement in memory ninety minutes later, most likely due to the improved responses of slow learners.[20] If you combine choline with other smart nutrients such as pyroglutamate, you can achieve the same memory-boosting effect at lower doses (see Chapter 35).

DMAE: A Natural Brain Stimulant

DMAE (again, sardines are a rich source) is a precursor of choline that crosses much more easily from the blood into brain cells, accelerating the brain's production of acetylcholine. It reduces anxiety, stops the mind racing, improves concentration, promotes learning, and acts as a mild brain stimulant.

Slight chemical variations of DMAE have been marketed as the drug Deaner or Deanol, which have proven highly effective in numerous double-blind trials in helping those with learning problems, attention deficit disorder, memory problems, and behavior problems. In one survey by Dr. Bernard Rimland in California, Deaner was found to be almost twice as effective in treating children with attention deficit disorder as the drug Ritalin, and without the side effects. The ideal dose for memory enhancement is 100–1,000 mg, taken in the morning or midday, not in the evening. (Too much can overstimulate and is therefore not recommended for those diagnosed with schizophrenia, mania, and epilepsy.) Don't expect immediate results. DMAE can take two to three weeks to work, but it's worth waiting for.

The ability of DMAE to tune up your brain was well demonstrated in a German study from 1996 with a group of adults with cognitive problems.[21] The participants had their EEG brain waves measured and were then given either placebos or DMAE. There were no changes in EEG for those on the placebos, but those taking DMAE showed improvements in their brain wave patterns in those parts of the brain that play an important role in memory, attention, and flexibility of thinking.

Here are some reports from people supplementing DMAE:

"I've been taking DMAE for several weeks, and I've noticed an amazing difference in mood and concentration level." A.F.B., Austin, Texas

"I am currently taking 100 mg of DMAE per day and notice a real difference in my alertness, energy level, and decreased need for sleep." R.S., Seattle, Washington

"I've been using DMAE with pantothenic acid and a good multivitamin for two months now. One of the first things I noticed was that I fall asleep faster and wake up with a clearer mind. I experience a much sounder, more restful sleep. I constantly feel more attuned to my creative potential and I'm always in a good mood. I truly feel alive and awake." P.W. [22]

Phosphatidyl Serine: Highly Receptive

The ability of neurotransmitters to deliver messages depends on having a fully functioning "docking port", or receptor site. These receptor sites are built out of phospholipids, essential fats, and protein. The predominant phospholipid is phosphatidyl serine, or PS. The secret of the memory-boosting properties of PS is probably due to its key role in brain cell communication.

Supplementing PS is particularly helpful for those with learning difficulties or age-related memory decline. In one study by Dr. Thomas Crook, 149 people with age-associated memory impairment were given a daily dose of 300 mg of PS or a placebo. When tested after twelve weeks, the ability of those on the PS to match names to faces (a recognized measure of memory and mental function) improved to equal that of people twelve years younger. [23]

Pyroglutamate: Master of Communication

A key brain chemical in enhancing memory and mental function is the amino acid pyroglutamate. The discovery that the brain and cerebrospinal fluid contain large amounts of pyroglutamate led to its investigation as an essential brain nutrient. One extraordinary finding was that pyroglutamate promotes the flow of information between the right and left hemispheres of the brain. A study published in 1988 by Dr. H. Pilch and colleagues suggests that pyroglutamate may increase the number of acetylcholine receptors in the brain. Older mice were given piracetam, a pyroglutamate derivative, for two weeks. The researchers found that these older mice had a 30 to 40 p higher density of receptors than before.[24] This suggests that pyroglutamate molecules do not only maximize mental performance but may also have a regenerative effect on the nervous system.

Pyroglutamate does three things that help improve your memory and mental alertness:

- Increases acetylcholine production

- Boosts the number of receptors for acetylcholine

- Improves communication between the left and right hemispheres of the brain

In other words, it improves both the brain's talking and listening, plus cooperation between the two sides. As a result it improves learning, memory, concentration, and the speed of reflexes. In fact, so powerful are its effects that there are now many slight variations of this key brain chemical being marketed as drugs for learning and memory-related problems. Numerous studies using these "smart drugs" have proven to enhance memory and mental function, not only in those with pronounced memory decline but also people with so-called normal memory function.[25]

Researchers at the University of Catania, Sicily, tested forty patients with age-related memory decline. Twenty were given pyroglutamate and twenty a placebo. After two months, various memory tests revealed that those on pyroglutamate had significantly improving memory compared to those on the placebo.[26]

Pyroglutamate is found in many foods, including fish, dairy products, fruit, and vegetables. The most common supplemental form is arginine pyroglutamate. You need about 400–1,000 mg a day for a mind-enhancing effect.

Glutamine: Amazing Brain Fuel

While acetylcholine is the major player as far as memory is concerned, many neurotransmitters are also involved. Some stimulate mental processes, while others prevent information overload. You need a balance. For example, the stimulating neurotransmitter glutamate helps forge links between memories, but too much can literally overexcite neurons to death. This is how MSG (monosodium glutamate) turns up the volume on tastes, but can be a bad thing in large quantities. Pyroglutamate greatly enhances learning, while GABA, a close relative of glutamate, calms down the nervous system. The right balance of these neurotransmitters is important for learning, memory, and mental function in general. So supplementing glutamine, an amino acid from which the brain can build and balance these neurotransmitters, can help promote memory.

Glutamine is the most abundant amino acid in the cerebrospinal fluid that surrounds the brain. Glutamine can be used directly as fuel for the brain and has been shown to enhance mood and mental performance and decrease addictive tendencies.[27] In studies designed to test whether glutamine proved safe in large doses, researchers from Boston Women's Hospital, Massachusetts, gave healthy volunteers between 40 and 60 g a day. Not only was it shown to be safe, but one of the "side effects" was enhanced ability to solve problems on continuous performance tests. This study was only five days long, showing that glutamine has an immediate effect, and possibly a greater effect over time.[28] In another study, this time on bone marrow transplant patients, large amounts of glutamine were reported to make patients more "vigorous, and less angry and fatigued."[29]

Glutamine is an important nutrient for the brain and there is good logic to adding 5–10 g, which can be bought as a powder, to your daily supplement program. This equates to 1–2 heaping teaspoons a day.

Another amino acid, carnitine, can be used directly by the brain as fuel. Acetyl-l-carnitine, often abbreviated ALC , is an especially useful form of this amino acid, since the "acetyl" part helps to make acetylcholine—the brain's memory neurotransmitter. Together with an antioxidant called alpha lipoic acid, acetyl-l-carnitine can reverse aging and promote memory in animals, according to research by Professor Bruce Ames at the University of California, Berkeley.[30] Not only did the rats in this study have improved memory after only a month on these supplements, they also become more active.

You need between 250 and 1,500 mg of ALC a day to get any benefit. Unfortunately, it is very expensive and is perhaps not my smart nutrient of choice for this reason. It's best to take it some time before or after eating to maximize absorption.

The Memory Herbs

Ginkgo Biloba: Ancient Wisdom

Ginkgo biloba is an herbal remedy that has been used for memory enhancement in the East for thousands of years and comes from one of the oldest species of tree known. Research has shown that it improves short-term and age-related memory loss, slow thinking, depression, and circulation, and it improves blood flow to the brain. It has also been seen to significantly improve Parkinson's and Alzheimer's diseases in one year. A review of ten studies testing ginkgo's effects on people with circulation problems, carried out at the University of Limburg in the Netherlands, found significant improvement in memory, concentration, energy, and mood.[31] A more comprehensive double-blind, placebo-controlled trial carried out in France found remarkable improvement in speed of cognitive processing of sixty- to eighty-year-olds, almost comparable to those of healthy young people, when given 320 mg a day.[32]

Ginkgo contains two phytochemicals called ginkgo flavone glycosides and terpene lactones, which give it its remarkable healing properties. It usually comes in capsule form, and you should look for a brand that shows the flavonoid concentration, which determines strength. The recommended flavonoid concentration is 24 percent, and you should take 30–50 mg of such a supplement, three times a day. You need to try ginkgo for at least three months before evaluating the results.

Vinpocetine: Secret of the Periwinkle

Much like the herb Ginkgo biloba, vinpocetine is another herb that improves blood flow and circulation, thus helping deliver oxygen to the brain. Vinpocetine is actually an extract from the periwinkle plant (*Vinca minor*).

Research carried out at the University of Surrey gave 203 people with memory problems either a placebo or vinpocetine. This and other studies have shown that those on vinpocetine experience a significant improvement in their cognitive performance.[33 34] Remarkably, improvements in concentration, memory recall, and learning have been reported after just one dose. One double-blind crossover study showed a significant improvement in memory after just one hour of taking 40mg of vinpocetine.[35]

Vinpocetine is recommended for those who've noticed a decline in memory, concentration, learning speed, neuromuscular coordination, and reaction time, or deficits in hearing or vision.

However, research shows that vinpocetine is particularly protective in cases where blood flow to the brain is diminished, usually by cerebral atherosclerosis (a condition in which a build-up of plaque clogs the arteries that supply oxygen to the brain), as well as during mini-strokes or situations where the blood supply to the brain is temporarily shut off. Like ginkgo, it may also help people with tinnitus, which can be caused by such circulation problems.

The secrets to vinpocetine's success in enhancing mind and memory are many. First, it definitely improves circulation in the brain, helping to deliver nutrients more effectively. Studies show that it widens blood vessels in the brain. Because of this action, red blood cells are better able to pass through narrow passages, meaning better oxygen delivery. Vinpocetine also inhibits platelet aggregation, stopping blood cells from clumping together and clogging the blood vessels.

Brain cells not only need a constant, good supply of oxygen, they also need energy, and vinpocetine has been shown to enhance energy production in brain cells.

By speeding up the transport of glucose and oxygen to the brain and their use once they get there, vinpocetine may reduce the effects of both strokes and the less dramatic mini-strokes that can lead to dementia.

Finally, vinpocetine has been found to stimulate noradrenergic neurons in an area of the brain called the locus coeruleus. These neurons affect the function of the cerebral cortex—the part of the brain we use to think, plan, and act. The number of these neurons declines with age, impairing concentration, alertness, and the speed with which we process information.

You need about 10–40 mg of vinpocetine a day for these positive effects. To date, no negative effects have been reported.

Don't Forget B Vitamins and Zinc

While I've already extolled the virtues of B vitamins, there are three that need special mention in relation to memory. Niacin, or vitamin B_3, is particularly good for memory enhancement. In one study, 141 mg of niacin was given daily to a group of subjects of various ages. Memory was improved by 10 to 40 percent in all age groups.[36] B_5 (pantothenic acid) is essential for the brain to make acetylcholine—it adds on the "acetyl" part. It is also essential for the formation of steroid hormones, including the stress hormone cortisol, so it is particularly important for people under stress.[37] An optimal intake is probably as much as 200 mg, although some people respond better to 500 mg. Compare this with the RDA, which is just 6mg in Europe!

B_{12} has also been shown to accelerate learning in rats[38] and is very important for the health of brain cells. B vitamins work together in many ways to help the brain make and use neurotransmitters. It is important to remember that B vitamins should be taken together, so if you wish to concentrate on a specific B vitamin, take this in conjunction with a B complex or multivitamin.

Zinc is another brain-friendly nutrient thought to be involved in memory. One theory is that memories are encoded by changing protein molecules in the brain, involving RNA, which is the master builder of proteins in the body. RNA is itself highly dependent on zinc. Deficiencies of zinc are well known to lead to an inability to recall dreams. Children with serious learning difficulties often have low zinc levels, and low zinc is also thought to be involved in the severe memory loss of dementia. As you'll see later in this book, correcting low zinc levels can also have remarkable results for people with depression and schizophrenia. The chances are you are low in zinc because it is the mineral in which we're generally most deficient. The RDA is 15 mg, more if you're pregnant or breast-feeding. Yet, according to government surveys, the average intake is 7.6 mg a day. That means that almost half the British population achieve less than half the recommended intake.

Seeds and seed foods are rich in zinc. Why seeds? Basically, if you can plant it and it grows, it's zinc-rich, because zinc is vital for the growth of both plants and animals. This means that seeds, beans, peas, and lentils are all rich in zinc. So are nuts, meat, and fish, and especially oysters. Eating these foods, as well as supplementing 10 mg of zinc every day, is the best way to ensure optimal amounts of this essential nutrient.

The Synergy Effect

The effects of enhancing mental performance through supplementation of "smart nutrients" such as phosphatidyl choline, pantothenic acid, DMAE, and pyroglutamate are likely to be far greater when taken in combination than individually. For example, a team of researchers led by Raymond Bartus gave choline and piracetam, a pyroglutamate derivative (see page 98), to some old lab rats with age-related memory decline, and piracetam alone to others.[39] They found that rats given the combination showed better memory retention than those that took piracetam alone. Results also showed that half the dose was needed when piracetam and choline were combined. Dr. S. Ferris and associates at New York University School of Medicine then carried out a study on humans. These researchers, too, found dramatic clinical improvements, way beyond those of people who were given either choline or piracetam separately.[40]

Since nutrients are more powerful in combination, my daily brain plan, in addition to a healthy diet and basic supplement program, consists of taking a teaspoon of hiPC lecithin every day plus a combination of the following mind- and memory-enhancing nutrients, which can be found in combination supplements.

Nutrient	Daily Amount
Phosphatidyl choline	250 mg–400 mg
DMAE	200 mg–300 mg
Phosphatidyl serine	20 mg–45 mg
Arginine pyroglutamate	300 mg–450 mg
Ginkgo	200 mg–300 mg
Vinpocetine	10 mg–20 mg
Plus B vitamins including	
Niacin (B$_3$)	10 mg–15 mg
B$_{12}$	10 μg–30 μg
Pantothenic acid	200 mg–300 mg

If you are over 50 or suffering from age-related memory decline, I recommend you add the following every day:

Phosphatidyl serine	100 mg
DHA	250 mg
Glutamine powder	5,000 mg (one heaping teaspoon)

In summary, here are some top tips to enhance your memory, in addition to the diet and supplement recommendations in Part 1:

- Add a heaping teaspoon of lecithin high in phosphatidyl choline to your cereal each morning, or a teaspoon of regular lecithin, or supplement the phospholipids phosphatidyl serine and phosphatidyl choline.

- Supplement a brain nutrient formula containing the nutrients and herbs listed above.

- Learn something new every day. Keep your brain active. If you don't use it, you lose it.

These nutrients are your first line of defense against memory decline. There are some other smart nutrients, drugs, and hormones that have proven memory-boosting effects. These are discussed in Part 7, "Mental Health in Old Age," because they are most effective later in life and for reversing more serious memory deficit diseases such as Alzheimer's.

Chapter 14

BEATING THE BLUES

Depression isn't a disease that you've either got or you haven't. We are all somewhere along a sliding scale that ranges from generally happy to completely depressed. Officially, 3 million people in Britain, or one in twenty, are depressed, with three times as many women suffering as men. They swallow 20 million antidepressants every week, take 80 million days off work each year because of it, and cost the nation between $5 and $8 billion.

But many more people feel blue a lot of the time. According to the mynutrition.co.uk survey of 22,000 people, 52 percent of people feel apathetic and unmotivated a lot of the time, while 42 percent feel depressed a lot of the time. This number goes up in the winter as millions suffer from SAD—seasonal affective disorder, commonly known as the winter blues.

Many of us sell ourselves short on mood. We may be consistently quite low but would never consider ourselves depressed or go to the doctor for treatment. Unless you feel relatively consistently happy and motivated, the odds are you can improve how you feel, just as the last two chapters explained how you can improve how you think. Check yourself out on the questionnaire below to see if there's room for improvement.

Mood Check

Score 1 for each "yes" answer.

☐ Do you often feel downhearted or sad?

☐ Do you often feel worse in the morning?

☐ Do you find it difficult to face the day?

☐ Do you sometimes have crying spells, or feel like it?

☐ Do you have trouble falling asleep or sleeping through the night?

☐ Is your appetite, or desire to eat, poor?

☐ Are you losing weight without trying?

☐ Do you feel unattractive and unlovable?

☐ Do you shun company and prefer to be alone?

☐ Do you often feel fearful?

☐ Are you often irritable or angry?

☐ Do you find it difficult to make decisions?

☐ Is it an effort to motivate yourself to do the things you used to do?

☐ Do you feel hopeless about the future?

☐ Do you feel less enjoyment from activities that once gave you pleasure?

If your score is:

Below 5: You are basically normal, even if you do occasionally feel a bit blue. Following the advice in this chapter will help keep your mood good and balanced.

5 to 10: Your mood needs a boost. The advice in this chapter will help improve how you feel.

10 or more: You are depressed and could use some help. As well as following the advice in this chapter, read Chapter 22 and consider seeing both a clinical nutritionist and a psychotherapist.

Depression: Anger without Enthusiam?

If your mood is often low, there are two avenues to explore—your mind frame and your chemistry. Many people taking antidepressants really need to deal with something that isn't working in their lives. For example, depression is often anger without enthusiasm. Ask yourself honestly whether you are angry about something. Make a list. Maybe there's a relationship that didn't work out, a job that's selling you short, a dream that didn't come true. Much of grief is often anger, but if you were brought up unable to express anger, you may be bottling it up inside in the form of depression. You may be depressed because you have unfinished business.

Many people become depressed because they are betraying themselves. Ask yourself in what way you are betraying yourself, not living your life true to who you are or who you could be. Does your work, your relationship, your life give you the opportunity to express yourself and your true feelings?

If all this is ringing big bells, you may benefit greatly from seeing a psychotherapist or counselor (see pages 367–368) or doing a life-enhancing course. My favorites are listed in Resources on pages 368–369. You may also benefit from tuning up your brain and neurotransmitters because your mood and motivation aren't only in your mind, they're in the chemistry of your mind.

Anatomy of Low Mood and Motivation

One of the greatest unrecognized truths is that ensuring optimum nutrition for your mind not only improves mood, but gives you the energy and motivation to make changes in your life. Few psychotherapists recognize how much better their results would be if they helped their clients tune up their brain biochemistry.

These are the common imbalances connected to nutrition that can worsen your mood and motivation:

- Blood sugar imbalances (often associated with excessive sugar and stimulant intake)

- Deficiencies of nutrients (vitamin B_3, B_6, folate, B_{12}, C, zinc, magnesium, essential fatty acids)

- Deficiencies of tryptophan and tyrosine (precursors of neurotransmitters)

- Allergies and sensitivities

One factor that underlies most depression is poor control of blood glucose levels. Keeping blood sugar levels more even can be achieved by eating small regular meals of natural, unprocessed foods, including protein and fiber at each one, and taking a combination of B vitamins and the mineral chromium. All this is explained in Chapter 3.

The most promising nutrients for improving mood are vitamins B_3, B_{12}, and folic acid, then vitamin B_6, zinc and magnesium, and essential fatty acids (EFAs). The first three are involved in the vital biochemical process known as methylation, which is critical for balancing the neurotransmitters dopamine and adrenaline. A study at Kings College Hospital in London found that giving folic acid supplements to people with borderline or low folic acid levels alongside standard drug treatment significantly improved recovery in patients with depression.[41] Their research found that a third of all people with depression and other psychiatric disorders were deficient in folic acid. Giving vitamin C has also been proven to enhance recovery.[42]

Chemical Blues

There are often two sides to feeling blue—feeling miserable, and feeling apathetic and unmotivated. The most prevalent theory for the cause of these imbalances is a brain imbalance in two families of neurotransmitters, the molecules of emotion. These are:

• Serotonin, which influences your mood, and

• Adrenaline and noradrenaline, made from dopamine, which influence your motivation.

All the major antidepressant drugs are designed to influence the balance and function of these neurotransmitters. These include selective serotonin re-uptake inhibitors (SSRIs) such as Prozac, Lustral, and Seroxat, which are designed to keep serotonin in circulation; adrenaline re-uptake inhibitors such as Edronax; a noradrenaline re-uptake inhibitor (NARI), designed to keep adrenaline in circulation; monoamine oxidase inhibitors, which help maintain adrenaline and dopamine levels; and the tricyclic antidepressants such as amitriptyline which also prevent adrenaline breakdown. All of these neurotransmitters are, however, directly influenced by nutrition.[43]

The major focus of attention has been on noradrenaline/adrenaline and serotonin. To test the theory that serotonin primarily controlled mood, and adrenaline and noradrenaline control motivation, Antonella Dubini, from the Pharmacia and Upjohn Medical Department in Milan, Italy, gave 203 people suffering from low mood and motivation either an SSRI drug, promoting serotonin, or a NARI drug, promoting noradrenaline. Sure enough, the former was more effective at improving mood, while the latter was more effective at improving motivation.[44]

If this theory is correct, that low mood is often a serotonin deficiency symptom and that low motivation is an adrenaline/noradrenaline deficiency symptom, then that begs two questions. Why are some people deficient, and which nutrients would correct these deficiencies?

I believe that, for many people, the pace of life and the speed at which we are having to adapt and change is stressing us out. The brain responds by producing more and more adrenaline and serotonin in response to our too frequent ups and downs, stresses, and strains. This is akin to the body producing more and more insulin to even out frequently fluctuating blood sugar levels. This increases our need for the building blocks, the nutrients from which we make these mood-enhancing neurotransmitters. So we end up suboptimally nourished in the nutrients from which we make these neuro-transmitters—partly because our diets are inadequate and partly because our demand for these nutrients is higher. Just as the stress of pollution in-creases our need for vitamin C, the stress of life increases our demand for tryptophan.

The figure below shows those nutrients that are needed for the brain and body to make enough serotonin, adrenaline, and noradrenaline.

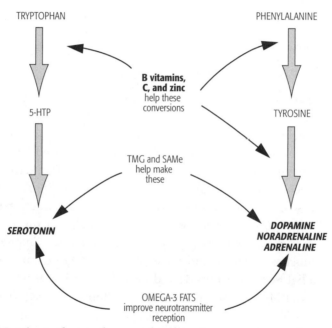

Fig 19 Nutrients that make mood-enhancing neurotransmitters

Depression in Women

Women are three times as prone to low moods as men. Many theories as to why this is have been proposed, some psychological, some social, but the truth is that women and men are biochemically very different. The research of Mirko Diksic and colleagues at McGill University in Montreal demon-strates this. They developed a technique using PET neuroimaging to meas-ure the rate at which we make serotonin in the brain.[45] What they found was that men's average synthesis rate of serotonin was 52 percent higher than in women. This, and other research, has clearly shown that women are more prone to low serotonin. They also react differently. In women, low serotonin is associated with depression and anxiety, while in men, low serotonin is related to aggression and alcoholism. One possibility is our social conditioning: Men "act out" their moods, while women are more conditioned to "act in" their moods. Another example of depression being the flipside of anger.

What has been learned about serotonin in the last few years is that there are six main reasons for deficiency, in addition to a lack of tryptophan:

• Not enough estrogen (in women)

• Not enough testosterone (in men)

• Not enough light

• Not enough exercise

• Too much stress, especially in women

• Not enough co-factor vitamins and minerals

If you are suffering from low mood, feel tense and irritable, are low in energy, tend to comfort eat, have sleeping problems and a reduced interest in sex, and the above apply to you, the chances are you are short on serotonin.

Low estrogen means low serotonin and low moods.[46][47] This is because estrogen blocks the breakdown of serotonin. This may largely explain why women are more prone to depression premenstrually, in menopause, and thereafter. Low testosterone has a similar effect in men (see Chapter 15.)

Light stimulates estrogen, and most of us don't get enough of it. The difference in light exposure outside and inside is massive. Most of us spend twenty-three out of twenty-four hours a day indoors, exposed to an average of 100 units (called lux) of light. That's compared to 20,000 lux on a sunny day and 7,000 lux on an overcast day. Now, more than ever before, many of us rarely expose ourselves to direct sunlight, and certainly not enough to maximize serotonin production. Of course, light deficiency is worse in the winter.

Stress also rapidly reduces serotonin levels. Physical exercise improves stress response, and therefore reduces stress-induced depletion of serotonin.

Each of these reasons for serotonin depletion affects women more than men. Men produce serotonin twice as fast as women, allowing them to rebalance from any of these serotonin depleters without prolonged blues, provided there's enough tryptophan in their diet.

Now we need to take a closer look at both serotonin and tryptophan.

The Blues Busters

Is Depression a Tryptophan Deficiency?

Antidepressant drugs like Prozac work by stopping the body from breaking down the neurotransmitter serotonin, therefore keeping more circulating in the brain. The trouble is that these kinds of drugs induce unpleasant side effects in about a quarter of those who take them and severe reactions in a minority (see Chapter 21). The natural alternative is to eat your way to happiness by choosing foods from which the body makes serotonin.

Serotonin is made from a constituent of protein, the amino acid tryptophan. Dr. Philip Cowen from Oxford University's psychiatry department wondered what would happen if you deprived people of tryptophan. He gave fifteen volunteers who had a history of depression, but were currently fine, a nutritionally balanced drink that excluded tryptophan. Within seven hours ten out of fifteen noticed a worsening of their mood and started to show signs of depression. On being given the same drink, but this time with tryptophan added, their mood improved.[48] Tryptophan is especially rich in fish, turkey, chicken, cheese, beans, tofu, oats, and eggs.

Supplementing the amino acid tryptophan* is already well proven to improve mood. Donald Ecclestone, professor of medicine at the Royal Victoria Infirmary in Newcastle in the United Kingdom, reviewed the available studies and concluded that supplementing tryptophan leads to an increase in the synthesis of serotonin in the brain, improving mood as well as some antidepressant drugs. You need 1 g for low mood, and up to 3 g a day for actual depression, taken either on an empty stomach or preferably with a carbohydrate food such as fruit, since carbohydrates help its absorption. Tryptophan promotes sleep, so it's best taken before bed.

As well as supplementing tryptophan, make sure your diet gives you at least 1 g a day by eating any two of the following meals, each giving 500 mg of tryptophan.

Five Ways of Eating 500 mg of Tryptophan

Oatmeal, soy milk, and two scrambled eggs
Baked potato with cottage cheese and tuna salad
Chicken breast, potatoes *au gratin*, and green beans
Whole wheat spaghetti with beans, tofu, or meat sauce
Salmon fillet, quinoa and lentil pilaf, and green salad with yogurt dressing

---

*Tryptophan is unavailable for sale in the United States.

However, ironically, eating a meal containing tryptophan doesn't raise brain levels of tryptophan as high as eating a carbohydrate meal does. This anomaly was discovered by Professor Richard Wurtman at MIT. He fed people standard American high-protein breakfasts versus high-carbohydrate breakfasts and found that only the latter caused increases in brain serotonin levels, despite containing no tryptophan![49] The reason for this anomaly is that tryptophan in the bloodstream competes badly with all the other amino acids in protein, so little gets across into the brain. However, when you eat a carbohydrate food such as a banana, this causes insulin to be released into the bloodstream, which carries tryptophan into the brain.

This may be why depressed people instinctly crave sweet foods to give them a lift. This causes a surge of insulin, which carries tryptophan into the brain, causing serotonin levels to rise! So, if you find sugar gives you a mood lift, you are probably low in serotonin. The trouble is, most carbohydrate snacks are high in refined sugar and fat, and make you fat, which is depressing. The solution is to supplement tryptophan with carbohydrates. This not only improves your mood, but also will reduce your appetite, especially for sugary foods. That's why tryptophan can also help you lose weight.

The Tryptophan Controversy

So why don't we supplement tryptophan? Thousands of people did, up to 1989, with tremendous results both for depression and for promoting sleep (see Chapter 17). But then a terrible thing happened. A Japanese company, Showa Denko, developed a way of producing cheaper tryptophan, but something was badly wrong, and the resulting product caused a condition called eosonophilia myalgia syndrome. Thousands were affected and thirty-seven people died. Many suspected the genetic modification used in its manufacture was the cause of the problem, though other shortcuts were also used by Showa Denko, and the GM link is not clear. The problem was, however, limited to this single source of tryptophan and the methods of production they employed.

Quite rightly, tryptophan supplements were withdrawn while this was investigated. But for no good reason, it is still not allowed in Britain except under prescription as Optimax. No adverse effects have been reported from taking this. While some countries, such as Holland, allow tryptophan supplements to be freely sold, Britain's Food Standards Agency continues to ban it for no good reason (for more details and to help the campaign to return tryptophan to free sale read *The Tryptophan Scandal,* under "Features," on www.patrickholford.com).

Another Way to Serotonin: 5-HTP

While supplementing tryptophan itself has proven an effective blues buster, even more effective is a derivative of tryptophan that is one step closer to serotonin. This is called 5-hydroxytryptophan, or 5-HTP for short, and is derived from an African plant called griffonia. The first study proving the mood-boosting power of 5-HTP was done in the 1970s in Japan under the direction of Professor Isamu Sano of the Osaka University Medical School.[50] He gave 107 patients 50–300 mg of 5-HTP per day, and within two weeks, more than half experienced improvements in their symptoms. By the end of the four weeks of the study, nearly three-quarters of the patients reported either complete relief or significant improvement, with no side effects. This study was repeated by other researchers who also found that 69 percent of patients improved their mood.[51]

Since then, studies have proven that this nutrient is as effective as the best antidepressants with a fraction, if any, of the side effects. One double-blind trial headed by Dr. Poldinger at the Basel University of Psychiatry gave thirty-four depressed volunteers either the SSRI antidepressant fluvoxamine, or 300mg of 5-HTP. Each patient was assessed for his degree of depression using the widely accepted Hamilton Rating Scale, plus his own subjective self-assessment. At the end of the six weeks, both groups of patients had had a significant improvement in their depression. However, those taking 5-HTP had a greater improvement in each of the four criteria assessed—depression, anxiety, insomnia, and physical symptoms, as well as the patient's self-assessment.[52]

While previous studies had shown 5-HTP to be as effective as the tricyclic antidepressant imipramine,[53] in this study 5-HTP had outperformed the best antidepressant. Given that 5-HTP is less expensive and has significantly fewer side effects, it is extraordinary that psychiatrists, virtually never prescribe it despite plenty of scientific evidence that it helps restore normal mood and normal serotonin levels.[54]

The recommended dosage of this natural supplement, available in any health food shop, is 100 mg of 5-HTP, twice a day, for depression. Some supplements also provide various vitamins and minerals such as vitamin B_3, B_6, and folic acid, which may be even more effective because these nutrients help to turn 5-HTP into serotonin. A small percentage of people, less than 5 percent, experience nausea on 5-HTP, especially the first time. This is because 5-HTP can be converted into serotonin in the gut, as well as the brain. Since there are serotonin receptors in the gut, which don't normally expect to get the real thing so easily, they can overreact if the amount is too high and cause nausea. If so, just lower the dose. Your body soon adjusts.

If you get very sleepy on 5-HTP, you probably don't need it. The same applies with tryptophan. 5-HTP is best absorbed on an empty stomach.

Is Apathy a Tyrosine Deficiency?

Another neurotransmitter deficiency associated with depression and lack of motivation is adrenaline and its brother, noradrenaline. As you can see in Figure 20, adrenaline and noradrenaline are made from a neurotransmitter called dopamine, which is made from the amino acid tyrosine, which is made from the amino acid phenylalanine. Now that we understand the "family tree" of adrenaline, it is logical to assume that if drugs that block the breakdown of these neurotransmitters do elevate mood, albeit with undesirable side effects, then supplementing the amino acid phenylalanine or tyrosine might work, too. And they do.

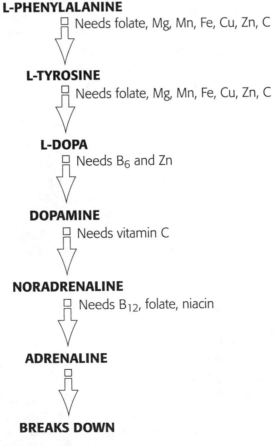

L-PHENYLALANINE
Needs folate, Mg, Mn, Fe, Cu, Zn, C

L-TYROSINE
Needs folate, Mg, Mn, Fe, Cu, Zn, C

L-DOPA
Needs B_6 and Zn

DOPAMINE
Needs vitamin C

NORADRENALINE
Needs B_{12}, folate, niacin

ADRENALINE

BREAKS DOWN

Fig 20   The catecholamine pathway

In a double-blind study by Helmut Beckmann and colleagues at the University of Wurzburg, Germany, 150–200 mg of the amino acid phenylalanine, or the antidepressant drug imipramine, were administered to forty depressed patients for one month. Both groups had the same degree of positive results— less depression, anxiety, and sleep disturbance.[55] A group of researchers at the Rush Medical Center, Chicago, screened depressed patients by testing phenythylamine in the blood; low levels mean you need more phenylalanine. They then gave forty depressed patients supplements of phenylalanine, and thirty-one of them improved.[56]

Tyrosine has been shown to work well in those with dopamine-dependent depression. In a pilot study administering 3,200 mg of tyrosine per day to twelve patients at the Hopital du Vinatier, France, a significant improvement in mood and sleep was observed on the very first day.[57]

The military has long known that tyrosine improves mental and physical performance under stress. Recent research from the Netherlands demonstrates how tyrosine gives you the edge in conditions of stress. Twenty-one cadets were put through a demanding one-week military combat training course. Ten cadets were given a drink containing 2 g of tyrosine a day, while the remaining eleven were given an identical drink without the tyrosine. Those on tyrosine consistently performed better, both in memorizing the task at hand and in tracking the tasks they had performed.[58]

The best results of all are achieved by supplementing all of these amino acids—5-HTP, phenylalanine and tyrosine—together with the B vitamins that help turn them into neurotransmitters, which are B_3, B_6, B_{12}, and folic acid.

SAMe and TMG: The Master Tuners

In Figure 19 you might have noticed these two strange-sounding nutrients. Both are kinds of amino acids. TMG stands for tri-methyl-glycine and SAMe stands for s-adenosyl methionine. They help to keep the brain and nervous system well tuned by donating "methyl groups." For example, noradrenaline turns into adrenaline by having a methyl group added. This process of adding on methyl groups, and sometimes taking them away, is totally critical to keeping the brain in balance. In fact, as you'll see in Chapter 25, many people with schizophrenia go crazy because their brains don't do this properly. These nutrients, plus B vitamins, can make all the difference.

SAMe is one of the most comprehensively studied natural antidepressants. Over 100 placebo-controlled, double-blind studies show that SAMe is equal to or superior to antidepressants, works faster, most often within a few days (most pharmaceutical antidepressants may take three to six weeks to take effect), and has few side effects.[59][60][61] (As with all anti depressants, there is a small risk of a rapid switch to mania in bipolar disorder with SAMe, so it should be used under supervision in these cases.)

Instead of side effects, SAMe has side benefits, including being an effective treatment for degenerative joint disease, fibromyalgia, and liver problems. According to one comprehensive review of all the studies, 92 percent of depressive patients responded to SAMe, compared with 85 percent to the medications.[62]

You need 200–600 mg a day, but the trouble is it's both very expensive and very unstable. A lot of SAMe sold in health food shops is pretty ineffective. Look for SAMe in the form of butanedisulfonate, which is more stable. Buy it and keep it refrigerated.

An alternative that is much more stable and less costly is tri-methyl glycine (TMG). In the body it turns into SAMe, but you need to supplement three times as much. Try supplementing 600–2,000 mg a day, again on an empty stomach or with fruit.

Mood-Boosting Fats

We've already encountered omega-3 fish oils. They are very much part of the equation for happiness. The higher your blood levels of omega-3 fats, the higher your levels of serotonin are likely to be. The reason for this is that omega-3 fats help build receptor sites, as well as improving reception. According to Dr. J. R. Hibbeln, who discovered that fish eaters are less prone to depression, "It's like building more serotonin factories, instead of just increasing the efficiency of the serotonin you have." [63]

A recent trial published in the *American Journal of Psychiatry* tested the effects of giving twenty people suffering from depression, who were already on antidepressants but still depressed, a highly concentrated form of omega-3 fat called ethyl-EPA, versus a placebo. By the third week, the depressed patients were showing major improvement in their moods, while those on the placebo were not.[64] Similar results are now being reported in England. Dr. Basant Puri from London's Hammersmith Hospital decided to try ethyl-EPA on one of his patients, a twenty-one-year-old student who had been on a variety of antidepressants, to no avail. He had a very low sense of self-esteem, sleeping problems, poor appetite, found it hard to socialize, and often thought of killing himself. After one month of supplementing the omega-3 fats he was no longer having suicidal thoughts and after nine months no longer had any depression.[65]

Let There Be Light

If you are particularly prone to the winter blues, technically known as Seasonal Affective Disorder (SAD), all the above will help, but there's one more nutrient you need: light. There are two likely reasons for the tendency to feel blue in the winter. The first is that brain levels of serotonin, the "happy" neurotransmitter, tend to fall partly because light stimulates the brain to produce this and other important brain chemicals. The second is that you may not be eating well and getting enough mood-boosting nutrients.

So, how do you get more light without emigrating in the winter? First, that's not such a bad idea: More and more people are having "summer vacations" in midwinter. But there's another way, involving a 60-watt lightbulb.

Light Exercise

Here's a simple exercise you can do with a regular lightbulb to increase your serotonin levels.

- Sit down in a quiet place, on the floor or on a chair. It is best to choose a place that you can completely darken. If not, you will need a blindfold.

- Place an anglepoise lamp, containing a 60-watt opaque (not clear) bulb, preferably with no writing on it, three feet away and directly in line with your line of vision.

- Make sure you can turn the light on and off without moving your head position.

- Turn the light on and look directly at the bulb for one minute, no longer.

- After one minute, turn the light off, close your eyes (put on your blindfold if the room is not completely dark), and focus on the afterimage, the phosphene, without moving your head, until it completely vanishes. This usually takes three to four minutes.

- This exercise is best done at dusk, effectively extending daylight hours.

It is also well worth investing in "full spectrum" lighting. These are lightbulbs that have the same quality of light as the sun, determined by the spread of different wavelengths. That's why sunlight and full-spectrum lighting is a much whiter light than a normal artificial light, which is yellower. Full-spectrum bulbs, although more expensive to start with, last ten times longer and use a quarter of the electricity. See the Resources section on page 369.

Melatonin, another tryptophan-derived brain chemical, helps balance the brain in the absence of light. Supplementing melatonin has also proven helpful for those with SAD.

Good Mood Foods and Supplements

If you want to eat your way to happiness, the key is to follow a diet that keeps your blood sugar level even and provides plenty of tryptophan, phenylalanine, B vitamins, and omega-3 fats. It's also worth supplementing these nutrients, and they can be found together in some supplements.

In summary, what this means, in addition to the basics in Part 1 including omega-3 fats, is supplementing:

- 2 g of phenylalanine or tyrosine, or 1 g of both

- 150 mg of 5-HTP

- A good multivitamin providing all the B vitamins

- Either 200 mg of SAMe or 600 mg of trimethyl glycine

These can be found together in some supplements. Combinations are the most effective, as KH found:

> "For years my girlfriend had suffered from depression, low self-esteem, and lack of energy. Since discovering your recommendations, she has really started to become herself once more. The heavy cloud that used to hang over her at the start of every day has gone, and in its place is a ray of sunshine. Thank you."

If you choose to take them separately, phenylalanine or tyrosine are best taken in the morning before breakfast because they increase motivation. Tryptophan and 5-HTP are best taken in the evening because they help promote a good night's sleep. Tryptophan needs to be taken on an empty stomach or with some fruit, while 5-HTP does not.

However, there are other causes for low moods and other cures for depression. These include hormonal imbalances, which are discussed in the next chapter, and can be helped by herbs such as St. John's wort and sceletium. These are discussed more fully in Chapter 22, which explores nutritional solutions to chronic depression, as opposed to low moods.

Chapter 15

BALANCING OUT
HORMONAL MOOD SWINGS

A common reason for mood swings is a hormone imbalance. This doesn't just affect women, and it isn't only related to premenstrual syndrome. Hormones are little different from neurotransmitters. They are both chemicals of communication that tell the body and brain cells how to behave. If out of balance, your mood goes out of balance too.

Here are the common imbalances that wreak havoc on how you feel:

- **Estrogen and progesterone deficiency** in menopause, for example, can cause depression.

- **Testosterone deficiency** in both men and women can cause depression, loss of motivation, and sex drive.

- **Testosterone excess** can lead to hyperactivity and aggression.

- **DHEA deficiency** can lead to depression and loss of motivation.

- **High estrogen and low progesterone** can lead to premenstrual syndrome, with cyclic depression and anxiety.

- **Melatonin** deficiency can lead to depression and insomnia (see Chapter 17).

- **Thyroxine deficiency**, the hormone of the thyroid gland, can cause depression and lack of motivation (see Chapter 22), while excess can lead to hyperactivity and even mania.

All of these hormones are produced in both men and women. Unlike the neurotransmitters we've spoken about already, which are made from protein, these hormones, with the exception of melatonin and thyroxine, are made from fat (stearic acid) and are thus called steroid hormones.

That's why people on very low-fat diets often develop hormonal imbalances. We need essential fats for the body to make its own cholesterol, from which it can make all these hormones. The chart below shows the "family tree" of all these hormones.

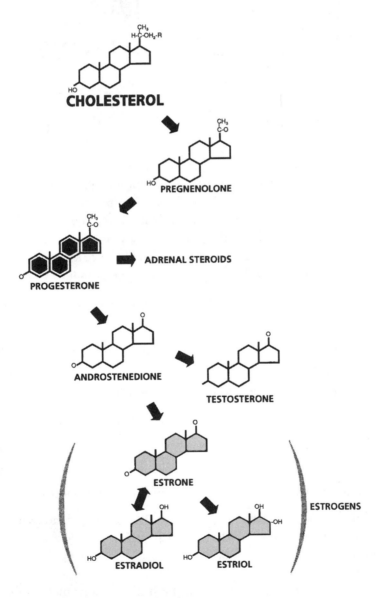

Fig 21   The family tree of steroid hormones

Banishing the Premenstrual Blues

More than a third of all menstruating women suffer from premenstrual syndrome (PMS), with ten percent suffering severely. Common symptoms include depression, anxiety, irritability, fluid retention, mood swings, bloating, breast tenderness, weight gain, acne, fatigue, sweet cravings, and forgetfulness, most often experienced in the week before menstruation and stopping within hours of the start of the period. Some women get symptoms at ovulation, halfway through their cycle.

As you can see from the figure below, these two times, ovulation and the days leading up to menstruation, are the times when there is the greatest changes in estrogen and progesterone levels. It's the balance between these hormones that is thought to be mainly responsible for the symptoms of PMS. The less adaptive capacity you've got, the worse you respond to these hormonal changes and others, such as the drop-off in estrogen and progesterone at menopause and the equivalent drop-off in testosterone at male menopause. Yes, men have a menopause too—it's called the andropause.

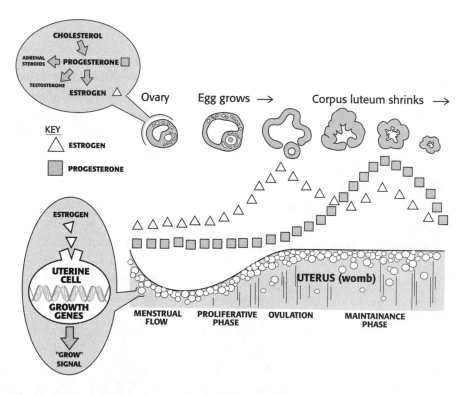

Fig 22   Hormone levels in a normal menstrual cycle

If you're deficient in vitamins, lacking in essential fats, and have poor blood sugar control, you are likely to suffer with mood swings when your hormones go up and down. Stress is also a big factor that can also upset hormonal balance. So the first tip to banishing those monthly blues is to follow the advice in Parts 1 and 2 of this book.

There are also different kinds of PMS. Some women get breast tenderness and water retention, some don't. Some get food cravings, some don't. Breast tenderness, probably a symptom of water retention, can be helped by supplementing 300 milligrams (mg) of magnesium a day, plus 100 mg of vitamin B_6, which is a natural diuretic. It is also wise to avoid salt, although there is one high in magnesium and potassium, and low-sodium salt called Solo, which is OK.

Women suffering from PMS often crave high-sugar, high-calorie foods. These are almost certainly linked to disglycemia, so stabilize blood sugar levels by avoiding sugar and stimulants throughout the month and "grazing" on slow-releasing carbohydrates, with some protein. They may also be connected to serotonin deficiency, corrected by increasing your intake of tryptophan or 5-HTP.

An Overload of Estrogen?

An estimated 75 percent of PMS sufferers have high estrogen levels in relation to progesterone. This may be partly due to our exposure to so many estrogen-mimicking chemicals, found in anything from detergents, plastics and pesticides, and to stress, which raises estrogen levels. The antidote is optimum nutrition with the right supplements. One clinical trial found that taking B_6 in the range of 200–800 mg reduced blood estrogen, increased progesterone, and reduced symptoms.[66] A simple saliva test can help identify whether you are estrogen dominant.

Following all the recommendations in this book, including eating organically grown produce, reducing consumption of high-fat meat and dairy produce, and eating foods rich in "phytoestrogens" such as beans and lentils, especially soy, can help balance excess estrogen. Paradoxical as it sounds, phytoestrogens lower excessive estrogen signals in the body and raise very low levels, as found in menopause. They do this by blocking the estrogen receptors, thereby preventing all those harmful estrogen-mimicking chemicals from wreaking havoc. They are very weak estrogens themselves, so they have little impact on overloading or imbalancing the system. These plant-based phytoestrogens are best thought of as hormone regulators.

Too much estrogen has many effects in the body that could explain an increased risk of mood swings and depression. High levels of the stress hormone cortisol are associated with depression and anxiety. Estrogen stops the body from breaking down cortisol, hence prolonging its effects. This may explain why women tend to be more greatly affected by stress and traumatic events. Estrogen increases copper levels, and high copper can deplete the body of zinc, while both high copper and low zinc are associated with depression. Zinc also helps vitamin B_6 to work, so make sure you supplement at least 15 mg a day if you suffer from PMS.

The four most important nutrients for banishing PMS-related mood swings are vitamin B_6, zinc, magnesium, and essential fats. Each has been proven to reduce symptoms of PMS on its own, but they are much more powerful in combination. Researchers at St. Thomas's Hospital in London gave 630 women up to 200 mg of vitamin B_6 as long ago as 1976 and found up to 88 percent had a significant improvement in their PMS.[67]

PMS sufferers have been shown to have significantly lower magnesium levels than women who do not have PMS,[68] and French researchers who gave 192 women up to 6 g of magnesium daily for the week before and the first two days of their period achieved amazing results—nervous tension was relieved in 89 percent, weight gain in 95 percent, breast tenderness in 96 percent and headaches in 43 percent of sufferers.[69]

The key, though, may be evening primrose oil (EPO). Numerous studies, including one large open study on women for whom other kinds of PMS therapy had failed, and several double-blind, placebo-controlled trials, have all demonstrated that EPO is a highly effective treatment for the depression and irritability, the breast pain and tenderness, and the fluid retention associated with PMS.[70] Nutrients known to increase the utilization and effectiveness of EPO include, you guessed it, vitamin B_6, zinc, and magnesium. So the clinical success obtained with some of these nutrients may in part relate to their effects on EPO (i.e. essential fatty acid) metabolism.

Women with PMS are often deficient in these nutrients, which can help banish mood swings and depression, not only premenstrually, but also during menopause. Some women do benefit from natural progesterone, given as a transdermal skin cream, but I don't recommend this for premenstrual women unless these diet and supplement recommendations haven't worked and a hormone test confirms progesterone deficiency. This can occur because a woman isn't ovulating. When the egg isn't released from the ovum, the ovum no longer produces progesterone in the second half of the cycle, which leads to relative estrogen dominance.

There is a worrisome trend in medicine to treat PMS with antidepressant drugs. While this can help, demonstrating the importance of adequate serotonin in relation to all mood-related problems, in my experience the optimum nutrition approach works better, without the associated risks inherent with these drugs (see Chapter 21). In fact, I have never seen a PMS sufferer who didn't improve dramatically with the right diet and supplements.

Preventing Menopausal Mood Swings and Depression

Mental health problems during the menopausal phase are exceedingly common. The most widespread are depression, anxiety, insomnia, and worsening memory. In one survey, 45 percent of women experienced minor depressive symptoms during menopause, while 27 percent complained of nervousness or irritability.

The same nutrients—B$_6$, zinc, magnesium, and essential fats—all greatly help to reduce menopausal symptoms and allow the body to better adapt to changing hormonal levels. Serotonin deficiency is also very common in menopausal women, who often benefit greatly from additional tryptophan or 5-HTP (see Chapter 14).

Menopausal depression and worsening mental acuity can occur due to estrogen and progesterone deficiency. According to John Lee, a doctor from California who pioneered research using "natural" progesterone, mood, mental clarity, and concentration frequently improve with the use of transdermal progesterone skin creams. Most conventional HRT includes synthetic progestins, sometimes called progestogens. These not only don't work very well, they've been linked to increasing risk of breast cancer.[71]

The good thing about natural progesterone is that the body can also make estrogen from it (follow the arrows in Figure 21). However, that being said, some women find greater relief with both estrogen and natural progesterone therapy. The combination of the two prevents the cancer risks associated with unopposed estrogen.

Andropause and Depression in Men

The effects of testosterone deficiency are not unlike the effects of estrogen and progesterone deficiency. Around a third of men in the forty to sixty-nine age group complain of a range of symptoms that commonly include, in order of importance, loss of libido, erectile dysfunction (inability to get or maintain an erection), depression, and worsening memory and concentration. These are the classic symptoms of andropause.

Despite years of research pioneered in Britain by Dr. Malcolm Carruthers, who wrote *The Testosterone Revolution*, many doctors still deny the existence of male menopause. However, these symptoms, especially depression, should be taken seriously. Depression in men is harder to diagnose since men tend to get angry rather than sad. They are also more likely to commit suicide. Andropause can be helped by supplementing the hormone testosterone.

If the symptoms above do sound like you, it is well worth having your testosterone levels measured. If low, meaning below 12 nmol/l, then you may benefit from testosterone replacement therapy. However, symptoms are as important, if not more so, than testosterone levels in the blood. This is because most testosterone in the blood is not "free," but bound and unavailable. The "free" testosterone is much harder to measure. Salivary testosterone levels may be a better indicator, backed up by symptoms. You can both test your symptoms and get a salivary testosterone test by visiting www.andropause.com. The salivary test also measures your DHEA levels (see below). These tests are also available through clinical nutritionists.

If you do have low testosterone, supplementing extra can really help. Dr. Elizabeth Barrett-Connor studied 680 men aged between 50 and 89 and found a direct relationship between testosterone levels and mood.[72] In the United Kingdom, Dr. Carruthers has treated 1,500 men and found a consistent elevation in mood once testosterone levels become normal.

From a nutritional point of view, make sure you are eating adequate protein and slow-releasing carbohydrates. Essential fats are required for healthy sperm and prostate function, antioxidant nutrients protect testosterone from being destroyed, and zinc helps everything to do with male sexual health and hormonal balance. So make sure you are getting enough of all these nutrients.

DHEA Deficiency and Adrenal Exhaustion

Sometimes mood swings and depression can be a result of too much stress and adrenal exhaustion. The adrenal glands, on top of the kidneys, produce a number of hormones—cortisol, adrenaline, noradrenaline, and DHEA. Prolonged stress can result in an inability to produce sufficient amounts of these motivating molecules. DHEA levels are frequently low in both anxious and depressed people and have been associated with aggressive and cynical attitudes and loss of enjoyment of life. Without sufficient adrenal hormones, especially DHEA, you lose your "get up and go" and ability to cope with the normal stresses of life, becoming more anxious, on edge, and depressed. Of course, the answer is to decrease stress, but how do you get your adrenal function up to par?

The answer can be to supplement DHEA. A study at the University of California psychiatry department in 1997 gave depressed, middle-aged, and elderly people 30–90 mg of DHEA and found a clear improvement in their moods.[73]

I never recommend DHEA, from which the body can make other adrenal hormones (follow the arrows in Figure 21), without first running a saliva test to determine whether you have low levels of this hormone. If they are low, I recommend 25 mg a day for women and 50 mg a day for men until these levels are normalized. DHEA isn't available over the counter in Britain but is in the United States. You and I can buy it by mail order for our own use. A clinical nutritionist can both determine your DHEA levels and let you know how you can order this supplement.

If you do suffer from mood swings and depression, and basic changes to your diet, including supplements, hasn't helped, you can check for hormonal imbalances quite simply. A simple saliva test can measure your estrogen, progesterone, testosterone, and DHEA levels. These tests are available through clinical nutritionists who can then advise you about how to bring your hormones back into balance.

In the meantime, here are a few things you can do for yourself:

- Ensure your diet is giving you plenty of essential fats and supplement 200 mg of GLA (either a borage oil 1,000 mg supplement a day, or 4 evening primrose oil 500 mg supplements).

- Supplement 100 mg of vitamin B_6, 20 mg of zinc, and 300 mg of magnesium.

- Eat little and often, choosing slow-releasing carbohydrate foods, combined with protein.

- Try adding 100 mg of 5-HTP if all the above doesn't help.

Chapter 16

UNWINDING ANXIETY
WITH NATURAL RELAXANTS

It's great to feel calm and centered, but too many of us are all wound up: stress and anxiety are, sad to relate, the hallmarks of twenty-first century living. A survey of 22,000 people in Britain found that one in two people frequently experience anxiety. You are not alone. Feelings and symptoms of stress affect most of us. These include headaches, muscle tension, dry mouth, excessive perspiration, pounding heart, insomnia, and fatigue.

In the long run, stress and anxiety age you. This is because they put the body into emergency mode, known as the "fight-or-flight syndrome," in which the body's energy is channelled away from maintenance and repair, and towards reacting physically to a stressful event. Adrenaline and cortisol start pumping, blood sugar levels go up, pupils dilate to let in more light, we huff and puff to take in more oxygen—but, unlike our ancestors, we don't (often) fight or take flight. The most we do is toot the car horn, raise our voice, or bottle it up inside.

Most people, when faced with an intense or constant feeling of anxiety, will either "self-medicate" with alcohol or cannabis, or see their doctors, possibly to be given a prescription for a tranquilizer. In one week in Britain, we pop 10 million tranquilizers, puff 10 million cannabis joints, and drink 120 million alcoholic drinks.

GABA: The Antidote to Anxiety

The choice of these three drugs—alcohol, cannabis, and tranquilizers—is no coincidence. They all promote the neurotransmitter GABA, which is the brain's peacemaker, helping to turn off excess adrenaline and calm you down.

That's why that beer or glass of wine makes you feel sociable, relaxed, happy, and less serious, at least for an hour as GABA levels rise. But after an hour or so GABA starts to fall and you feel irritable and disconnected, so you have another one, and another one. The trouble is that after a session of drinking, GABA levels become very suppressed, leaving you grumpy and irritable. So many of us avoid this by drinking in the evening and going to sleep under the influence. What we don't realize is that alcohol also disturbs the normal cycle of dreaming, and it's dreaming that regenerates the mind. So, when you wake up in the morning, you're mentally tired, grumpy and irritable because of the low GABA, dehydrated, and feeling sluggish as your body detoxifies the alcohol from the night before. The net effect is that alcohol, in the long run, makes you more anxious, not less. The same is essentially true for cannabis which, if habitually smoked, reduces drive and motivation.

Tranquilizer Addiction

The most common antianxiety drugs are the benzodiazepine tranquilizers, such as Valium, Librium, and Ativan. These are highly effective at reducing anxiety in the short term, but highly addictive in as little as four weeks. For this reason doctors are strongly advised not to prescribe these for more than four weeks.

Despite this, a poll carried out by *Panorama* found that 3 percent of people polled, equivalent to one and a half million people nationally, have been on tranquilizers for more than four months. Of these, 28 percent had been on them for more than ten years![74]

These tranquilizers are more addictive than heroin, and coming off them is no joke. Withdrawal can lead to insomnia, anxiety, irritability, sweating, blurred vision, diarrhoea, tremors, mental impairment, and headaches. Abrupt withdrawal from high doses can lead to seizures or even death.

The sad truth is that tranquilizers, much like alcohol, increase anxiety and depression in the long run, as well as being addictive. With tranquilizers, however, the reason is slightly different. Tranquilizers open up the brain's receptor sites for GABA, making the brain more sensitive to its effects. So you feel more relaxed, less anxious. The next day, however, you can feel "hung over." The more often you take them the more you need to get the same effect, and without them, you can get rebound anxiety and insomnia. Knowing all this, it's shocking that these drugs are still prescribed for anything other than short-term traumas, especially when we now know there are natural, nonaddictive and more effective alternatives.

Natural Relaxants

States of anxiety are associated with the stress hormones adrenaline and cortisol. In Chapters 3, 9, and 10 we discussed how blood sugar ups and downs and overuse of stimulants such as caffeine and nicotine can stress us out. So, the step to reducing anxiety is to balance your blood sugar by eating slow-releasing carbohydrates and avoid or, at least considerably reduce, your use of stimulants.

Then there are natural GABA promoters that ensure you produce and release GABA when you need a healthy relaxation response. These include both amino acids, minerals, and herbs, the most effective being:

- GABA

- Taurine

- Kava

- Valerian

- Hops

- Passion flower

- Magnesium

Let's explore how these can reduce your anxiety level.

GABA: The Antidote to Stress

As we saw above, GABA (gamma-amino-butyric acid) is the main inhibitory or calming neurotransmitter. It not only calms down excess adrenaline, noradrenaline, and dopamine, it also effects serotonin, thereby affecting your mood. For these reasons, having enough GABA in your brain is associated with being relaxed and happy, while having too little is associated with anxiety, tension, depression, and insomnia.[75]

GABA is not only a neurotransmitter, it's also an amino acid. This means it's a nutrient, and by supplementing it, you can help to promote normal healthy levels of GABA in the brain. Supplementing 500–1,000 mg, once or twice a day, is a highly effective natural relaxant.

While it is not addictive, that doesn't mean there are no side effects in large amounts. While up to 2 g a day has no reported downside, supplementing 10 g a day can induce nausea, vomiting, and increases in blood pressure. So use GABA wisely, especially if you already have high blood pressure, starting with no more than 1 g a day, and do not exceed 3 g a day.

Taurine: GABA's Best Friend

Taurine is another relaxing amino acid, similar in structure and effect to GABA. Many people think taurine is a stimulant because it is used in so-called "energy drinks," but it is not. It helps you relax and unwind from high levels of adrenaline, much like GABA.

Taurine has many other uses as well, including insomnia, depression, and even mania, the "high" phase manic depression, discussed in Chapter 23.

Taurine is highly concentrated in animal foods such as fish, eggs, and meat. Vegetarians are therefore more likely to be at risk of deficiency. While the body can make taurine from the amino acids, L-cysteine and L-methionine (provided you've got enough vitamin B_6), if you are prone to high levels of anxiety, you may benefit from supplementing this relaxing amino acid. Try 500–1,000 mg of taurine, twice daily. There are no known cautions or adverse effects at reasonable doses.

Kava kava: A Pacific Herb

Kava is a native Polynesian vine that has been consumed as a social and ceremonial nonalcoholic drink by Pacific Islanders for over 3,000 years. The first description of this member of the pepper family came to the West from Captain James Cook on his celebrated voyages through the South Seas. The root is used both for the drink and dried to make the supplements available in the West, where it is being used increasingly to counteract stress, anxiety, and insomnia.

Kava is excellent at reducing anxiety. One four-week study of patients diagnosed with anxiety found that participants experienced dramatic improvements in their symptoms of anxiety after just one week, with improvement continuing through week four.[76] In the longest (six-month) study to date, by Dr. H. P. Volz in Germany, kava provided significant relief of anxiety versus a placebo, and with minimal side effects[77]. Numerous studies have compared the effectiveness of kava not just with placebos but also with the leading tranquilizer medications and found it just as effective but without the side effects common in those on the drugs.[78 79 80] Kava relaxes both emotions and muscles, making it useful for headaches, backaches, and other symptoms caused by muscular tension. It also reduces excessive mental chatter and increases mental focus. But, most important of all, it is non-addictive.

The reason kava works is because it contains a unique resin made up of kavalactones and other compounds acting both on the limbic system, which is the emotional center of the brain (most likely through an indirect action on GABA receptors), and directly on muscles, thus promoting relaxation in two different ways, while causing no habituation, tolerance, addiction, or hangover as alcohol does.

You need 60–75 mg of kavalactones, taken two to three times daily, to get this antianxiety effect. As a sedative to aid sleep, take 120–200 mg before retiring. Different forms of kava have different concentrations of kavalactones, so it is always best to work out the dose from the kavalactones rather than the total amount of kava in any given powder, capsule, or tincture. Sadly, however, kava is banned in a number of countries.

Can Kava Be Liver Toxic?

Taken in these typical doses, kava has no known side effects except for exceedingly rare skin rashes in sensitive individuals, headache, or mild stomach upset. Recent investigations in Germany have focused on the potential liver-toxic effects of excessively concentrated extracts, which may make it difficult for the liver to process the fatlike kavalactones. This means that the liver has to "biotransform" kavalactone residues to eliminate them from the body. This is done with a series of enzymes in the liver that are dependent on a nutrient called glutathione. The whole kava root contains both kavalactones and glutathione, but some kava extracts (especially those giving 60 percent or more kavalactones) concentrate the kavalactones and eliminate the glutathione. Under normal circumstances this isn't a problem. But alcohol and many prescription drugs, for example paracetamol, use the same detoxification enzymes. So, if you drink a lot of alcohol and are on liver-toxic drugs including benzodiazepine tranquilizers, kava adds to your liver's burden. There were some cases in Germany where just this happened.[81] For this reason, I don't recommend using kava extracts if you are a heavy drinker, or are on prescription medication, without your doctor's approval.

Valerian: Nature's Valium

Another excellent antianxiety herb is valerian (*Valeriana officinalis*). Derived from the dried rhizomes and roots of an attractive perennial with pretty pink flowers, it grows throughout Europe in wet soils. As a natural relaxant it is useful for several disorders such as restlessness, nervousness, insomnia, and hysteria, and it has also been used as a sedative for "nervous" stomach. Valerian acts on the brain's GABA receptors, enhancing their activity and thus offering a similar tranquilizing action as the Valium-type drugs but without the same side effects. As a relaxant you need 50–100 mg twice a day, and twice this amount 45 minutes before retiring for a good night's sleep.

Since valerian potentiates sedative drugs, including muscle relaxants and antihistamines, don't take it if you are on prescribed medication without your doctor's consent. Valerian can also interact with alcohol, as well as certain psychotropic drugs and narcotics.

Hops and Passion Flower: Favorites of the Aztecs

Hops (*Humulus lupulus*) is an ancient remedy for a good night's sleep and probably included in beer for that reason. Hops helps to calm nerves by acting directly on the central nervous system, rather than affecting GABA receptors. You need about 200 mg per day, but the effect is much less than kava or valerian and most effective when taken in combination with these and other herbs such as passion flower.

Passion flower (*Passiflora incarnata*) was a favorite of the Aztecs, who used it to make relaxing drinks. It has a mild sedative effect and promotes sleep much like hops, with no known side effects at normal doses. Passion flower can also be helpful for hyperactive kids. You need around 100–200 mg a day.

Combinations of these herbs are particularly effective for relieving anxiety and can really help break the pattern of reacting stressfully to life's challenges.

Magnesium: Relaxing Mind and Muscle

Magnesium is another important nutrient that helps you relax. It's also commonly deficient. Magnesium not only relaxes your mind, it relaxes your muscles. Symptoms of deficiency therefore include muscle aches, cramps, and spasms, as well as anxiety and insomnia. Low levels are commonly found in anxious people, and supplementation can often help. You need about 500 mg of magnesium a day. Seeds and nuts are rich in it, as are vegetables and fruit, but especially dark green leafy vegetables such as kale or spinach. I recommend eating these magnesium-rich foods every day and supplementing an additional 300 mg. But, if you are especially anxious and can't sleep, supplement 500 mg in the evening.

Cutting Out the Culprits

Supplementing to alleviate anxiety is vital. But we also need to look at substances in the body that you might need to control to feel calmer.

The Histamine-Copper Connection

While blood sugar problems and low magnesium levels are common reasons for reacting stressfully, they are not the only biochemical imbalances that can lead to anxiety. Dr. Carl Pfeiffer found that many of his patients who experienced extreme fears, phobias, and paranoia had very low histamine levels. Many also had high copper levels, a toxic element in excess, which can depress histamine levels.

These low-histamine patients, Pfeiffer found, had many characteristics that were opposite to the high-histamine types described later in Chapter 22. These included more body hair, more likelihood of being overweight, rare headaches or allergies, a high pain threshold, and a suspicious nature. He found that these people also did really well on large amounts of niacin, folic acid, and B_{12}, plus vitamin C, zinc, and manganese, which help to lower high levels of copper.

If these symptoms sound like you, it's well worth having your mineral levels checked, and if you do have high levels of copper or any other toxic minerals, then taking the necessary steps, described in Chapter 10, to lower your levels. If you do experience extreme fears and anxiety, you may also benefit from supplementing large amounts of niacin, folic acid, and vitamin B_{12}. This should, however, only be done under the guidance of a clinical nutritionist.

Lactic Acid: Pushing the Panic Button

Some people experience panic attacks, characterized by extreme feelings of fear. These are not at all uncommon. Symptoms often experienced during a panic attack include palpitations, rapid breathing, dizziness, unsteadiness, and a feeling of impending death. Those with agoraphobia, a fear of being alone or of public places, often know that they can go out or can be alone, but are afraid of having a panic attack.

As "psychological" as this sounds, there is a biochemical imbalance behind many people's anxiety attacks, apart from, or as well as, any psychological factors. It's too much lactic acid. When muscles don't get enough oxygen, they make energy from glucose without it. The trouble is there's a byproduct called lactic acid. As strange as this might seem, giving those prone to anxiety attacks lactic acid can induce an anxiety attack.[82]

One way to increase lactic acid levels is to hyperventilate. Many people will do this when they're experiencing anxiety attacks. Hyperventilation changes the acid level of the blood by altering the balance of carbon dioxide. The body responds by producing more lactic acid. The solution is to breathe into a paper bag during a hyperventilation attack and concentrate on breathing deeply for a minute. This helps redress the balance. Moments of blood sugar dips can also both bring on hyperventilation and increase lactic acid. So, keep your blood sugar level even by eating little and often. Finally, deficiency in vitamin B_1 stops the body from breaking down glucose properly, again promoting lactic acid. So, make sure you are supplementing with a good B complex or multivitamin. Also, check yourself out for food allergies. These are the most common biochemical imbalances that can lead to panic attacks.

Combinations of Herbs and Nutrients Work Best

The combination of relaxing amino acids and herbs is the most effective for reducing high levels of anxiety. The synergistic action of nutrients and herbs such as GABA, taurine, kava, valerian, hops, and passion flower also means the doses for each can be lower.

While the causes for high levels of anxiety are often psychological, by balancing blood sugar, reducing stimulants, ensuring optimum nutrition, plus judiciously using these natural antianxiety herbs and nutrients, you can break the habit of reacting with fear and anxiety to life's inevitable stresses.

Here's one man's experience on a combination of these natural relaxants, which are available in combination in some supplements:

"They certainly seem to take the 'sharp edges' off daily stresses. I am conscious of the detrimental effects of relying on alcohol to 'wind down' at the end of the day and feel I have found a good substitute. The effect is quite subtle, although still very noticeable."

In summary, to beat stress and reduce anxiety:

- Keep your blood sugar even by eating slow-releasing carbohydrates and avoiding stimulants and sugar.

- Deal with the underlying causes of your stress and anxiety, perhaps by working with a counselor or psychotherapist.

- Supplement kava or valerian, or the amino acids GABA or taurine, or a combination of these relaxing herbs and amino acids, plus magnesium.

Chapter 17

SOLVING SLEEPING PROBLEMS

None of us can live without it. We need it every day. And most of us are deficient in it. It's not a vitamin or a mineral—it's sleep. An alarming 47 percent of people have difficulty falling asleep or staying asleep throughout the night, but many more are simply not getting enough for optimal health.

Before the electric lightbulb extended our days, most people slept for up to ten hours a night. The figure now hovers around seven and continues to fall. Not only are we sleeping less in the twenty-first century because we've learned how to extend our daytime, but we also sleep less to get more done. Yet research clearly shows that it's a rare person who can survive on a great deal less than seven or eight hours' sleep a night.

One of the great mysteries is why we need sleep at all. Without it, even for a night, the body shows clear signs of stress—mood and concentration go, defenses drop, levels of vital nutrients such as zinc and magnesium fall, vitamin C is used up at an alarming rate. Sleep rejuvenates both the body and the mind. During the first three hours of sleep, the body goes into rapid repair mode. This is one of the reasons why, if you are injured or sick, nothing is better than a good night's sleep.

The Importance of Dreaming

After a couple of hours, we enter the dream-state sleep, known as rapid eye movement, or REM, Stage 1. REM sleep normally occurs ninety minutes after the onset of sleep, but if we are sleep deprived, it may occur within thirty minutes.

Dreaming occurs during REM sleep, and most of us have four or more REM periods per night, even though many people have difficulty remembering the dreams that occur in them. As well as providing physical rest, sleep may provide the chance to make a "back-up tape" of the day's events for our large computer, the brain. While Westerners pay little heed to dreams, one African tribe believes "real life" is lived in dreams and daytime is the illusion. The Bolivian philosopher Oscar Ichazo describes dream reality like the stars at night: Dream thoughts are always happening, but the brightness of the sun, daytime consciousness, blots them out. Many scientists believe that nutritional deficiency is one reason why poor or no dream recall can occur.

In a survey at the Institute for Optimum Nutrition we found that more than 40 percent of people had no or very infrequent dream recall. When researching the signs and symptoms of vitamin B_6 and zinc deficiency, we found that an alarming proportion of deficient people couldn't recall their dreams. After supplementation with B_6 and zinc their dream recall returned, and they reported their dreams as more vivid.

So if you don't think you dream, it's worth supplementing B_6 and zinc, gradually increasing the dose up to 200 mg B_6 and 30 mg of zinc. (It is best not to take more than this without the advice of a nutritionist.) Combinations of sleep-promoting herbs and amino acids, discussed below, are also excellent for promoting good-quality sleep and dreams.

One woman told me she hadn't slept more than five hours a night for at least ten years. After supplementing a combination of kava, hops, passion flower, GABA, and taurine, she slept for twelve hours straight and woke up feeling fantastic. Another woman reported great benefits from the same combination, but not in promoting sleep. Her problem was in waking up. After supplementing these sleep-promoting nutrients she started waking up at 8:00 A.M. full of energy, rather than at 10:00 A.M. still tired. Another reported that after supplementing a combination of kava and 5-HTP, she started dreaming in color for the first time in her life! Many others have reported more lucid dreams and improved dream recall, as well as deeper sleep without waking.

Given that it is an essential way of resting, recharging, and nourishing both your body and mind, sustained, unbroken sleep, and dreaming, is part of the lifestyle package that determines the quality of our lives and our health.

Are You Sleep Deprived?

Sleep specialists at Loughborough University have carried out a series of tests into how the brain functions when it is deprived of sleep. And the results are very clear: Sleepy people have problems finding the right words, coming up with ideas, and coping with rapidly changing situations. So cutting back on sleep may make you less efficient, not more.

Even if you're not involved in any particularly brain-taxing work, a lack of sleep is likely to lower your mood and your general ability to cope with what life throws at you. How much easier is it to deal with a mistake by your bank or a late train if you're feeling alert and well rather than half awake? Sleep deprivation makes us moody and irritable, and in the long term, even depressed. Scientists have measured the body's ability to fight off infections when it is tired, and research has shown that sleep-deprived individuals have a reduction in natural killer cells, a type of immune cell needed for resistance against invaders.

Six Steps to Supersleep

If you are having problems getting to sleep, staying asleep, or getting enough sleep, there are six steps you can take to improve your sleep life:

- Get to the bottom of any factors interrupting your sleep.

- Manage your stress levels.

- Maintain even blood sugar levels throughout the day.

- Balance your minerals, supplementing magnesium.

- Balance your sleep neurotransmitters—serotonin and melatonin.

- If necessary, use a natural sleep aid such as kava kava or valerian.

There is always a reason why you have sleep problems—whether it's getting to sleep, waking in the night, or waking too early, emotional or physical. Dealing with the cause must be the first step before you reach for the sleeping tablets—even the natural ones. So first, look at the box on the next page to see whether there are any triggers you can deal with right away.

Perpetuating sleeplessness—which apply to you?

- stress
- noise
- heat or cold
- irregular sleeping hours
- shift work
- medication side effects (e.g., some bronchodilators for asthma, some antidepressants)
- eating too close to bedtime
- excessive/late caffeine intake
- excessive/late alcohol intake
- late cigarette smoking
- indigestion
- pain
- depression
- widely fluctuating blood sugar levels
- breathing problems
- recreational drugs
- excessive afternoon napping
- uncomfortable or old bed
- expecting to have problems sleeping

Most people at some time in their lives have experienced the frustration, restlessness, and exhaustion of not being able to get enough sleep or waking up too early and not getting back to sleep. Although this is usually linked to an anxious time or to the factors listed above, it is also very much affected by what you eat.

Stress, Sugar, and Stimulants Keep You Awake

Many of our bodies' daily rhythms, including those that dictate our energy and sleepiness, are finely tuned mechanisms that depend on certain hormonal patterns, body chemicals, and nutrients. At night time, the levels of the stress hormone cortisol should dip, calming your body and preparing it for sleep. If, however, your cortisol levels are out of kilter for any reason (usually stress or a diet high in stimulants or sugar), your ability to get to sleep, to sleep through the night, or to wake up refreshed are likely to be impaired. If cortisol levels are high at night, this suppresses the release of growth hormone, which is essential for daily tissue repair and growth. This effectively speeds up the rate at which your body ages. A nutritionist can run a saliva test for you to determine whether your cortisol rhythm is out of sync.

Dealing with underlying causes of stress is clearly important. So too is keeping your blood sugar levels balanced by eating regular meals throughout the day, including some protein-rich food at each meal (such as fish, eggs, lean meat, or a form of soy), avoiding refined foods, coffee, sugary foods and drinks, and minimizing alcohol. Many people who wake in the night and then can't get back to sleep find that keeping blood sugar levels even during the day sets the scene for the correct patterns at night, giving more chance of a good night's sleep.

How Serotonin and Melatonin Help You Sleep

During the daytime, adrenaline levels are higher and keep you stimulated. As you start to wind down, serotonin levels rise and adrenaline levels fall. As it gets darker, another neurotransmitter, melatonin, kicks in. Melatonin is an almost identical molecule to serotonin, from which it is made, and both are made from the amino acid tryptophan. Melatonin's main role in the brain is to regulate the sleep/wake cycle. Interestingly, melatonin is produced in the light-sensitive pineal gland in the center of the brain, also known as the third eye and considered by René Descartes to be the seat of the soul. Have you ever thought about where the light comes from when you dream?

As we learned earlier, many people, especially women, become serotonin deficient. Without enough serotonin you don't make enough melatonin. Without melatonin it is difficult to get to sleep and stay asleep. Waking far too early in the morning and not being able to get back to sleep is a classic symptom of deficiency of these essential brain chemicals.

Adequate amounts of B_6 and tryptophan are needed for you to get sleepy. Foods that are particularly high in tryptophan are chicken, cheese, tuna, tofu, eggs, nuts, seeds, and milk. As usual, a traditional remedy—drinking a glass of milk before bed—becomes grounded in science. Other foods associated with inducing sleep are lettuce and oats.

Most effective of all is supplementing 5-HTP or melatonin itself. 5-HTP (hydroxytryptophan) is the direct precursor of serotonin, and by supplementing it you can increase levels of melatonin and serotonin. 5-HTP is very highly concentrated in the seeds of the African griffonia plant. Supplementing 100 mg–200 mg of 5-HTP half an hour before sleep helps you get a good night's sleep. Tryptophan, 2,000 mg a night, also works but is not available over the counter. It is, however, available on prescription from your doctor.

Melatonin, which is a neurotransmitter, not a nutrient, can also be helpful but needs to be used much more cautiously. This is because supplementing too much can have undesirable effects such as diarrhea, constipation, nausea, dizziness, reduced libido, headaches, depression, and nightmares. However, if you do sleep badly, you may want to try 3 mg before bedtime.

Sometimes supplementing 5-HTP or melatonin for a month can bring you back into balance, reestablishing proper sleep patterns, after which the supplements become unnecessary to continue. This is a great way to wean yourself of more harmful sleeping pills.

Melatonin is also very useful for jetlag, when your body clock goes out of sync with the earth. The best way to bring yourself back into balance is to supplement 1 mg of melatonin for every one-hour time difference, just before your new bedtime. So, if you fly from London to Los Angeles, which is eight hours behind, you take 8 mg on the first night, then halve it to 4 mg for the second night, 2 mg for the third, then 1 mg, then stop. Always take it just before you want to go to sleep and halve the dose each night. Melatonin cannot be bought over the counter in Britain, but can be bought for your own personal use by mail order or on the Web from the United States where these restrictions don't apply.

Calming Minerals

A lack of the minerals calcium and magnesium can trigger or exacerbate sleep difficulties because they work together to calm the body and help relax nerves and muscles. Magnesium levels may well be low if you are particularly stressed or consume too much sugar. Including some magnesium in the evening, perhaps even in a supplement, may help. Your diet is more likely to be low in magnesium than calcium—so make sure you are eating plenty of magnesium-rich foods such as seeds, nuts, green vegetables, whole grains, and seafood. Milk products, green vegetables, nuts, seafood, and molasses are particularly good sources of calcium. Some people find it helpful to supplement 600 mg of calcium and 400 mg of magnesium at bedtime. Ensuring adequate B vitamins daily help support the body in many ways, including its ability to deal with stress—take B-complex vitamins earlier in the day rather than in the evening, though, as they are also involved in energy production and keep some people awake.

Herbal Nightcaps

It's really best to resort to sleeping aids—natural or pharmaceutical—only as a last resort. Medicinal sedatives are generally bad news in that they are usually addictive and your tolerance increases, making higher and higher doses necessary for any effect. They have a range of side effects such as daytime drowsiness, memory problems, confusion, depression, dry mouth, sluggishness, and all sorts of other unpleasant symptoms. They are also strong chemicals which need to be detoxified by the body, placing a burden on your liver.

There are many natural substances that can help you sleep, although again, they should be used when other avenues have been exhausted and then only occasionally. You'll find many of them, especially the herbs, are sold in blended formulas.

Valerian is sometimes referred to as "nature's Valium." As such, it can interact with alcohol and other sedative drugs and should therefore be taken in combination with them only under careful medical supervision.
Dosage: 150–300 mg about forty-five minutes before bedtime.

Passion flower's mild sedative effect has been well substantiated in numerous animal and human studies. The herb encourages deep, restful, uninterrupted sleep, with no side effects.
Dosage: varies with the formula, generally 100–200 mg of a standardized extract.

Kava kava is a relaxant for both mind and body. If taken twenty minutes before bedtime, kava can help promote a deeper sleep with no drowsiness on waking. See the cautions on page 131.
Dosage: 250 mg an hour before bed (standardized to 30 percent kava-lactones).

St. John's wort, also called Hypericum, has both serotonin- and melatonin-enhancing effects, making it an excellent sleep regulator.
Dosage: 300 mg (standardised to 0.3 percent hypericin).

Hops has been used for centuries as a mild sedative and sleeping aid. Its sedative action works directly on the central nervous system.
Dosage: varies, but around 200 mg per day.

Combinations of these herbs, together with 5-HTP, are the most effective natural sleep promoters of all. Here are a couple of reports from people who found them of benefit:

"I was suffering from chronic insomnia for a year and a half and was not keen to take sleeping pills. I decided to try a certain combination of relaxing herbs and nutrients, seeing that they were 100 percent natural. I took one an hour before bed and they actually work. Over the last two weeks I have fallen straight to sleep. At long last I can feel refreshed in the morning."

"My problem isn't getting to sleep—it's waking up! I have two alarm clocks and left to my own devices, I don't wake up before 11:00 A.M. I'm the girlfriend from hell in the morning! Then I tried taking a combination of kava, GABA, taurine, and hops before bed. The next morning I woke up at 8:30 A.M. happy and awake. I've tried this several times, and it always works."

Sleep is not the only time that we relax and recharge. Regular exercise, doing relaxation exercises such as yoga, t'ai chi, meditation or breathing exercises, enjoying a pastime such as painting or playing an instrument, spending fun time with a partner, children or a pet—all these can help to divert attention from work and worries, leaving bedtime for sleeping, and maybe sex, if you're not too tired!

In summary, if you want to ensure you get a good night's sleep, with some dreaming thrown in:

- Avoid sugar and stimulants, especially after 4:00 P.M.

- Find ways of relaxing and de-stressing in the evening.

- Make sure your supplement program includes vitamin B_6 100 mg and zinc 10 mg (up to 30 mg if no dream recall).

- Supplement 400 mg of calcium and 300 mg of magnesium in the evening and eat calcium- and magnesium-rich foods, such as seeds and crunchy or dark green vegetables.

- If you suffer from insomnia, supplement either 200 mg of 5-HTP or two 2,000 mg capsules of l-tryptophan before bed, or herbs such as kava or valerian or a combination of these herbs and nutrients.

PART 4

WHAT IS MENTAL ILLNESS?

Mental illness, more than any other disease, is a stigma in modern society. Yet as with many diseases, we know a lot about what causes, prevents, and improves problems from depression to schizophrenia. Often the cause is biochemical, and with the right nutrition, many people make complete recoveries. In this part you will discover what mental illness means, how to get the right diagnosis, why long-term drug therapy is rarely the answer, and all about more effective alternatives.

Chapter 18

UNDERSTANDING MENTAL ILLNESS

Before discussing what to do to alleviate certain types of mental illness, it is important to understand what we mean by this term. It is often used, by layman and specialist alike, as an identity tag with no apparent clear-cut definition or understanding. In fact, the United Kingdom Mental Health Act of 1983 contains no definition. Instead it states,

"In practice the decision as to whether a person is mentally ill is a clinical one, and the expression invariably has to be defined by reference to what the doctor says it means in a particular case rather than to any precise legal criteria."

In other words, it's up to your doctor or psychiatrist.

What we commonly understand by the term "mental illness" is a state of being that falls short of what we consider normal or acceptable. We have all experienced some degree of this. At one end of the spectrum we become unhappy for no apparent reason or find ourselves reacting explosively to the smallest stress or insult. At the other extreme, we hear voices that just won't go away, or feel that we can't go on any more.

In practice, what tends to happen is that a person who continuously suffers from less than normal mental states is labeled depressed, manic depressive, schizophrenic, or with some other mental disorder. He may then carry this label for life and be tagged as a less than normal human being. Such labels do nothing of actual benefit for the individual, so in defining what we mean by mental illness it is important to avoid a label that in itself could contribute to more mental turmoil.

It might therefore be more useful to define our terms in reference to the concept of mental well-being. If a good state of mental health refers to a condition of feeling stable, happy, and satisfied that one is coping adequately with the inevitable problems of day-to-day living, then a mental health problem would refer to a condition where one is *not* coping, where a person is unhappy a lot of the time, frequently feels distressed, and is unnaturally and frequently afraid.

With that in mind, what I call mental illness is a state of mind in which one is unable to cope with some aspect of life to the point where one's ability to lead a fulfilling life is seriously impaired.

Mind and Body: A Self-Organizing Jungle

Every thought and feeling we have can both alter, and is altered by, the chemistry of our body. The mind and body are completely interconnected. One does not exist without the other. The Western concept that we are our minds (I think therefore I am) and that our body is a machine has created this false idea of separation. This idea generated the notion that mental illness is a result of that part of the machine responsible for thinking and feeling, the brain, going wrong. This led to the notion of mental illness as something that must be destroyed by drugs, or surgical procedures such as lobotomies and electroconvulsive shock treatment, both of which damage the brain.

The other avenue that emerged from this concept of separation was a blind belief in psychoanalysis and the notion that mental illness is purely the result of problems in the abstract mind, not the physical brain. This false separation continues today.

Instead of the concept of trying to fix the part that doesn't work, be it the physical brain or the abstract psyche, I prefer to conceive of us human beings as "complex adaptive systems," more like a self-organizing jungle than a complicated computer. Rather than trying to "control" a person's health by playing God with hi-tech medicine, there's a new way of looking at health that considers a human being as a whole, with an interconnected mind and body that is designed to adapt to health if the circumstances are right. We have this amazing drive toward health and happiness, and an extraordinary ability to restore balance when health is lost.

Of course, this "adaptive capacity" is not the same for all. We all have different strengths and weaknesses. So, in this new model, our health is a result of the interaction between our inherited adaptive capacity and our circumstances. For example, on a physical/chemical level that would be

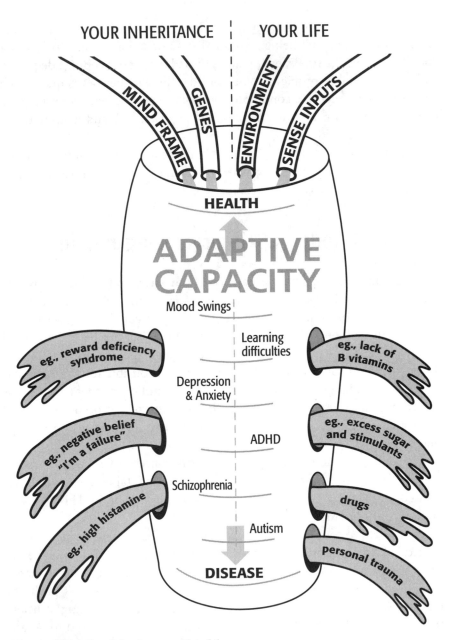

Fig 23   New model of mental health

between our genes and our environment (see Figure 23). If our environment is sufficiently hostile (poor diet, pollution, allergens, and so on), we exceed our ability to adapt and become unwell.

We can apply the same model on a psychological level. Our psychological "environment" is literally everything we see, hear, smell, touch, and taste—

the total sum of all our sense inputs. Our psychological "genes" are our mental constructs, our mind frame, that interprets whatever comes in through the senses in order to make sense of our world. We don't see reality as it actually is, we interpret all we see based on our mental constructs, which are the result of reactions we've had to past similar experiences, which makes up the basis of our childhood conditioning. In this way we form likes and dislikes, attractions and aversions, and so on.

In this new model of health there are four aspects to mental health and four contributors to mental illness:

Environment—This includes all the nutrients and antinutrients we take in. As we learned in Parts 1 and 2, deficiencies in certain vitamins, minerals, essential fats, phospholipids, and amino acids can cause mental health problems, as can excesses in antinutrients. These can be corrected by improving your nutrition and making lifestyle changes to minimize the effects of anti-nutrients.

Genes—In some conditions, including Down's syndrome and schizophrenia, there is clear evidence of genetic differences, which means that a particular aspect of a person's brain chemistry is in a state of imbalance. This too can be vastly improved by specific nutritional strategies. This is also why some people need much more of a nutrient to stay well than others. We are all unique.

Sense input—In many cases, mental health problems develop in times of high stress, when there is more going on than a person can cope with. Adjusting your life to minimize stress is part of the equation. The other is changing the way you interpret what is happening in your life. Although it is of less importance in this part of the equation, once again nutrition does make a difference in how you perceive. For example, zinc deficiency alters perceptions about body size and appetite, both of which can contribute to eating disorders (see Chapter 32).

Mind frame—It's important to realize that we don't perceive reality as it actually is. We all interpret what is happening in our lives. "Don't change the world. Change the prescription of your glasses," says Swami Muktananda, a master of meditation. Most forms of psychotherapy are nothing more or less than techniques to help a person develop self-observation and become aware of negative mental patterns that lead to self-destructive behavior. Developing a more expanded and positive mind frame promotes mental well-being.

While nutrition would seem to have little to do with your mind frame, the two are related. When we cannot cope with our interpretation of reality, we have to "let off steam," to dissipate the fear, anxiety, or pain, which we sometimes do by eating too much or by consuming toxic substances such as sugar, alcohol, and cigarettes—or even more harmful drugs such as heroin or cocaine. These compensating behaviors leave us drained of energy and nutrients, which makes matters worse. To cope with the tiredness we then use stimulants, which further deplete us, leading to more and more addiction, and worsening mental health. It's a vicious downward spiral.

Imagine this scenario. Peter has blood sugar problems, is lacking B vitamins, and has "reward deficiency syndrome." This is a genetic predisposition to underproducing dopamine, the motivating neurotransmitter. All of these factors make him tired and unmotivated. He therefore craves stimulation and stimulants, such as sugar and caffeine, to make him feel good. Unfortunately, these make him more mentally hyperactive, with excessive thoughts. He can't switch off. So he starts drinking alcohol every day. This makes him more depressed. His doctor prescribes antidepressants. His wife leaves him, and he loses his job. He feels useless, worthless, and hopelessly inadequate. He can't cope with what's happening in his life and escapes into his own world. He has a breakdown. He is prescribed major tranquilizers and, although "stable," or at least not harmful to others, he is clearly suffering from mental illness.

This example shows the complex interplay between genes, environment, sense input, and mind frame, depicted in Figure 23. Drugs alone will not restore his health. He needs to rebalance his brain's chemistry with optimum nutrition, rebalance his psyche with good psychological guidance and support, and, most of all, he needs the willingness to change his diet, his lifestyle, and his mind frame. This total approach is likely to be much more effective than just drugs, psychotherapy, or nutritional therapy alone.

A Common and Growing Problem

Whatever the cause, mental health problems are incredibly common and very much on the increase. Currently, diagnosis with a mental health problem is as common as heart disease and three times more common than cancer. Official figures suggest that 6 million people in Britain, one in ten, are sufferers at any one point in time.[1] In the course of a year 12 million adults attending GPs' surgeries have symptoms of mental illness. Every five years the number of children up to the age of fourteen seen by psychiatric services is doubling.[2] In fact, out of 100 people who you know, up to 20 will be affected at any point in time.

As unwelcome as the thought may be, any one of us is a potential sufferer of a mental health problem. We are all subject, to a greater or lesser degree, to the stresses and strains of daily life, which for many people may be in addition to a much deeper source of stress or unhappiness coming from a particularly difficult past or present experience. The vast majority (80 percent) of disorders appear in the form of either anxiety states, depression, or stress-related disorders, with the remaining 20 percent being made up of alcohol and drug dependency, dementia, and personality and psychotic disorders such as schizophrenia.

There is no question that mental health problems are more common in those who are socially deprived. Suicide rates are eleven times higher among the unemployed, and fifty-three people per thousand are being admitted to psychiatric hospitals from deprived areas, as opposed to nineteen per thousand as a national average.[3] However, this still begs the question as to why some people seem to cope reasonably well with a given situation while others will start to manifest the symptoms of mental illness.

Mental illness costs all of us a small fortune. In Britain, almost 10 percent of the National Health Service budget is spent on mental illness. This, plus sickness and invalidity benefit, plus the cost of informal care in the community, exceeds $17 billion, or approximately $335 per person per year.[3] We desperately need a new way of dealing with mental health problems that is both more effective and more cost-effective. The good news is that the optimum nutrition approach is both.

Chapter 19

Getting the Right Diagnosis

There's an old saying: "Neurotics build castles in the sky, psychotics live in them, and psychiatrists collect the rent." Neurotics was the term for those anxious or depressed, while psychotics referred to those who had lost touch with reality.

Nowadays the diagnosis of a mental health problem is much more complex, but still based largely on a subjective judgment of a person's condition, rather than objective tests. The "categories" are defined in a book called the *Diagnostic and Statistical Manual of Mental Disorders*, generally referred to as "DSM-IV," which has seventeen categories for mental health problems. The main ones are shown below:

- **Disorders first diagnosed in childhood and adolescence:** retardation, learning disorders, attention deficit disorder, autism, and so on.

- **Delirium, dementia, amnestic, and other cognitive disorders:** delirium, dementia, Alzheimer's disease, and so on.

- **Substance-related disorders:** alcohol, amphetamine, caffeine, cocaine, and so on.

- **Schizophrenia and other psychotic disorders:** schizophrenia, various subtypes.

- **Mood disorders:** manic depression, depression.

- **Anxiety disorders:** phobias, anxiety, and so on.

- **Personality disorders:** paranoid, schizotypal, histrionic, and so on.

- **Eating disorders:** anorexia, bulimia, and so on.

- **Sleep disorders:** insomnia, and so on.

The Trouble with Diagnoses

The trouble with this categorization is that it completely ignores the many physical/biochemical factors that lead people into mental illness. A landmark study in 1980 found that 46 percent of people diagnosed with psychiatric disorders had a physical ailment, such as a nutritional deficiency.[4] Far too few psychiatrists test their patients for nutritional deficiencies, stimulant addictions, or hormone imbalances, all of which can bring on symptoms of mental illness.

Also, not everybody makes the same diagnosis, as this study by a Stanford University professor of law and psychology, Dr. Rosenhan, clearly demonstrates.

Dr. Rosenhan and seven others, including three psychologists and a psychiatrist, gained admission to twelve hospitals on the East and West Coasts of the United States by faking mental illness (eleven of the hospitals were totally funded by public money). The story they told to gain admission was that they "heard voices." Asked what the voices said they replied that they were often unclear but as far as he could tell they said "empty," "hollow," and "thud." However, once admitted to the hospital, they acted in a normal manner. In therapy, they answered all questions truthfully, including those about their childhoods and their current areas of interest. They engaged in normal activities in the hospitals, and, short of revealing their true purpose, they did everything possible to gain their release. Yet, only the other patients in the hospitals were able to tell that these "pseudopatients" were sane. The first three pseudopatients to be hospitalized took careful notes. Their accurate accounts show that 35 of a total of 118 regular patients were suspicious of them. Referring to their continual note-taking, one regular patient remarked: "You're not crazy. You're a journalist or a professor. You're checking up on the hospital."

The hospital staff, however, were not able to detect the pseudopatients' sanity. One nurse saw the note-taking as a symptom of a sick compulsion: "Engages in writing behavior," she put on the patient's chart. This led Dr. Rosenhan to conclude that, "Once a patient is designated as abnormal, all their other behaviors and characteristics are colored by that label." Whether this generalization is true or not, the inability of the hospitals to diagnose properly, or even suspect something, shows how the thin line between sanity and insanity may be blurred. Proper use of the medical model entails careful differential diagnosis, which draws this line firmly in view for both the staff and patient.

None of the pseudopatients were discharged as cured; all bore the label "schizophrenia in remission." In other words, it would seem they were still "insane." With the word "schizophrenia" on their records they would have to bear this stigma and even be expected to behave as a schizophrenic again, concluded Dr. Rosenhan.

The uniform and simple disperception that the pseudopatients reported in their first interview at the hospitals was the only "evidence" of schizophrenia—an example of waste-basket diagnosis (if it won't fit in anywhere else, they throw it in there!). Psychiatrists assume that no one would actually want to report a disperception unless so afflicted. The error, of course, is the lack of diagnosis based on proper tests. In one such test, the EWI (Experiential World Inventory), the patient can report disperceptions in a setting where he has no fear of recrimination, in a more or less objective fashion. There is no possibility that 200 answers can be faked.

One observation that Dr. Rosenhan made, as a result of this study, was that mental illness carries with it a connotation entirely different from that of a physical disorder. The *Diagnostic and Statistical Manual of Mental Disorders*, the official bible of psychiatric diagnoses, might have one believe that the sane are always clearly distinguished from the insane, and that "schizophrenia" (that phrase of the waste basket) is always treated as objectively and straightforwardly as a broken leg. Rosenhan found that, in actual practice, this was not the case. For example, sensible questions asked by the pseudopatients were frequently ignored. One patient stopped a doctor and asked, "Excuse me, Dr. .... , could you tell me when I am eligible for grounds privileges?" The doctor replied, "Good morning, Dave. How are you today?" and moved on without waiting for an answer or answering the patient's question. Not only was the credibility of the patients impaired in this way (presumably because of their diagnostic labels), but also they were denied privacy even in matters of personal hygiene. They reported feeling depersonalized, even though they knew they did not belong in the mental hospital.

Not Really Sick?

Dr. Rosenhan further wondered whether the atrocious diagnostic performance of the hospital staff merely reflected their professional caution. Having once been informed that a patient was hearing voices, perhaps the psychiatrists felt obliged to alert all future doctors to the possibility of trouble. Thus, Rosenhan wondered if his findings resulted from the greater inclination of physicians to call a healthy person sick than a sick person healthy. To check on this, he provided an esteemed psychiatric hospital, one of those involved in his first study, with yet another opportunity to redeem its reputation for adequate and proper diagnosis. The staff was informed that at some time during the next three months, one or more pseudopatients would once again attempt to be admitted into their hospital. The staff members were asked to rate each person who presented himself for admission as to the likelihood that the patient was a pseudopatient. Of the succeeding 193 patients admitted, 41 (or 21 percent) of them were judged, with a high degree of confidence, to be pseudopatients by at least one member of staff. The joke, again, was on the hospital staff. No pseudopatients at all had been sent to the hospital!

The study proved, basically, that insanity can easily be faked in front of professionals who do not use objective diagnostic tools such as psychometric assessments and biochemical tests. Although I hope diagnosis has improved substantially since this study, which was performed in 1973, we can conclude that psychiatric diagnosis, without objective laboratory tests and psychometric tests, are frequently erroneous; and that without an accurate diagnostic method, a label should not be applied. After all, labels tell you nothing about the underlying causes of a person's problem. We badly need a fresh approach to psychiatric diagnosis and treatment.

What Divides Abnormal Behavior from Mental Illness?

A valid point for debate is whether certain abnormal behavior qualifies as mental illness. Patients who have certain mental symptoms after strokes or infections of the brain present no problem in being considered ill. In contrast, there is a group of disorders listed as "personality disorders." There is nothing in this term to suggest any organic or physiological derangement, so to call them mental illness is highly debatable. Similarly, how many are inappropriately diagnosed with ADHD? The now commonplace diagnosis of attention deficit hyperactivity disorder is another "waste-basket" diagnosis used to classify and treat children with a wide variety of symptoms and behaviors. A conference held by the National Institutes of Health in the United States in 1988 failed to find any substantial evidence that there is a single condition called ADHD. Some are simply super-intelligent, bored, and understimulated children, exacerbated by poor diet. Others are probably suffering from manic depression, a diagnosis that doesn't exist in children. The worst thing you can do is give these children stimulant drugs such as Ritalin. Others are dyslexic, dyspraxic, and unable to concentrate, often due to a deficiency in essential fats.

Diagnosing Manic Depression and Schizophrenia

Somewhere beyond the extremes of eccentric behavior are patients with two major psychoses: the schizophrenias and manic-depressive psychosis. It has become popular also to regard manic-depressive psychosis as "better" than schizophrenia. Manic-depressive psychosis has long been felt to have a biochemical basis, and anyway, doctors claim "it is only a disorder of emotions, the patient isn't really crazy." Perhaps this is, in part, because intellectual functioning may be less impaired than in one of the severe schizophrenias.

Schizophrenia has become a dirty word, a diagnosis to be whispered, and often to be concealed from patient, family, or friends. Again, a broken leg or even blindness would be more bearable because it is visible, explicable, and being plainly physical, is something one can live with. Schizophrenia, about which some people have such strong and irrational feelings (no doubt because of their own fears or other emotional reactions), strikes everywhere in the world. This led some researchers to believe that there may be a genetic cause, creating a biochemical weakness, in many people with schizophrenia and that the genetic twist occurred very early in humanity's evolution, back in Africa. Hence, the equal spread throughout all cultures, a pattern unseen in almost all diseases.

The commonly quoted figure for schizophrenia as 1 percent of all humanity is certainly far short of the actual incidence. We should add to this estimate the walking wounded who are never seen by any doctor, since only one-third of those afflicted need to be hospitalized. We must also add the teenager who commits suicide before an accurate diagnosis is made. Thus the problem is one that is important from the viewpoint of numbers, as well as individual misery. Heart disease may cause more deaths, but the schizophrenias cause more heartache.

There are many conflicting descriptions and explanations for the schizophrenias, but at a basic level, there is usually little difficulty in making a preliminary diagnosis; and there is usually agreement among doctors in making the diagnosis, even though they may disagree about the possible causes and the ultimate outcome for any given patient. Since the schizophrenias may vary from simple (but abnormal) feelings of disperception or persecution to complete loss of contact with reality, the doctor hesitates to apply the term schizophrenia to the mild forms of disorder. Instead he uses the terms "schizoid personality," "schizophrenic reaction," or other such words. The doctor really means "I am puzzled and will sit on the fence until I see what happens to you in the next year or so as you freewheel through life with or without medication."

The Indicators of Biochemical Imbalances

One way to differentiate between a "psychotic" condition and purely a mood disorder is the Hoffer-Osmond Diagnostic test. This test was developed to help identify those people with disorders of perception. Below are some of the items in the HOD test that are checked if applicable:

People's faces sometimes pulsate as I watch them.
People watch me all the time.
Now and then when I look in the mirror, my face changes and seems different.
Sometimes when I read, the words begin to look funny—they move around or grow faint.
Sometimes objects pulsate when I look at them.
My hands or feet sometimes seem much too large for me.
I sometimes feel that I have left my body.
I often hear or have heard voices.
I can no longer tell how much time has gone by.
I often hear thoughts inside my head.
I find that past, present, and future all seem muddled up.

The presence of these symptoms suggests that something isn't right in the way the brain is processing information, which is a good indicator that a person has a biochemical imbalance, not purely a psychological imbalance.

A New Classification of Mental Health Problems

The modern classification of mental health problems should be made, both from symptoms, objectively measured in questionnaire tests, and from physical and biochemical tests that help determine if any of the many kinds of biochemical imbalances are causing, or contributing to, a person's problems. Here are some of the more common biochemical imbalances that can result in symptoms of mental illness.

- Stimulant and drug intoxications

- Dysglycemia—blood sugar problems

- Allergy—especially wheat gluten

- Under- or overactive-thyroid

- Niacin/folic acid/B_{12} deficiency

- Essential fat and prostaglandin deficiency or imbalance

- Heavy metal toxicity—copper, lead, cadmium, and so on

- Pyroluria and porphyria—resulting in zinc deficiency

- Histamine imbalance—excess or deficiency

- Serotonin imbalance—excess or deficiency

- Dopamine/adrenaline imbalance—excess or deficiency

- Acetylcholine deficiency

- High homocysteine

- Detoxification overload leading to inflammation

The good news is that all these can now be tested and, as a result, a more accurate assessment of their contribution to a person's mental health problems can be evaluated. The modern approach to mental illness involves keeping an open mind to all the possible contributory causes, understanding that, in most cases, more than one apply. Diagnoses are made on the basis of objective biochemical tests and subjective symptom assessment. The treatment is more often specific nutritional therapy, together with psychotherapy.

Once symptoms are gone and test results are normalized, the patient can be declared better. Dr. Abram Hoffer, a psychiatrist who has pioneered this approach since the 1950s, claims a 90 percent success rate in acute schizophrenia, with thousands of cases to prove it. His definition of cure is threefold: free from symptoms, able to socialize with family and community, and paying income tax! This, of course, is a tremendous step forward in the most debilitating of all mental health problems, for which many psychiatrists still believe there is no cure.

The next chapter explains the most common biochemical causes of mental health problems, how to identify whether a person has them, and what to do if you do.

Chapter 20

What's Your Problem?

If you've got a strange set of physical symptoms, your doctor is probably going to run a basic biochemical screening blood test, just to see if anything abnormal shows up. The same is rarely done for those with mental health problems: The belief seems to be that biochemical imbalances don't manifest as psychological symptoms. Of course, the reverse is true. The brain is far more sensitive to biochemical imbalances than any other organ of the body. The very fact that most treatment of mental illness involves chemical drugs proves the direct link between a person's biochemical state and his psychological state.

So, if you do have mental health problems, it is well worth checking out the most common biochemical imbalances that can cause mental illness. Each has a clear set of symptoms. If you score high on these, then an objective biochemical test can be run to prove whether or not this imbalance is present. Then, a nutritional strategy can help bring you back into balance.

The easiest way to find out if there's a high probability that one or more of these is contributing to your problems is by completing the "Mental Health Questionnaire" at the website www.mentalhealthproject.com. This is a free service and gives you a printout that you can copy and give to your nutritionist, doctor, or psychiatrist so they know what tests to run and what to do if the results are positive. To find a nutritionist, see Useful Addresses on page 366.

Biochemical Imbalances: 13 Common Causes of Mental Health Problems

Blood Sugar Problems

The most common underlying imbalance in many types of mental health problems is fluctuating blood sugar levels, called dysglycemia. If you've got this, the chances are you crave sweet foods or stimulants such as tea, coffee, and cigarettes, all of which affect your blood sugar levels. Here are the most common symptoms:

Difficulty concentrating
Palpitations or blackouts
Fainting or dizziness or trembling
Excessive or night sweats
Excessive thirst
Chronic fatigue
Frequent mood swings
Forgetfulness or confusion
Tendency to depression
Anxiety and irritability
Feeling weak
Aggressive outbursts or crying spells
Cravings for sweets or stimulants
Drowsiness after meals

If you've got five or more of these, the chances are you have dysglycemia. The best way to confirm this is a blood test measuring "glycosylated haemoglobin." Hemoglobin is a red blood cell. Glycosylated simply means "sugar-coated." If your blood sugar level goes up and down like a yo-yo along with your mood, the red blood cells get sugar-coated. In the old days we used to measure your blood sugar level every half hour for five hours (the five-hour glucose tolerance test). Now there's this single test, and it's much more accurate than simply measuring your blood glucose level, which can vary from moment to moment.

Meanwhile, follow the guidelines in Chapter 3 for stabilizing your blood sugar level.

Stimulant and Drug Dependence

If you've read this far, the chances are you already know if you are suffering from stimulant or drug intoxication. But many people don't because they assume that drinking lots of tea, coffee, caffeinated drinks or alcohol, eating sugar, and smoking cigarettes, while not good for their health, is hardly going to make them crazy. This is far from the truth. Intoxication with stimulants or drugs (amphetamines, cocaine and crack, heroin, cannabis in excess, Ecstasy) can and does bring on symptoms of mental illness. The symptoms are very similar to those for dysglycemia, coupled with a craving for any of these substances. In addition, you can experience disperceptions, extreme anxiety, paranoia, and depression through the excessive use of some of the substances.

Complete the "stimulant inventory" below for a week.

	Unit	Sun	Mon	Tue	Wed	Thu	Fri	Sat
Green Tea	2 cups							
Tea	1 cup							
Coffee	1 cup							
Cola or Caffeinated Drinks	1 can							
Caffeine pills (e.g., No-Doz, Excedrin, Dexatrim)	1 pill							
Chocolate	2 oz							
Alcohol (units) Glass of wine is 1 Bottle of beer is ½ Shot of spirit is 1	1 unit							
Added sugar	1 teaspoon							
Hidden sugar (see sugar contents on ingredients lists)	1 teaspoon/5 g							
Cigarettes	1 cigarette							
Cannabis	½ joint							
Amphetamines	½ pill							
Ecstasy	½ pill							
Cocaine	½ line							
Heroin	½ hit							

Add up your total number of "units." The ideal is five or fewer per week. If you are having more than ten stimulant units a week, this is going to have an effect on your mental well-being. If you score thirty or more, this could well be contributing to mental health problems. I strongly recommend you quit all these substances for at least a month (see Chapter 10) and see how that helps your mental health.

If you are currently taking prescription drugs, please read the next chapter carefully because many of the side effects of prescription drugs get mistaken for symptoms of a person's mental health problem.

Food and Chemical Allergies and Intolerances

If you suffer from daily mood swings, or are fine sometimes and not others, for no apparent reason, one possibility is that you are reacting to something you're eating. The most common single food that's been linked to mental health problems is wheat, which is a rich source of gluten. Wheat gluten allergy can make some people feel crazy. Other foods that can cause allergic reactions include milk products, oranges, eggs, grains other than wheat, foods with yeast, shellfish, nuts, beef, pork, and onions. Food colorings such as tartrazine and other chemical additives can also cause problems. Some people also develop intolerances to tea and coffee, while alcohol, which irritates the gut wall and makes it more leaky, often increases allergic sensitivity to anything eaten. Check yourself out on the symptoms below:

Child history of colic, eczema, asthma, rashes, or ear infections
Daily mood swings
Deep depressions for no particular reason
Frequent, rapid colds or blocked nose
Difficulty sleeping
Facial puffiness, circles, or discoloration around eyes
Hyperactivity
Dyslexia or learning difficulties
Aggressive outbursts or crying spells

If you score five or more, or know you feel better off certain foods, then food or chemical allergies may be contributing to your problem. See a nutritionist, who can show you how to do a two-week "avoidance," then "challenge" test with your suspect foods. Alternatively, have a quantitative IgG ELISA allergy test. This involves taking a single blood sample and testing your allergic potential to some fifty different foods and chemicals. For more details, read Chapter 11.

Under- or Overactive Thyroid

If your mind and body feel sluggish most of the time, you may have an underactive thyroid, referred to as hypothyroidism. If your thyroid is clinically underactive, your doctor may prescribe thyroid hormones to be taken directly. However, blood tests are often unable to detect sub-clinical hypothyroid, so it may be better to go by the symptoms. You can also test your thyroid function yourself with the Broda Barnes Temperature Test. If your temperature before rising in the morning is consistently below 97.7°F, this suggests your thyroid may be underactive. Check yourself out on the symptoms below:

Physical or mental fatigue or lethargy
Depression or irritability
Dry skin and/or hair
Intolerance to cold or cold hands and feet
Constipation, gas, bloating, or indigestion
Gain weight easily
Painful periods
Muscle pain
Poor memory
Sore throat or nasal congestion

If you score five or more, an underactive thyroid may be contributing to your problem. Get it tested by your doctor and also see a clinical nutritionist who can show you which foods to eat and which foods to avoid to support your thyroid. Chronic stress can deplete thyroid function, as the stress hormone cortisol inhibits it. Thyroid health is also dependent on specific nutrients in the diet, most importantly iodine, which is abundant in seafood and seaweed, and tyrosine, an amino acid found in all protein-rich foods, plus zinc and selenium. (See also How's your Thyroid? on page 187 in Chapter 22, and do the home test.)

Niacin, Pyridoxine, Folic Acid, or B₁₂ Deficiency

These four B vitamins are your brain's best friends. They "oil the wheels" of the brain's neurotransmitters, especially dopamine, adrenaline, noradrenaline, and serotonin. Without enough of these vital B vitamins the brain can produce chemicals that make you crazy. They help to control "methylation," which is how the brain keeps everything in balance. They also stop the body from producing homocysteine. This causes inflammation in the brain and body, now thought to be a potential underlying cause for a variety of mental health problems. Some people need a lot more B vitamins than others, so it's best to be guided by symptoms, rather than blood tests. Here are the more common symptoms:

Feeling "unreal"
Hearing your own thoughts
Anxiety and inner tension
Inability to think straight
Suspicious of people
Good pain tolerance
Seeing or hearing things abnormally
Having delusions or illusions
Loose bowels or skin problems at onset of mental health problems
Difficult orgasm with sex
Tendency to be overweight
Frequent mood swings

If you have five or more of these symptoms, it may be worth your while to increase your intake of these nutrients for two months. See Chapter 25 for more details and guidance on the amounts to take.

Essential Fats Deficiencies or Imbalances

Essential fats are intimately involved in brain function, and imbalances in brain fats are now known to be associated with everything from dyslexia, hyperactivity, and depression to schizophrenia and manic depression. Changes in our intakes of essential fats, especially during pregnancy, could easily explain the rapid increases in mental health problems. In short, it is essential to assess your need for essential fats if you have a mental health problem. Common symptoms are the following:

Excessive thirst
Chronic fatigue
Dry or rough skin
Dry hair, loss of hair, or dandruff
PMS or breast pain
Eczema, asthma, or joint aches
Dyslexia or learning difficulties
Hyperactivity
Depression or manic depression
Schizophrenia

If you have five or more of these symptoms and you have a mental health problem, it may be worth your while to have a blood test to determine your essential fat status. Your nutritionist or possibly your doctor can let you know how.

Heavy Metal Toxicity

Although high levels of lead are less common since the advent of lead-free gas, some people have very high copper levels, mainly from copper plumbing in soft water areas. Copper suppresses histamine and, in excess, can exacerbate anxiety, fears, and paranoia. It is also a zinc antagonist, making zinc deficiency worse. High levels of cadmium are often found in smokers, as tobacco is relatively rich in it. Check yourself out on the symptoms below:

Anxiety, extreme fears, or paranoia
Phobias
Poor concentration or confusion
Poor memory
Angry or aggressive feelings
Hyperactivity
Emotional instability
Headaches or migraines
Joint pain
Nervousness

If you score five or more, I'd recommend a hair mineral analysis to test whether you've got an excess of toxic minerals. This inexpensive, non-invasive test can also highlight deficiencies in important minerals such as zinc, magnesium, and manganese. Your nutritionist can arrange this test for you.

Pyroluria and Porphyria

Some people produce more of the proteinlike chemicals kryptopyrroles and porphyrins than is healthy. An excess of them is linked to mental illness. The madness of King George III, for example, was almost certainly caused by porphyria. This, and probably pyroluria, are genetically inherited tendencies that increase a person's need for zinc. Stress also depletes zinc. So, if your mental health problems are strongly stress-related and the symptoms below apply to you, you may be pyroluric, or even porphyric, although the latter is much less common:

Nausea or constipation
White spots on fingernails
Pale skin that burns easily
Frequent colds and infections
Stretch marks
Irregular menstruation
Impotency
Crowded upper front teeth
Poor tolerance of alcohol or drugs
Poor dream recall

If you score five or more you may be pyroluric. You can test this by having a urine test for kryptopyrroles. If high, you need more zinc and B_6.

Histamine Imbalance

Histamine is an often overlooked neurotransmitter. Some people are genetically preprogrammed to produce more histamine, a condition known as histadelia, and this can make a person excessively compulsive and obsessive. High histamine types have a faster metabolism and therefore use up nutrients at a fast rate. Without good nutrition, they can easily become deficient, which can precipitate patches of deep depression. These are some of the symptoms associated with excess histamine:

Headaches or migraines
Sneeze in sunlight
Cry, salivate, or feel nauseated easily
Easy orgasm with sex
Abnormal fears, compulsions, rituals
Light sleeper
Fast metabolism
Depression or suicidal thoughts
Produces a lot of body heat
Little body hair and lean build
Large ears or long fingers and toes
Good tolerance of alcohol
Inner tension or "driven" feeling
Shy or over-sensitive as child
Seasonal allergies (e.g., hayfever)
Obsessive or compulsive tendencies

If you have five or more of these symptoms, you may be a high histamine type. You can check this out by having a blood test for histamine. If your blood levels are high, you will benefit from supplementing vitamin C, plus the amino acid methionine, together with calcium. But don't take large amounts of folic acid. For more details on histadelia read Chapter 22.

Low levels of histamine are associated with the same kind of symptoms of B_3/B_{12} and folic acid deficiency, and respond well to supplementing these nutrients.

Histamine levels can also be determined as part of an overall Neurotransmitter Screening Test. See below.

Serotonin Imbalance

Serotonin deficiency is one of the most common findings in people with mental health problems. It is associated with sleeping problems, mood disturbance, and aggressive and compulsive behavior. Check yourself out on the symptoms below:

Depression, especially post-menopausal
Anxiety
Aggressive or suicidal thoughts
Violent or impulsive behavior
Mood swings, including PMS
Obsessive or compulsive tendencies
Alcohol or drug abuse
Sensitive to pain (low pain threshold)
Craves sweet foods
Sleeping problems

If you score five or more, you may be low in serotonin. A Neurotransmitter Screening Test can help confirm this. Your nutritionist can arrange this blood test for you. If you're low, there are specific nutrients, including the amino acids tryptophan or 5-hydroxytryptophan (5-HTP), which can help restore normal mental health.

Adrenal Imbalance

The adrenal glands and the brain produce three motivating neurotransmitters called dopamine, adrenaline, and noradrenaline. The adrenal glands also produce cortisol. Excesses of adrenaline can result in states of high stress and anxiety, while deficiency results in the opposite—low energy, no motivation, and poor concentration. There is evidence that some people may abnormally turn excessive amounts into toxins that induce disperceptions and even hallucinations. Check yourself out on the symptoms below:

Irritability
Nervousness or anxiety
Extreme fears
Raised blood pressure
Rapid or irregular heartbeat
Insomnia
Cold hands and feet
Excessive sweating
Teeth grinding
Headaches or migraine
Muscle tension
Restlessness
Seeing or hearing things

If you score five or more, you may have excessive levels of adrenaline or cortisol. If, on the other hand, you have the following symptoms, you may have adrenal insufficiency:

Depression
Difficulty concentrating
Short attention span
Lack of drive or motivation
Rarely initiates or completes tasks
Frequently tired
Can't deal with stress
Socially withdrawn

Both excess and deficiency can be tested with either an Adrenal Stress Index, using saliva samples, or as part of a Neurotransmitter Screening Test. Your nutritionist can arrange these tests. For high adrenaline levels, cut back on stimulants and sugar and up your intake of vitamins B and C (also see Chapter 16, page 127). For low adrenaline levels, you may benefit from supplementing the amino acid tyrosine. "Adaptogenic" herbs such as Asian ginseng, eleuthero (formerly nicknamed "Siberian ginseng"), or rhodiola can also help.

Acetylcholine Imbalance

Acetylcholine is the brain's learning neurotransmitter. Low levels are associated with memory loss and even Alzheimer's disease. Levels tend to decline with age, but they don't have to if you are optimally nourished. Check yourself out on the symptoms below:

Poor dream recall
Infrequent dreaming
Difficulty visualizing
Dry mouth
Poor memory or forgetfulness
Mental exhaustion
Poor concentration
Difficulty learning new things

If you score five or more, chances are you might be low in acetylcholine. A Neurotransmitter Screening Test can help confirm this. Your nutritionist can arrange this blood test for you. Alternatively, you can simply supplement brain-friendly nutrients, as explained in Chapter 13.

Detoxification Overload and Inflammation

Inflammation, externally characterized by pain, redness, or swelling, is the body's alarm signal when things get out of hand. It is a natural response to too many insults and not enough nutrients. Omega-3 fats, one of the nutrients we're most deficient in, are especially important in preventing inflammation.

New evidence is now emerging that many mental health problems, as well as heart disease, cancer, and diabetes, have excessive inflammation as part of the root cause. Alzheimer's disease is certainly an inflammatory disease, but so too can be autism, depression, Parkinson's disease and possibly schizophrenia. We are beginning to learn that inflammation upsets the brain as much as the body. The most common cause of inflammation is faulty digestion, leading to an overload of substances for the liver to detoxify. We also produce toxins, such as homocysteine, in the absence of the right nutrients.

Check yourself out on the symptoms below:

Headaches or migraine
Watery, itchy eyes, red eyelids, or dark circles under the eyes
Itchy ears, frequent ear infections, or ringing in the ears

Excessive mucus, a stuffy nose, or sinus problems
Excess sweating and strong body odor
Indigestion or bloating
Constipation or diarrhea
History of eczema, asthma
Joint or muscle aches or pains or arthritis
Mental health symptoms are often worse after eating

If you score five or more, you may have detoxification problems and be "inflamed." Your doctor can check this by running a standard blood test, measuring your ESR rate. If raised, you have excessive inflammation. A clinical nutritionist can also assess whether you have digestion and detoxification problems. The antidote is more omega-3 fats, more antioxidants, and fewer oxidants (especially saturated, processed, and fried fats), and solving any underlying digestive problems.

In summary, these are thirteen reasonably common biochemical imbalances that can lead to a whole host of mental health problems, both major and minor. Most mental health problems are down to a number of factors, however. The next part of this book looks specifically at the most common mental health problems and what we know about their causes and treatment, using optimum nutrition principles.

Chapter 21

THE DANGERS OF DRUGS
AND HOW TO GET OFF THEM

Since the 1950s, the treatment of mental illness with drugs has become the major therapeutic tool of psychiatrists the world over. There are three main types of such drugs: antidepressants (such as Prozac), stimulants (such as Ritalin), and tranquilizers (such as Valium). Tranquilizers can be further divided into minor tranquilizers for the treatment of anxiety and sleeping problems, and major tranquilizers (such as chlorpromazine, sold as Thorazine) for the treatment of psychotic conditions, including schizophrenia.

Perilous Prescriptions

Antidepressants: They Work, but the Side Effects Are Depressing

Antidepressant drugs may work, but they are not without considerable risk. Tricyclic antidepressants such as amitriptyline, Anafranil, and Prothiadin have over twenty side effects listed in the doctors' drug guide, the *British National Formulary*, including dry mouth, blurred vision, nausea, confusion, cardiovascular problems, sweating, tremors, and behavioral disturbance.[5] Monoamine oxidase inhibitors (MAOIs) such as Nardil and Parstelin have even worse side effects and can be very difficult to come off: They're highly addictive. Some patients have died after taking MAOIs and failing to avoid alcohol or certain foods, like cheese and yeast, which are both found hidden in many convenience foods.

Selective serotonin reuptake inhibitors (SSRIs), a class of antidepressants that work by keeping levels of serotonin relatively high, are touted as having less side effects for most people. But they can create profound problems in a significant minority. Prozac, the market leader, prescribed to more than 38 million people worldwide, has forty-five side effects listed in the *British National Formulary*. According to psychiatrist David Richman, between 10 and 25 percent of people experienced: nausea, nervousness, insomnia, headache, tremors, anxiety, drowsiness, dry mouth, excessive sweating, and diarrhea. These drugs also tend to flatten moods, sometimes to the point of zombie like emotionlessness, and reduce libido and sexual performance.

Prozac and Seroxat, two of the most frequently prescribed anti-depressants, show clear evidence of agitation leading to potential aggressive and suicidal behavior in as many as a quarter of patients in a number of clinical trials. There have now been ninety legal actions and one recent successful litigation with $6.4 million dollars being awarded against the pharmaceuticals company. "I estimate that about one person a day has committed suicide as a direct result of taking Prozac since it was introduced," declares Dr. David Healy of the North Wales Department of Psychological Medicine in Bangor, who has been petitioning the government's Medicine Control Agency to take action to warn users about these potential adverse reactions. In the United Kingdom that means about 1,000 suicides and 10,000 attempts.[6] With ten times as many prescriptions in the U.S., this could mean up to 10,000 suicides and 100,000 attempts.

SSRI antidepressants are also addictive. There is now considerable evidence that some 50 percent of those who try to quit get alarming withdrawal effects. One study testing withdrawal showed that as many as 85 percent of the volunteers, people with no previous hint of depression, suffered agitation, abnormal dreams, insomnia, and other adverse effects.[7] Antidepressants should be used only as a last resort, and even then only for a short period of time (see Chapters 14 and 22 for equally effective, much safer alternatives).

If you are currently on antidepressants and would like to come off them, the best strategy is to phase out the antidepressant and phase in the nutrients and herbs that help promote a good mood, but without the side effects. I recommend you do this only with the guidance of a nutritionist (see Useful Addresses, pages 366–367) and the support of your doctor.

Stimulants: 10 Million Children Are on Ritalin

Sadly, many hyperactive children are not evaluated for chemical, nutritional, and allergic factors, nor are they treated nutritionally. Instead, they're quickly put on drugs such as Ritalin, a habit-forming amphetamine with similar properties to cocaine. Diagnoses of hyperactivity and ADHD have risen more than fifteen-fold in the last decade, and prescriptions for Ritalin and other stimulant drugs are not far behind. Now it is given to around 10 percent of boys in United States schools, and researchers looking at its effectiveness have found that it can worsen the behavior of more children than it helps.

According to the U.S. Drug Enforcement Agency, the harmful side effects of taking Ritalin can include increased blood pressure, heart rate, respiration and temperature, appetite suppression, stomach pains, weight loss, growth retardation, facial tics, muscle twitching, insomnia, euphoria, nervousness, irritability, agitation, psychotic episodes, violent behavior, paranoid delusions, hallucinations, bizarre behaviors, heart arrhythmias and palpitations, tolerance, psychological dependence, and even death. Some of these symptoms do not go away on stopping the drug.

Structurally and pharmacologically similar to cocaine, Ritalin has a similar dependency profile and may be even more potent. Researchers have found that it is chosen over cocaine in self-administered preference studies with nonhuman primates. Using brain imaging, Dr. Nora Volkow of the Brookhaven National Laboratory in Upton, New York, has shown that Ritalin occupies more of the neural transporters responsible for the high experienced by addicts than smoked or injected cocaine. The only reason Ritalin has not produced an army of addicted schoolchildren, she concludes, is that it takes about an hour for Ritalin in pill form to raise dopamine levels in the brain, while smoked or injected cocaine does this in seconds.[8] There are now growing reports of teenagers and others abusing Ritalin by snorting or injecting it to get a faster rush.

But it doesn't end there. Dr. Joan Baizer, Professor of Physiology and Biophysics at the University of Buffalo, has shown how Ritalin, which physicians considered to have only short-term effects, may initiate changes in brain structure and function that remain long after the therapeutic effects have dissipated.[9] This can in turn lead to a greater susceptibility to drug dependence in later life.

As you'll see in Chapter 27, nutritional approaches to the multitude of problems lumped together as ADHD have already proven to be more effective than these drugs. However, as with any stimulant, coming off Ritalin does result in withdrawal symptoms. These can best be minimized by keeping blood sugar levels even. Follow the strategy given in Chapters 3 and 9.

Tranquilizers: The False Calm

As I mentioned earlier, every week in Britain we take 10 million tranquilizers. These are often prescribed for sleeping problems and anxiety. Major tranquilizers are also prescribed for people with schizophrenia, to calm them down.

The most frequently prescribed tranquilizers are benzodiazepines such as diazepam (Valium), chlordiazepoxide (Librium), clonazapine (Klonopin), and the shorter-acting alprazolam (Xanax) or temazepam (Restoril). In the United States around 25 million prescriptions are written annually to treat anxiety and insomnia.[10] They work because they open up the receptor sites for GABA, the inhibitory neurotransmitter that acts as the brain's peace-maker. By increasing GABA activity, the benzodiazepines dull both aware-ness and overall brain function, calming your anxiety but also dulling your mind.

The big problem is that they are highly addictive. In fact, they are as addictive as heroin, and dependence on them can occur within two weeks of use.[11] Doctors are specifically instructed not to prescribe more than a four-week supply, yet a MORI poll in the 1980s found that 35 percent of those prescribed benzodiazepines had been on them, not for four weeks, but for over four months! The poll estimated than 1.5 million people in Britain are addicted to tranquilizers.[12]

In the late 1980s, thousands of tranquilizer addicts sued the drug com-panies. The case was, however, abandoned in 1994 due to lack of funding.

Tranquilizers are highly addictive, and long-term use can make you become more forgetful, drowsy, accident-prone, and antisocial. Withdrawal can make you anxious, irritable, confused, and unable to sleep. These symptoms can go on for months but, with the right nutritional support, can be greatly reduced (see www.mentalhealthproject.com/comingofftranquilizers.) Mary's story, from the book *Natural Highs* (case generously supplied by coauthor Dr. Hyla Cass at www.cassmd.com), is a case in point:

> When Mary was in her thirties, she found herself stuck in an unhappy marriage, and with a young child. Seeing no escape, she was taking large doses of Valium to shut out the pain. One day, while filling yet another prescription for Mary, the pharmacist said, "In case you don't know it, you're addicted. Speak to me when you're ready to stop." This was Mary's wake-up call.
>
> In shocked response, she simply stopped the drug cold. She was too ashamed to face the pharmacist, who would have advised a slow with-drawal program under medical supervision. Then, not knowing she was suffering from withdrawal symptoms, she simply, in her words, "went crazy" for the next two months or so. It took that long for her brain to readjust itself.
>
> What had happened was that the Valium had caused Mary's brain to

down-regulate. It had adjusted to Valium's relaxing action. This led to extreme agitation (withdrawal) when she stopped it, until, in time, her brain readjusted. "When I finally got my mind back, I decided to leave my husband. I never looked back. Nor did I ever dare take another tranquilizer," declares Mary, now at forty-eight, a successful writer and a proud grandmother.

If you have become dependent and want to quit, it is essential that you seek professional support and guidance. I'd also recommend seeing a psychotherapist to help deal with the underlying issues for your anxieties. As well as following all the advice in Parts 1 and 2, the relaxing herbs valerian and kava can be gradually substituted, but only under the guidance and support of a clinical nutritionist and your doctor. You can also get some great support and guidance from the charitable self-help group CITA. Their details are in the Useful Addresses section on page 359.

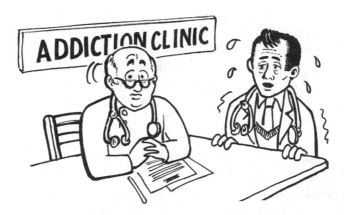

Fig 24 "Doctor, I seem to have become addicted to prescribing drugs."

Antipsychotic Drugs: Chemical Straitjackets

The first antipsychotic drug, reserpine, was introduced into psychiatric practice in 1952, shortly followed by chlorpromazine (Thorazine) in 1954. The perfecting of this type of antipsychotic drug was achieved in the 1960s with the introduction of fluphenazine (Prolixin) and haloperidol (Haldol). Most other antipsychotic drugs introduced since 1970 have been "me too" drugs which have little advantage over these two standard and now cheaper drugs.

For patients who will not take these medications by mouth, oil-soluble decanoate salts are available for intramuscular injection. These weekly injections—Depixol for example—do not give as smooth a result as the daily use of the drug by mouth. Most patients can have the daily dose they need by taking the pills at bedtime with dephenhydramine (Benadryl). If they develop muscle shakes from taking the drug, a small dose of Cogentin, Artane or Kemadrin is often given each morning (see also below).

Drugs such as the major tranquilizers should only be considered as temporary crutches, to be used until the biochemical imbalances are slowly corrected by nutritional therapy. According to Dr. Abram Hoffer, a psychiatrist with fifty years of experience in treating mental illness, tranquilizers never cure mental illness—they just replace one psychosis with another. No normal person can function under the influence of tranquilizers. Yet even today, one unfortunate consequence of understaffing at public mental hospitals is that excessive doses of chlorpromazine are routinely prescribed to keep a difficult patient quiet.

When a columnist with the *San Francisco Examiner*, Bill Mandel, tried 50 mg of Thorazine, he reported,

> *"Simply put, it made me stupid. Because Thorazine and related drugs are called 'liquid lobotomy' in the mental health business, I'd expected a great grey cloud to descend over my faculties. There was no grey cloud, just small, unsettling patches of fog. My mental gears slipped. I had no intellectual traction. It was difficult, for example, to remember simple words."*

Most patients are prescribed 2 to 16 times the amount taken by Mandel. Tranquilizers such as these should only be used as a last resort, and even then, phased out as the patient improves on the right diet and treatment with specific nutrients, based on a proper diagnosis.

Side Effects of Antipsychotic Drugs

A major problem in treating mental disorders with pharmaceutical drugs, which is often played down, is the immense discomfort caused by some of the side effects. Drugs such as the now antiquated chlorpromazine (Thorazine or Largactil) can have some annoying and sometimes serious side effects. Patients taking these drugs may find themselves unable to steady their hands. Their facial muscles may twitch involuntarily. They may try to read but find their vision is too blurred to decipher the printed lines. The eyes may turn up and refuse to come down. The patients may be restless and pace the floor until they have blistered feet. A severe skin reaction may follow even a brief exposure to the sun, so that patients on the drug are compelled to spend much of their time indoors. After long-term drug therapy, a patient may look in the mirror one morning to discover that his face has acquired a purplish-gray hue, a very slowly reversible condition. This pigment can also lodge in the heart muscle and may cause sudden death, as several studies have shown.

Imagine the agony of an intelligent young man or woman, particularly the artistic or intellectual type, who is forced to take this medication—only to find, at some point, that his or her imaginative facilities are simply no longer available. Is it ethical, twenty-five years after the introduction of chlorpromazine, to increase the agony of the suffering schizophrenic by giving him this drug, when safer drugs and treatments are available?

If needed, a drug such as haloperidol or fluphenazine may be substituted for chlorpromazine. These produce fewer side effects, but should only be used as "holding drugs" until the nutrients begin to take effect. A "pharmacological lobotomy" is not at all necessary, nor is the frustrating disruption of patients' imaginative resources.

These antipsychotic drugs, if given at high doses for many months, may produce tardive dyskinesia—a delayed impairment of voluntary motion causing incomplete or partial movement. The risk of getting this side effect after long-term use is around 75 percent, according to Dr. William Glazer, an expert on the condition.

Since the drugs, called phenothiazines, have been found to attach to manganese, making it less available for use in the brain, one researcher hypothesized that manganese might be useful for preventing the side effects caused by the drugs. Out of fifteen people given manganese supplements, seven were cured outright of their involuntary muscle twitches, three were much improved, and four were improved. Only one person did not respond.[13] Manganese taken daily in doses of 25 mg is helpful, as is the daily use of phosphatidyl choline or DMAE, which builds up acetylcholine, the neurotransmitter involved in brain and muscle function. Vitamin E may also help, at a level of 800ius per day.[14]

The "neuroleptic malignant syndrome" is yet another, sometimes lethal, side-effect of antischizophrenic medication. More than twenty publications have depicted the sad effects of prolonged use of the antischizophrenic drugs. Patients may get elevated temperature, sweating, rapid pulse, panting, soiling, rigidity, dazed mutism, stupor, and coma. If the drug is not withdrawn, death can occur within twenty-four hours.

Problems with Multi-Drug Use

Another problem is multiple drug interactions. Many psychiatric patients simultaneously take daily doses of one or more antipsychotics, antidepressants, a minor tranquilizer, and a hypnotic to make them sleep at night. In addition, because of certain Parkinson's-like side effects of these drugs, most patients are also given drugs used to treat Parkinson's disease, such as Cogentin or Kemadrin. These make reading even more difficult. Then there are drugs for coexisting illnesses prescribed by other doctors, and self-medication with over-the-counter drugs, all of which the patient could conceivably take simultaneously. Taken together, this adds up to a potentially dangerous constellation of pharmacological interaction and personal neglect of the patient which might prolong suffering and delay rehabilitation.

While antipsychotic drugs can have beneficial short-term effects, the lethargic, asocial, odd behavior of some patients, which is usually attributed to illness, is more often than not the result of medication. Every avenue of treatment, including nutrition, should be thoroughly explored before sentencing a person to the chemical straitjacket of long-term tranquilizer use.

In summary, in almost all cases, with the right guidance, the right nutritional program and support, it is possible to get off medication. This is desirable since almost all drugs currently used for mental health problems do have unwanted side effects, especially in the long term.

However, coming off medication should never be done too quickly, nor without the full support of your doctor and nutritionist or other health professional who can support you with less toxic nutritional approaches for keeping you in a good state of mind.

PART 5

Solving Depression, Manic Depression, and Schizophrenia

More people suffer from depression and schizophrenia than any other mental health problem. In Britain, 1 in 20, or around 3 million people, are diagnosed with depression. One in 40 are diagnosed with schizophrenia. Both conditions can be a living hell. But it needn't be this way, as both conditions are, for the most part, curable with the right nutrition, plus psychotherapy. Yet more often than not, the only treatment given is far less effective drugs. In this part you will find out about the proven biochemical imbalances that can cause these conditions and how to solve them.

_____

Chapter 22

OVERCOMING DEPRESSION

In Chapter 14 we explored how blood sugar imbalances, allergies, and deficiencies in vitamins, minerals, essential fats, and amino acids have all been linked to low mood. If you suffer from depression, it's best to start by correcting these. But there is much more that you can do, and that's what this chapter explores in depth.

There's no doubt that there is a need to counteract depression: It's ten times more common today than it was in the 1950s. Depression is also the primary cause of suicide, claiming 3,000 lives a year, and is now the second most common cause of death in young people aged 15 to 24. As depressing as all this sounds, there is a lot that can be done, both with nutrition and proper counseling.

The classic symptoms of depression include:

- Feelings of worthlessness or guilt

- Poor concentration

- Loss of energy and fatigue

- Thoughts of suicide or preoccupation with death

- Loss or increase of appetite and weight

- A disturbed sleep pattern

- Slowing down (both physically and mentally)

- Agitation (restlessness or anxiety)

If you are experiencing four or more of these, this chapter is for you. It's important to realize that there is rarely one cause for a set of symptoms that we call "depression," nor a single cure.

As a general rule, however, it's a good idea to keep crucial neurotransmitters in balance. You may remember from Chapter 14 that low levels of serotonin are strongly associated with states of depression, while low levels of dopamine, adrenaline, or noradrenaline are associated with a lack of motivation. Most prescription drugs aim to correct these imbalances but have undesirable side effects. Instead, I recommend supplementing the amino acid 5-hydroxytryptophan (5-HTP) 100 mg–300 mg, twice a day, to boost your serotonin levels. Supplementing tyrosine, 500 mg–1,000 mg, twice a day, helps boost motivation. Tyrosine is best taken on an empty stomach.

Natural Ways to Beat the Blues

St. John's Wort: The Happiness Herb

Another highly effective natural remedy is the herb St. John's wort (*Hypericum perforatum*). It is one of the most thoroughly researched of all natural remedies.

St. John's wort works just as well as tricyclic antidepressants but has fewer side effects.[1] Tricyclic antidepressants such as imipramine are widely prescribed but often produce undesirable side effects. For instance, in a recent study published in the *British Medical Journal,* 324 patients were randomly assigned to treatment with either St. John's wort or imipramine. Both were equally effective in treating patients with mild to moderate depression. However, St. John's wort was better tolerated than imipramine, and fewer patients withdrew as a result of adverse effects.[2]

An analysis of twenty-three such "randomised" clinical trials on St. John's wort versus placebos, involving 1,757 people in total, proves that the herb is highly effective with minimal side effects.[3] In one German study using 300 mg of St. John's wort, 66 percent of patients with mild to moderately severe depression improved, with less depression and complaints of disturbed sleep, headache, and fatigue, compared to just 26 percent of those receiving a placebo.[4] It is not, however, as effective for severe depression. The same is true for SSRI antidepressants.

A 300 mg dose of St. John's wort (containing 0.3 percent hypericin) two or three times a day helps most people with mild depression, while twice this amount may help those who suffer severely. But don't expect instant results. It often takes a couple of weeks to work.

The Joy of Minimal Side Effects

One of the consistent findings in this research, and my clinical experience, is that St. John's wort has minimal side effects. It is much gentler than antidepressant drugs. That said, there are some side effects reported. About 2 percent of people report side effects including gastrointestinal symptoms, allergic reactions, anxiety, and dizziness. These have often been exaggerated in the media, possibly because more and more people are opting to take St. John's wort instead of antidepressant drugs, and the drugs companies are fighting back with scare stories in the popular press.

Concerns about St. John's wort causing photosensitivity (increased skin sensitivity to strong sunlight) should not be alarming, having only occurred at very high doses rather than the recommended 600–900 mg a day.[5]

St. John's wort does "up regulate" certain liver enzymes. This means that the liver works a bit harder. The same happens with almost all drugs and substances foreign to the body, as the liver tries to detoxify them.

The prominent psychiatrist Dr. Hyla Cass is one of the world's leading experts on St. John's wort. In her excellent book *St. John's wort: Nature's Blues Buster* (Avery Publishing, 1997), she gives ten reasons why she prefers St. John's wort to antidepressant drugs:

1. Its side effects are not nearly as severe or frequent.

2. Mixing with alcohol doesn't lead to adverse reactions, as with the other antidepressants.

3. It is not addictive.

4. It does not produce withdrawal symptoms when you stop.

5. It does not produce habituation or the need for increased dosages to maintain its effects.

6. It can be easily stopped and restarted without requiring a long build-up period.

7. It enhances sleep and dreaming.

8. It does not inhibit sex drive as SSRIs do in some people—and can actually enhance it in some people.

9. It does not make you sleepy in the daytime. In fact, it has shown in experiments to enhance alertness and driving reaction time.

10. According to one report, the annual rate of death by overdose on antidepressant drugs is 30.1 per 1 million prescriptions. No one has ever died from an overdose of St. John's wort. In fact, we don't think anyone has even tried to OD with it!

Exactly how St. John's wort works is still a bit of a mystery. However, a $6 million research grant in the United States means we'll be hearing a lot more about this herb in the near future. Recent research indicates that hypericin, thought to be one of the major active ingredients in this herb, may act by inhibiting the reuptake of serotonin and dopamine. This may explain some of its benefits, but not all. In another study where the purported active ingredient hypericin was removed, St. John's wort still raised levels of the brain chemicals. So we have to conclude that so far, we still don't know enough about the activities and synergistic abilities of the many compounds found in this and other herbs.[6]

Bump Up Your Folic Acid

If you're depressed, you may well be low in folic acid. In a study of 213 depressed patients at the Depression and Clinical Research Program at Massachusetts General Hospital in Boston, people with lower folic acid levels had more "melancholic" depression and were less likely to improve when given SSRI antidepressant drugs.[7] Very depressed people, and also those diagnosed with schizophrenia, are often deficient in folic acid. A survey of such patients at Kings College Hospital's psychiatry department in London found that one in three of them had borderline or definite folate deficiency.

These patients then took part in a double-blind, placebo-controlled trial of folic acid for six months in addition to their standard drug treatment. The longer they took the folic acid, the better it worked.[8] However, they were taking 15,000 mcg (the RDA is 300 mcg!) I recommend starting with 1,200 mcg if you suffer from chronic or severe depression, together with 100 mg of vitamin B_6. Folic acid is only available over the counter in supplements up to 400 mcg, so this means taking three a day. Both folic acid and vitamin B_6 help "tune up" the brain and increase production of SAMe,[9] another intelligent nutrient that helps the brain to work better. SAMe (or TMG, from which it is made) is itself a natural antidepressant, and well worth supplementing at 200 mg a day. All of these nutrients not only help the brain to make more serotonin, but they are the masters of "methylation."[10]

Methylation and Mood

You might have wondered why such large amounts of nutrients such as folic acid, way above what you can eat in a well-balanced diet, seem to be effective.

The answer is that we are biochemically unique, and there is growing evidence that some people, perhaps those prone to severe depression and also schizophrenia, don't "methylate" properly. Methylation is a chemical process that goes on throughout the brain and body, helping to turn one neurotransmitter into another. For example, noradrenaline turns into adrenaline by having a "methyl" group added. Nutrients that can donate or receive methyl groups help the brain to function better. Folic acid and SAMe, for example, help donate methyl groups. Depressed patients may have a particular weakness in this area and therefore benefit from more of these key nutrients.

Later on, in Chapter 25, you'll learn how megadoses of vitamin B_3, which receives methyl groups, are particularly helpful in some people diagnosed with schizophrenia. SAMe, while often very helpful for depression, can aggravate "manic" symptoms, both in schizophrenia[11] and manic depression. It's all one great, big balancing act, helping your brain's chemistry to be in sync.

The Right Fats to Keep You Happy

Talking of balancing acts, B_3, B_6, and folic acid also have a crucial role to play in how the brain makes its essential brain fats. Throughout this book I've extolled the virtues of the essential fats from fish and seeds. However, to turn these essential fats into building materials for the brain, for example in making the receptor sites for neurotransmitters, you need these B vitamins too. That's because they drive the enzymes that turn one essential fat into another. Essential fats are also converted into hormonelike prostaglandins by these B-vitamin-dependent enzymes. Both these enzymes and the prostaglandins themselves further promote the brain's production of serotonin and other key neurotransmitters. It's one big happy family of chemical reactions. Your job is simply to make sure that your brain gets enough of all the right pieces of the equation. These are:

- Essential fats, especially omega-3 fats

- B vitamins

- Amino acids such as 5-HTP, tyrosine, and SAMe or TMG

In fact, a recent study published in the *American Journal of Psychiatry* has confirmed that patients already on antidepressant medication who still have pronounced symptoms of depression experience major improvements in as little as three weeks when given daily supplements of omega-3 fats.[12] In fact, the higher your blood levels of omega-3 fats, which help build the brain's neurons, the more serotonin you are likely to make. According to Dr. Joseph Hibbeln, who discovered that fish eaters are less prone to depression, "It's like building more serotonin factories, instead of just increasing the efficiency of the serotonin you have." [13]

This also may explain why very low intakes of fat or cholesterol can lead to depression. According to a study of 121 healthy young women by Duke University psychologist Edward Suarez, low cholesterol is a potential predictor for depression and anxiety.[14] An eight-year Finnish study of 29,000 men aged 50–69, published in the *British Journal of Psychiatry*, found that those reporting depression had significantly lower average blood cholesterol levels than those who did not, despite a similar diet.[15] The best way to ensure adequate cholesterol and essential fats is to eat coldwater fish such as herring, tuna, salmon, sardines, and mackerel.

The Histamine Connection

Supplementing folic acid doesn't work for everybody. Dr. Carl Pfeiffer, founder of Princeton's Brain Bio Center, discovered that while many depressed patients get better with massive amounts of folic acid, some get worse. He wondered why, and found that those people who got worse had high blood histamine levels. These "histadelics," as he called them, are genetically preprogrammed to overproduce histamine. High-dose folic acid supplements further stimulate the production of histamine in these people, and this can lead to serious depression, as we'll see below.

Dr. Pfeiffer's discovery is yet another example of biochemical individuality, illustrating how each of us is unique. For this very reason, to diagnose depression purely on the basis of symptoms, and then treat everyone with the same drug, is to ignore the many potential underlying reasons for depression, both biochemical and psychological.

I know about high histamine types because I am one. I remember sitting in the waiting room of the Brain Bio Center at the age of twenty, about to meet Dr. Pfeiffer, this extraordinary pioneer in nutritional medicine and mental health. He took one look at me and my white, marked nails and said, "You're high histamine. You need more zinc and B$_6$. Do you wake up early, have a good appetite, an active mind, tend towards being compulsive and obsessive, suffer from allergies, and rarely gain weight?" Yes, that sounded like me.

As Dr. Pfeiffer spoke, all became clear. We all make histamine, but some more than others. This is a genetic trait nicknamed histadelia. Since histamine speeds up the body's metabolism, providing more heat, and since vitamin C is an antihistamine, we think that when our ancestors lost the ability to make vitamin C—a fate they share only with other primates, guinea pigs, and flying bats—this put them at an advantage in colder climates during and after the Ice Age.

But histamine also causes allergic reactions, increased production of mucus and saliva, a tendency to hyperactivity, compulsive behavior, and depression. Some of these traits can be an advantage, but when histamine levels become excessively high, they can lead to chronic depression and even suicide. Marilyn Monroe and Judy Garland are examples of likely high histamine types who died a suicidal death. High histamine types often love alcohol because it sedates an overactive mind. Many alcoholics are high histamine and commit a kind of slow suicide through drink.

But it's not all bad news. Many great artists, writers, and pioneers are high histamine types, passionate and compulsively driven to accomplish. High histamine types are, by nature, compulsive and obsessive people. Dr. Carl Pfeiffer, who identified this genetic trait, described the high histamine type as "built for the twenty-first century, complete with self-destruct." The point is that a faster metabolism means a greater need for nutrients, and insufficient nutrition leads the fast-burning high histamine type to "burn out" fast. Without the right nutrients, a high histamine person can end up severely depressed. If this all sounds familiar, you can check yourself out on the mini-questionnaire on pages 164–165, or online at www.mentalhealthproject.com.

Are You Histadelic?

Histadelics have certain obvious physical signs and symptoms. Histamine promotes the production of saliva, so the teeth are frequently cavity-free. They also produce more mucus and tears, and so can cry more easily. Since Marilyn Monroe was probably histadelic, we can, at this late date, understand better her remark to photographers, "You always take pictures of my body, but my most perfect feature is my teeth—I have no cavities." With good salivary flow, teeth are well bathed in saliva, and the histadelic may have the habit of wiping saliva from the corners of the mouth with thumb and index finger. High-histamine types are not hairy people and don't have excessive body or extremity hair. In men, the beard is usually light, and there are few chest hairs. They have a faster metabolism and are fast oxidizers, and the rapid oxidation of foods means a person can eat a lot and never gain weight.

Histadelics usually have relatively long fingers and toes, with the second toe longer than the big toe. When Monroe met her sister Berniece for the first time, at the age of twenty-five, Berniece said in an interview, "the most exciting thing was discovering our toes. See how the second toe is longer than the rest. Marilyn had the same thing." Their mother, Gladys, spent many years in a mental institution, diagnosed as a schizophrenic. Abraham Lincoln is another example of a high-histamine type, with his long, skinny fingers.

Histadelics usually have an easy and well-sustained orgasm and higher than usual sex drive. Histadelic patients often have the most severe insomnia. A history of allergies or periodic headache and sensitivity to pain is also common. Histadelics are often hooked on excess sugar in coffee or tea and like alcohol and other drugs, often having a high tolerance level.

Pfeiffer tested twelve hardcore drug addicts and found them all to be high in histamine. When histamine levels are too high, a person is more likely to be depressed, compulsive, and have abnormal thinking. Therefore heroin, methadone, uppers, downers, alcohol, and sugar are often craved to compensate for these feelings. The compulsive day-in-day-out drinker of alcohol is often found to be histadelic.

The Link to Depression, Suicide, and Schizophrenia

Dr. Pfeiffer found that histadelics comprise about 20 percent of so-called schizophrenics and a substantial proportion of depressed patients. This estimate was based on the thousands of patients who were treated at the Brain Bio Center over forty years. Here's how he described these patients:

"The histadelic person is often the problem patient at psychiatric clinics and hospitals. Our first contact with histadelia occurred in a biochemical and psychiatric study of outpatient schizophrenics. Two out of nine chronic patients on whom we had extensive data and repeated visits showed significant positive correlations between blood histamine and the Experimental World Inventory (EWI), a psychological measure of stability. In other words, both the highly elevated EWI score and the blood histamine decreased as the patient got better.

Histadelia usually runs in families, with the onset at around twenty years of age. The easily elicited history of suicide, depression, and allergies among near and distant relatives is a strong indication of possible histadelia. This disorder has probably been termed familial psychotic depression in the past. The undiagnosed histadelic patient is treated as a schizophrenic, but the patient does not respond to any of the usual drug therapies, electroshock, or insulin coma therapy. We have now treated over a thousand of these patients, and our experience provides many important signs that help in making early diagnosis.

The classic symptoms are disperceptions, obsessions, compulsions, thought disorder, abnormal fears, constant suicidal depression, easy crying, confusion, and blank mind. The symptom of blank mind is elicited by asking if the patient can visualize the face of her mother or visualize why, on a motorway, she might be directed to turn left though she actually wants to turn right on to a new motorway (clover leaf turn). She often cannot visualize these things.

The greatest problem in the severely depressed histadelic is the constant threat of suicide. We can never meet this degree of mental over-alertness with good nutrition. We can make the patient feel normal but not stop the hyperactive mind. For some of these compulsive patients normality is just not enough."

Optimum Nutrition for Histadelics

If you suspect you are a high-histamine type and are experiencing undesirable symptoms, the best thing to do is see a nutritionist who can recommend a blood test to determine your histamine status. If you've had a standard blood test and your "basophil count" was high, this is an indicator of high histamine status.

The ideal optimum nutrition for you depends on your histamine status. For all high histamine types it is best to eat a diet relatively low in protein and high in complex carbohydrates, emphasizing fruit and vegetables. Proteins like meat contain amino acids that further increase histamine levels. Vitamin C is a natural antihistamine and supplementing 2 g a day is wise. Also important is sufficient zinc, manganese, and B_6. Make sure you are supplementing 15 mg of zinc, 5 mg of manganese, and at least 50 mg of B_6. Some people need double these amounts.

If you are experiencing undesirable symptoms or have a high histamine level in your blood, go one step further and supplement 500 mg of calcium and 500 mg of the amino acid methionine, morning and evening, plus a basic supplement program. Calcium supplementation releases some of the body's stores of histamine, and the natural amino acid methionine helps to detoxify histamine by attaching methyl groups onto it—the usual mode of detoxification of histamine in the human body. Phenytoin, the antiepilepsy drug (trademarked Dilantin in the United States) in a dose of 100 mg, taken morning and afternoon, will usually provide some relief for the severely depressed or compulsive patient. However, the methionine plus calcium combined with zinc and manganese is often sufficient. It is also best to avoid doses of folic acid above 200 mcg until your histamine levels are under control, as large amounts of folic acid can further raise histamine. The same regimen of zinc, manganese, calcium, and methionine provides successful treatment in many severely allergic patients who are not depressed.

With the right nutrients, high-histamine types can lead a perfectly normal and productive life. Liz is a case in point.

Liz started suffering from depression at the age of fourteen. By the time she was seventeen she had become extremely anxious, fearful, and depressed and was hearing voices. She was put on three drugs—Sulpiride and Depixol injections, plus Kemadrin to offset the side effects of the other drugs. The drugs somewhat sedated her, but she continued to suffer from extreme depression and anxiety and continued to hear voices in her head. She also had psychotherapy, but neither this, nor the drugs, made any real difference.

She consulted a nutrition counselor who identified chronic nutritional deficiencies and an excessive level of histamine. Within six months she was no longer depressed, and rarely heard voices or became anxious. She came off all medication and continued to improve. She is now perfectly healthy and happy and recently gave birth to a baby girl. She experienced no post-natal depression.

How's Your Thyroid?

Another classic cause of depression is having an underactive thyroid. In the United States, thyroid medication is the fourth most commonly prescribed drug. The thyroid gland, in the base of the throat, makes the hormone thyroxine, which tells all brain and body cells to keep active. Often as a long-term consequence of stress and suboptimum nutrition, the thyroid gland can start to underproduce thyroxine. This is a classic cause of depression and lethargy, although symptoms of irritability, anxiety, and panic attacks have also been reported in those with low thyroxine levels.

The telltale signs of an underactive thyroid are lethargy, depression, indigestion or constipation, poor memory, and weight gain. Since thyroxine speeds up your metabolism, which produces heat, the definitive symptom is a drop in body temperature. This is something you can check yourself by taking your temperature with a thermometer. Here's how you do it:

Shake out a thermometer and keep it by your bed. When you wake in the morning, and before getting up, put the thermometer under your arm and lie there for ten minutes. Your basal temperature should be 97.7°F (36.5°C) to 98.06°F (36.7°C). Do this for at least two days. (Women should do this test on day two or three of their period as body temperature fluctuates during the cycle.) If either of your temperature readings are below 97.7°F (36.5°C), take it again over a longer period, say a week, to see if it is low on a fairly regular basis. If it's lower than 97.7°F, you probably have an underactive thyroid.

If you suspect you have a thyroid problem, your doctor can run a blood test to further investigate this possibility. However, an apparently normal thyroxine level, if at the low end of normal, backed up by lowered temperature and symptoms, may still be worth treating.

While the medical approach is to give you thyroxine, this hormone is made from tyrosine. Iodine is also needed to turn tyrosine into thyroxine. Recent research is indicating that both zinc and selenium are important too. So, try 1,000 mg of tyrosine on waking and at noon, taken on an empty stomach, together with a multimineral containing iodine, zinc, and selenium. Exercise also stimulates the thyroid. If you suspect that you have a thyroid problem you may also want to visit www.thyroiduk.org.

Building a Happy Lifestyle

There are many things you can do, other than nutrition, to improve your mood. Modest exercise is a good place to start. A recent German study has shown that a daily thirty-minute walking regimen can produce a significant drop in depression within ten days.[16] This confirms previous findings from Duke University showing that a brisk thirty-minute walk or jog three times a week was as effective as antidepressants and was more effective against relapse than the drugs.[17] However, you've got to keep exercising to stay happy. An eight-year follow-up study of people prone to depression found that their depression returned if they stopped exercising.[18]

Increasing your exposure to natural daylight and using full-spectrum lightbulbs for indoor lighting also helps. Light has a direct effect on the pineal gland, which produces melatonin, a close relative of serotonin. Exactly how light elevates mood isn't known, but we all know it to be true. There's a simple light exercise in Chapter 14 for elevating your mood, but it's a good idea to have a vacation somewhere sunny in the winter, and expose yourself to natural daylight. For indoor lighting use full-spectrum lightbulbs.

Being outside in nature may have more benefits than the light and the exercise. Air near waterfalls, mountains, beaches, and forests, places frequently associated with feelings of tranquillity, are among those places where there are more health-promoting ions in the air. (It's the negative ions that are good for you, and the positive ions that are not!) After a lightning storm, most of us feel invigorated and refreshed. This is because the electrical storm has generated trillions of negative ions that ease tensions and leave us energized. Researchers now believe that winter blues or seasonal affective disorder (SAD) may be caused, at least in part, by the depletion of negative ions in the air by winter winds. Researchers at Columbia University's Department of Psychiatry measuring the antidepressant effect of negative ions in the ambient air found that 58 percent of patients treated with high-density negative ions had significant relief from their symptoms, almost identical to the number improved with drugs but with no side effects. So, consider getting yourself an ioniser.

The right music can certainly elevate your mood, as can the right essential oils. Particularly uplifting are bergamot, geranium, petitgrain, or neroli oil. The book *Natural Highs*, which I coauthored with Dr. Hyla Cass, includes many ways to give yourself a mood boost.

Finally, consider seeing a counselor or psychotherapist. As complex as the biochemistry of mental health is, so too is the nature of the psyche. Psychotherapists exist to help you remove the inner blocks to leading a happy and fulfilling life. Useful Addresses on pages 359–368 lets you know how to find the right therapist for you.

In summary, if you are experiencing chronic or severe depression:

- See a clinical nutritionist who can check for any biochemical imbalances, and devise a nutritional program to improve your mood. This may include supplements of St. John's wort, 5-HTP, tyrosine, SAMe, folic acid, B_6, zinc, and manganese, plus a diet to stabilize your blood sugar and ensure enough omega-3 fats.

- If you have the signs of high histamine, have your histamine level checked.

- Change your lifestyle to consciously use light, color, sound, and smell to enhance your mood.

- Consider seeing a counselor or psychotherapist.

Chapter 23

MOOD SWINGS AND MANIC DEPRESSION

It's not at all uncommon to have mood swings. In fact, one in two people in Britain alone say they often get mood swings, according to an online survey of 22,000 people taken in 2001 at www.mynutrition.co.uk. These swings may be generated by a huge number of factors, including too much coffee, too much stress, hormone imbalances, food allergies, and nutritional deficiencies.

Most of the people who experience mood swings can fall into depression with symptoms such as low mood, loss of appetite or weight, feeling tired, poor sleep patterns, loss of interest in hobbies and/or sex, avoiding people, irritability, poor concentration, and feeling guilty or even suicidal. Of course, there are different degrees of mood swings. About 1 in every 100 people swing between marked depression, on the one hand, and mania or hypomania on the other. Those with marked symptoms are said to have manic depression, or as psychiatrists prefer to refer to it these days, bipolar disorder.

Manic depressives who have mild symptoms, in that they do not have a complete breakdown that leaves them incapable of coping outside a hospital or other supported living, can still be severely affected by the illness. They may, for instance, have exciting sex lives that get them into a broad variety of trouble, and then they may suddenly become unproductive and need to take time out. On the other hand, some of them become successful politicians or millionaires. Ironically, these people may suffer the most disruption to their lives with manic depression because, by virtue of their status or less obvious swings, they may completely avoid the medical profession or other forms of help and blame other people for their irritability and other eccentricities.

With no medication, their behavior may lead to divorce, loss of friends, prison, or worse.

The most severe form of manic depression carries the risk of breakdown, which can often lead to loss of job or home. Generally these sufferers spend time either living on the street, in prison, or in a hospital. They are often known to the local police for the trouble they cause when they lose touch with reality. Fortunately, the extent of their disruptive behavior often gets them some sort of medication, though that may bring its own problems.

In practice, psychiatric diagnoses frequently change with time. Schizophrenics may frequently appear to be manic depressive at first. The two diagnoses are often swapped and changed through the course of the disease. Some psychiatrists speculate that the two diagnoses are variants of the same disease. Patients showing signs of both conditions may be labeled schizoaffective (a cross between the two diseases).

Someone showing a pure bipolar mood disorder has a high probability of being either short of zinc and vitamin B_6, have blood sugar imbalances, or brain allergies, or any combination of the three. However, those with mood swings and perceptual problems (such as hearing or seeing things that are not there or experiencing strange sensations in their bodies) or have confused thought patterns (beyond simple elation or depression) may suffer from a range of chemical disorders that are often closer to the imbalances found in schizophrenia. These are fully explored in the next chapter.

Understanding Manic Depression

Most people with manic depression spend the majority of their time either in a normal mood or mildly depressed. Some do remain mildly high all the time. This makes clearly assessing their mood very difficult. Often sufferers can be unaware of how moody they are. Their closest friends may be used to their mood swings and assume they are normal. Worse still, it is possible to be both up and down at the same time! Low mood with racing thoughts and feeling a dire need to sleep but being incapable of "switching off" is a common scenario.

This makes treatment options that attempt to push sufferers out of one mood swing potentially dangerous because they may push them into the other one. A number of treatment options, including some complementary therapies, can cause this and should only be used with the guidance of knowledgeable and experienced practitioners.

Psychiatrists can be very wary about prescribing antidepressants to those with manic depression, even if they are suicidal, for fear that they will "go high." Fortunately most nutritional treatments do not fall into this potential trap as they treat and prevent both types of swing simultaneously.

Three Ways to Achieve Balance

There are three safe ways of helping a person with manic depression that can help minimize the risk of disruptive moods. The first is to take nutrients that help to stabilize mood. These can reduce swings in either direction. The second is to take nutrients and herbs that help reduce anxiety and promote relaxation. Many mood swings coincide with a buildup of stress. Finally, there are nutrients that promote healthy sleep patterns. Insomnia is a major source of stress that only makes matters worse.

Mood, Food, and Allergies

Many mood swings are triggered by blood sugar imbalances or food allergies. The brain is almost totally dependent on glucose for its supply of energy, so maintaining a stable level of glucose is important for improved mental health. People with elevated blood sugar levels may become high, whereas low blood sugar is associated with depression. Blood sugar balance is disrupted by too much sugar, stress, and stimulants, including cigarettes. Cigarette smoking is very harmful for manic depressives. One study conducted by Aidan Corvin and colleagues of St. James' Hospital, Dublin, studied ninety-two manic depressives. Fifty-three were smokers, of whom 70 percent were found to have psychotic symptoms, compared to 32 percent of non-smokers.[19]

According to the nutritional pioneer Dr. Carl Pfeiffer, daily or weekly swings in mood may be triggered by stress or regular consumption of meals containing ingredients that prompt an allergic reaction. He reported one patient who found that his blue Mondays came on because his family had chicken every Sunday. When he avoided chicken on Sunday, his Mondays were once again productive. Even sudden, large, and irregular swings in mood may be triggered by allergies. For example, sustained eating of gluten by celiacs causes nutrient malabsorption that may come to a crisis point, at which point a major mood swing occurs. (See Chapter 25, page 216, for more on how gluten affects the brain.)

Exploring the possibility of food allergies can be invaluable, as Janet's story shows:

Janet was diagnosed with manic depression at the age of fifteen. At times she would become completely hyperactive and manic, and at other times become completely depressed. She was put on three drugs—lithium, Tegretol, and Zirtek. These helped control the severity of her manic phases, but she was still frequently depressed and anxious. Two years later she consulted a nutrition counselor who found she was deficient in many nutrients, especially zinc, and allergic to wheat. As soon as her nutrient deficiencies were corrected and she stopped eating wheat her health rapidly improved. She was able to stop all medication and, provided she stays off wheat, no longer gets depressed. She is now doing her final degree exams and continues to feel good and achieve well. However, if she has any wheat, even inadvertently in a sauce, she becomes depressed, confused, forgetful, and anxious for three to four days. Her manic phases, however, have never returned.

Allergies can also be triggered by seasonal changes. Inhalant allergies are common in the spring with trees and grass pollen, and in the autumn with weed pollens. See Chapter 11 to check this possibility.

Lithium: Is It Essential?

One of the most successful drugs in psychiatry is lithium, usually prescribed in the range of 300–1,200 mg a day. Though some suffer from significant side effects or simply cannot tolerate the drug, for others it has caused a dramatic improvement in their lives. Now, lithium is being prescribed more frequently to those diagnosed with schizophrenia and depressed patients as well. Compared with other psychiatric drugs, it really is a "wonder drug."

Lithium may not be a drug at all. It may be an essential trace mineral. It is certainly essential for goats and some species of pig. Lithium is unusually low in British water supplies. Gerard Schrauzer and colleagues, by analyzing hair mineral samples from 2,648 people, found that nearly 20 percent of Americans had extremely low hair lithium content, and the same was true for samples from Germany and Austria. Hair lithium levels are low in people with certain conditions, including heart disease, learning disabilities and violent criminal tendencies.[20] So people may respond to lithium because they are deficient in it.

However, too much lithium does have the side effect of overdampening emotional expression, which is a common complaint against standard lithium therapy. These high doses force mood stabilization instead of restoring healthy emotions. Nutritionally orientated psychiatrists tend to use lithium in a variety of ways. It is very effective at doses at or above 300 mg a day, and often allows the reduction of other drugs. Dr. Abram Hoffer has had good results using 300 mg a day to improve patients' energy levels, eliminate depression, and stabilize mood. Lithium lowers folic acid levels in the blood, and supplementing folic acid may increase lithium's ability to stabilize mood.[21] However, high-histamine types should avoid increasing folic acid levels (see the previous chapter). Depressed patients are often found to have low hair lithium levels, so low-dose supplements are worth a try.

Low levels of lithium (up to 5 mg) might help us all, whether we are depressed or not. The mineral is found in kelp, dulse, and seafood, and supplements containing low doses of lithium are available from Higher Nature (www.highernature.co.uk).

Omega-3 Fats: Miraculous for Mood

Omega-3 fatty acids are now being intensively researched for their mood-stabilizing properties. The Institute of Psychiatry in London is currently running a large double-blind trial with fish oils.

The virtues of omega-3 fats for optimal mental health have been extolled throughout this book. Thanks to Dr. Andrew Stoll and colleagues at Harvard Medical School we now know that they can be extremely helpful for those with manic depression, too. They ran a double-blind, placebo-controlled trial of omega-3 fats, placing fourteen adult manic depressives on the fish oils EPA (eicosapentaenoic acid) and DHA (docosahexaenoic acid) and compared them with fourteen taking an olive oil placebo. Both took the supplement alongside their normal medications. Those taking the omega-3 fats had a substantially longer period in remission than the placebo group. The fish oil group also performed better than the placebo group for nearly every other symptom measured.[22]

In his book *The Omega-3 Connection*, Stoll quotes a mother of a woman with manic depression now taking fish oil:

"It has been seven days with no antidepressant. I never believed this could be possible—it is definitely a record for my daughter. She has not been off antidepressants for that many days in six years, in fact, going off for one day before fish oil led to immediate suicidal ideation with her screaming for me to kill her . . . For the first time in her entire life she is relaxed and her memory and cognitive abilities have returned— I cannot tell you how fortunate we feel."

Since his book and research were published, Dr. Stoll receives daily emails from around the world reporting "miraculous" responses to fish oil.

Not enough studies have been conducted to determine exactly how much is optimum, but the study used 6.2 g EPA and 3.4 g DHA, which is a good guide. However, the active ingredient in the capsules is now thought to be EPA, and Dr. Stoll finds that generally 1.5–4 g of EPA is adequate to improve mood in patients with mood disorders.

Fish oils have little or no side effects unless taken in enormous quantities. Gastrointestinal side effects may be a problem, but a reduction in the dose, spreading it out through the day or only taking the oil with a meal, should eliminate this problem. The high doses of EPA needed to treat mood disorders make fish liver oil supplements unsuitable for the task. Fish liver oils contain too much vitamin A, and if you take too much of this, it can lead to toxicity. Vegetarians may be able to substitute a vegetarian source of alpha-linolenic acid (such as flaxseed oil) for the fish oil, as long as they take the optimum amounts of magnesium, zinc, and vitamins B_3, B_6, biotin, and C that are needed to convert flaxseed oil into EPA and DHA. However, you are probably better off with fish oil concentrates of EPA and DHA, since the amount the body makes from flax can be very low in some people. Antioxidants are also needed to help protect these fats. Dr. Stoll suggests 1,000 mg vitamin E and a good general multivitamin and mineral including coenzyme Q_{10}. For more information on essential fats, see Chapter 4.

Magnesium: Finding Your Balance

Before the Second World War, magnesium was commonly used to stabilise mood. Since the introduction of lithium (see above) its use has faded, but interest in it has been increasing recently. One study of nine people with manic depression characterized by rapid mood swings found that half of them were stabilized by magnesium as least as well as would be expected with lithium.[23] Intravenous magnesium sulphate has also been used with some success for calming manic patients.[24]

Although these studies were small, magnesium does have an excellent reputation as a mild tranquilizer. Most of us are deficient in it. Diets provide around 200 mg on average, while the RDA is 300 mg. The following symptoms may indicate a deficiency: muscle tremors or spasm, muscle weakness, insomnia or nervousness, high blood pressure, irregular heartbeat, constipation, fits or convulsions, hyperactivity, depression, confusion, and lack of appetite. You can increase the levels of magnesium in your diet by increasing the amount of vegetables, fruit, nuts, and seeds.

More Minerals and Vitamins Too

While no specific nutrient has been proven to cause or cure manic depression, there are many that can make a difference. Dr. Carl Pfeiffer observed that many manic depressives that came to his Brain Bio Center in New Jersey were short of zinc and vitamin B_6 due to stress-induced pyroluria (see the next chapter). Their mood swings often follow a weekly pattern as they tend to become workaholic and then can't relax properly at weekends.

Niacin (vitamin B_3) is a key nutrient in many mental health conditions, including mania, as Sonia's story shows:

> Sonia was admitted to the hospital with mania, having previously been mildly depressed and prescribed the antidepressant paroxetine. The physical examination failed to pick up that she had severe diarrhea, had vomited, and her hand was turning bright red. She was prescribed the antipsychotic droperidol and the tranquilizer diazepam. She remained "high" and was detained under the Mental Health Act. She managed to "steal" some of her own B vitamins (including niacin) and swallowed twelve of them. She recovered almost completely in the next twenty-four hours and her detention was cancelled. But she couldn't obtain any more vitamins and relapsed. She was put on a longer detention and diagnosed with manic depression. It was more than two months and numerous doses of drugs including haloperidol, depixol, and lithium before she returned to normal. Today her mood is stable, and her chronic depression since childhood has cleared. She takes 3 g of niacin per day and has a low sugar and gluten-free diet, and is studying to become a nutrition consultant. Her psychiatrist concedes that niacin deficiency is a credible explanation for her symptoms, and her lithium dose is being reduced.

A study of 885 psychiatric patients found that about a third of them had blood vitamin C levels that were below the threshold that has been associated with behavioral problems.[25] Another large study of psychiatric inpatients found over 10 percent showing signs of borderline scurvy.[26] Both could be explained by poor diet rather than the direct effect of the condition. However, anxiety or excitement speeds up the breakdown of vitamin C.[27] Also a double-blind trial on 40 chronic male psychiatric patients (including four with manic depression) confirms that many psychiatric patients have borderline scurvy. Supplementation with just 1 g of vitamin C a day eliminates this possibility.[28]

The trace mineral vanadium is almost certainly an essential mineral. One study by Graham Naylor of the University of Dundee and colleagues showed that elevated levels of vanadium are found in the hair of manic patients and that they fall towards normal as the patient recovers.[29] Other studies confirmed that vanadium levels in various tissues are altered by mania or depression.[30] There is a credible but far from proven mechanism by which a particular form of vanadium might disrupt mood. However, it is not clear that there is enough vanadium in the human body to make such a dramatic difference to mood. Nor is it clear that vanadium changes are the cause rather than the effect of mood changes. Vitamin C disarms vanadium turning it into a form far less likely to disrupt mood, even if it could before. However, vanadium supplementation is probably inadvisable in those with manic depression.

The best place to start is by supplementing a multivitamin and mineral because nutrients do not work on their own but in conjunction with other nutrients. One study conducted by Bonnie Kaplan of the University of Calgary, Canada, has specifically demonstrated how effective this can be for manic depression. In this study, eleven manic depressive adults were given vitamins and trace minerals in addition to their prescribed medications. Over the next six months, on average, they halved their need for the medications, and every patient experienced between a 55 to 66 percent reduction in symptoms.[31]

Amino Acids: Use With Caution

Amino acids, from which the body makes neurotransmitters, can help in manic depression, but should only be supplemented under the guidance of a health professional. Dr. Abram Hoffer gives the amino acid L-tryptophan to assist his patients when in normal phase and finds it reduces the frequency of manic phases. However, he cautions against giving it during manic phases. L-tryptophan is best absorbed with a carbohydrate snack. In some countries L-tryptophan and/or 5-hydroxytryptophan are restricted nutrients. The recommended amount of L-tryptophan is 1 g twice a day, or 100 mg of 5-HTP twice a day. Unless under professional guidance, do not supplement these amino acids together with antidepressant medication.

The depressed phase following a period of mania may actually be "burnout," and can be virtually eliminated by optimum nutrition. Dr. Hoffer finds L-tyrosine, the amino acid from which we make dopamine, adrenaline, and noradrenaline, particularly effective during these depressed phases. However, it should be used with caution because high levels, in some people, can encourage mania. However, many people diagnosed with bipolar disorder do have low thyroxine levels in the depressed phase, and these people can be helped by tyrosine.[32]

Taurine, which helps the body make GABA, the relaxing neurotransmitter, can help reduce mania. It has many other uses as well, in treating migraine, insomnia, agitation, restlessness, irritability, alcoholism, obsessions, and depression.

Helpful Herbs

Herb–drug interactions can occur and, like drug–drug interactions, may not have been fully recognized yet. Also herbs can cause problems with specific conditions. St. John's wort is an example. Though it has great antidepressant effects, there have been cases of it inducing mania in those with manic depression.

One herb that may well be useful, if used under guidance, is kava. It is an excellent relaxant for both muscles and emotions. It reduces mental "chatter," increases mental focus, and promotes good sleep. However, it should not be used with diazepam (Valium) or any of the other benzodiazepine tranquilizers, unless under expert guidance, because the two potentiate each other. This can be used to advantage in weaning people off these addictive drugs. See Chapter 17 for more on kava.

Sleep and Vigilance

During manic phases sufferers tend to sleep less and less, which is a great stress on the body and mind, rapidly depleting nutrients such as magnesium, zinc, and vitamin C. Kava can help to promote sleep. During depressed phases sufferers tend to sleep too much, probably due to adrenal exhaustion and nutritional deficiency. Encouraging a regular pattern of seven hours of uninterrupted sleep can help to smooth out the curves.

The United Kingdom Manic Depression Fellowship (MDF) has pioneered a self-management training course for people diagnosed with manic depression in England and Wales. It encourages participants to detect warning signs and triggers prior to a mood swing, including loss of sleep, irritability, or changes in lifestyle, plus what steps they can take to prevent a mood swing from happening. Daily recording of mood, sleep, and medication are encouraged. This can give an early indication of a mood swing. These records can also assist when negotiating with medical professionals for a change in treatment. Mood monitoring can also easily be combined with a food diary to assist in detecting allergies. Feedback from the MDF training course has been encouraging. One participant said:

> *"The self-management program turned my life around. Now I'm better equipped to cope [self-manage] with most of my mood swings."*

Other therapies that encourage self-observation and help to undo negative behavior patterns can be most helpful for those with manic depression. Cognitive behavioral therapy (CBT) aims to improve mood and behavior by investigating and challenging unhelpful thought patterns. It aims to set up a "virtuous circle" where beneficial beliefs applied to real-life situations produce good thoughts and positive behavior that reinforces the beliefs. Having proven successful with depression, CBT is currently being researched for its efficacy with manic depression. A good book on the subject is *Think Your Way to Happiness* by Dr. Windy Dryden and Jack Gordon (see Recommended Reading, page 356).

In summary, here's what you can do to stabilize your mood swings:

- Avoid sugar, stimulants, cigarettes, and excess stress.

- Check yourself out for food allergies (see Chapter 11).

- Increase your magnesium intake by eating plenty of vegetables, fruit, nuts, and seeds, and consider supplementing 200 mg a day, found in good multivitamin/mineral formulas.

- Take fish oil supplements providing between 1.5 and 4 g EPA.

- Supplement a good multivitamin and mineral every day, plus 1,000 mg of vitamin C.

- Become more aware of what triggers your mood swings and how to control your thoughts to improve your stability.

- Consult a clinical nutritionist who can advise you about nutrients and herbs that can help keep you in balance, as well as explore potential food allergies or intolerances.

Chapter 24

DEMYSTIFYING SCHIZOPHRENIA

S chizophrenia is a loaded word, feared by patient and public alike. It conjures up images of dangerous and crazy people. In truth, most members of the public have no real idea what is meant by this word, often believing that sufferers have split personalities, like Jekyll and Hyde.

The diagnosis of schizophrenia is in fact a kind of "waste-basket" diagnosis for a collection of symptoms, most of which we've already covered. These include:

- Depression

- Anxiety

- Fears, phobias, and paranoia

- Disperceptions and thought disorders

- Illusions and delusions

- Auditory and visual hallucinations

- Antisocial behavior

A person labeled schizophrenic may have any or all of these, but at a level of severity that makes either them unable to cope or others unable to cope with them. The lack of firm, objective signs is perhaps the crux of the continuing argument as to whether schizophrenia has any physiological or biochemical basis or is just "in the mind." However, more and more evidence is emerging to suggest that most people with this label do have biochemical imbalances, or predispositions, sometimes also triggered by traumatic life events.

Most of us have, at some time or other, experienced some level of psychosis, a temporary losing touch with reality as we collectively know it. The experiences of schizophrenics are reproduced in certain toxic or feverish states. The normal person recovering from the delusions brought on by a high fever can breathe a great sigh of relief at the thought that his experience was only temporary. The person under the influence of the hallucinogenic drug LSD can at least rely on the clock, since the drug-induced schizophrenia will wear off with time. Some people's experience of so-called schizophrenia can be likened to a nightmare state from which they may awaken intermittently. For some, schizophrenia is like living in a nonstop nightmare.

Whose Problem Is It?

The symptoms that characterize people with schizophrenia can be separated into two classes: those that bother them, and those that bother the people around them. The two may not be the same, and there is often considerable friction between the patient and those around them.

Consider the case of the man who says he has visions and hears the voice of Jesus. Hallucinations are considered by doctors to be evidence of psychosis. But what if this man is a lay preacher to one of the churches teaching that if you only have enough faith, Christ will appear in person? To him, people who say he is mentally ill are simply nonbelievers. Many of the stresses and frustrations of everyday life could be relieved if one had a firm belief in being a chosen child or disciple of God. (Many people have this without being delusional about it, of course.)

This kind of discord creates certain practical difficulties. Take a young woman. We'll call her Kate. Kate keeps insisting to her family that she is carrying the new Christ-child in her abdomen because she hasn't had a menstrual period for three months. This failure to menstruate is actually owing to a lack of zinc in her body because of stress, and eating a zinc-deficient diet high in refined sugar. Her family is upset and annoyed by her continued delusion as well as by her untidiness, lack of cooperation, and general unpleasantness around the house. A complaint is then made to the family doctor—by the family, not by Kate. Kate refuses flatly to even talk to the doctor, insisting that she is in good health: "It's just that my family don't understand me and my new role in society." This kind of situation can create a dilemma for the doctor.

Although the diagnosis is reasonably clear, should the doctor insist on treating a patient who has not asked for help? Of course, if the patient asks for treatment, there is no problem. If the patient presents some clear evidence that he or she may harm someone, intervention is clearly justified. However, aside from the unethical taint of unsolicited treatment, a major goal should be to keep patients out of the hospital whenever possible. Sometimes that alone is a victory because with some of today's mental hospitals, there is the probability that the patient may be better off at home. One situation that creates great difficulty occurs when the doctor suspects that the patient may be suicidal or homicidal. Since the conservation of human life has high priority, the doctor must try to treat the patient. Being only human and acting on the basis of insufficient tests, the doctor is sometimes wrong, no matter how great his or her ability. Patients, after such a false alarm, are often bitter and unforgiving. Indeed, they frequently incorporate the memory of such a forced hospitalization into their delusional systems.

Spiritual Crisis or Awakening?

Some so-called schizophrenic breakdowns are spiritual awakenings. These can and do take the form of visions, inner voices, "electricity" shooting up the spine, clairvoyance, elation, and so on. For whatever reason, some people have such experiences, which are described in mystical traditions the world over. But often they lack an understanding or support to ground these experiences and end up in a mental hospital. To the unprepared, these experiences can shatter their beliefs about the nature of reality and be very scary indeed.

Whether real "schizophrenia" or something else, many people end up being given major tranquilizers, whether voluntarily or involuntarily. These drugs do not cure schizophrenia, although they can make extreme symptoms bearable. Most "psychotropic" drugs, as they are often classified, leave the patient drowsy and "drugged" and have nasty side effects (for which other drugs have to be given), as well as carrying the long-term risk of brain damage.

Route to a Cure

With 1 in 100 people diagnosed as suffering from schizophrenia, and many more suffering from depression, anxiety, extreme fears, and phobias, help is badly needed. But what treatment is available? For the seriously mentally ill, this means psychiatric help. Some psychiatrists still view mental illness as a psychologically based disease, a perplexing nightmare often intertwined with suspicious family interactions. The treatment may be endless psychoanalysis, and an enormous drain on financial resources with little more than a slim chance of help. (As one patient said after years of psychoanalysis, "I may know myself a lot better, but I'm still mentally ill!")

Other psychiatrists lean more heavily on drug treatments, but these too have only a small chance of really helping. At best, they can give partial relief, but virtually no one taking these major tranquilizers gets well enough to hold down a job. Fortunately, by understanding the biochemical imbalances that can lead to these symptoms and correcting them with specific nutrients rather than drugs, there is every reason to hope that people suffering from these extreme symptoms of mental illness can recover and lead productive lives.

The starting point is the recognition that "schizophrenia," as a specific disease, does not exist. Each person must be considered as an individual, with their own spread of symptoms and biochemical imbalances, determined by objective tests. These symptoms are not incurable. The nutritional approach to the so-called schizophrenias, especially if started before long-term drug therapy, gives sufferers an 80 percent chance of achieving a major recovery. As Dr. Abram Hoffer says, having successfully treated over 5,000 sufferers since the 1950s with optimum nutrition, this means freedom from symptoms, ability to socialize with family and friends, and paying income tax! Let's take a look at the approach Hoffer used in the following chapter.

Chapter 25

SCHIZOPHRENIA CAN BE CURED

There is no such single disease as schizophrenia, nor is there likely to be any single cure. It is more accurate to talk about "the schizophrenias," because there are many ways to end up with the symptoms and behaviors that will get you this label.

As we've seen, about 1 in 100 people develops so-called schizophrenia, which affects men and women equally. Remarkably, this is relatively true the world over. Since most diseases vary from place to place, one theory is that schizophrenia has a genetic origin that began before humanity migrated out of Africa. It also occurs far more commonly in "genius" families. There's an old saying that goes "What's the difference between genius and madness? Genius has limits." One theory for the leap in intelligence that occurred only in us humans is that, at some point in the evolution of our species, there was a biological shift in how our brains used fats—almost like a new microchip, so to speak. Indeed, one of the big differences in our brains, compared to less intelligent mammals, is the quantity of special essential fats. Those well placed to adapt to this evolution become super-intelligent while those with a slight variation in their brain chemistry flip over into schizophrenia. This fascinating theory is explained fully in David Horrobin's *The Madness of Adam and Eve* (see Recommended Reading, page 356).

Although, I'm sure, there are cases where people go crazy for purely psychological reasons, there is now overwhelming evidence that in most people so diagnosed, something isn't right in the brain. Researchers from the London Institute of Psychiatry have confirmed that the frontal cortex of the brain is involved in schizophrenia. Using functional magnetic resonance imaging (fMRI), they have also been able to show that the deterioration in brain function in schizophrenia is not irreversible.[33]

The best results I've seen in helping those with so-called schizophrenia are achieved by investigating a number of possible avenues, most of which we've already touched on in other chapters. These include:

- Blood sugar problems

- Essential fat imbalances

- Too many oxidants and not enough antioxidants

- Niacin, B_{12} and folic acid therapy

- Pyroluria and the need for zinc

- Wheat and other allergies

- Histadelia/histapenia

I am not saying that so-called schizophrenia is purely a result of nutritional deficiency, although we know that certain nutrients, if lacking, do cause these symptoms in anybody. I'm rather saying that the collection of biochemical imbalances that lead an individual to have a distorted experience of life can be minimized and, in many cases, completely corrected by providing the right intake of nutrients for that particular person. These nutrients "tune up" different aspects of our brain, and it is likely that the drugs currently used employ similar mechanisms, but with much more undesirable side effects. They are like sledge-hammers compared to nutrients, and although useful in the short-term are best avoided in the long-term.

I say this because the best, and most consistent, positive results in the treatment of this debilitating condition have been reported by the late Dr. Carl Pfeiffer and Dr. Abram Hoffer, who was formerly director of psychiatric research for Saskatchewan. Both assess a number of potential biochemical abnormalities, then devise a personalized regimen of diet and supplements. Pfeiffer reported that over 95 percent of their schizophrenic patients had at least one biochemical disorder, and that 90 percent of the patients whose biotype had been identified showed great improvement, even complete recovery, when they followed an appropriate nutrition-based program. Hoffer also claims a 90 percent cure of acute schizophrenia, meaning recently diagnosed patients with no more than two years of the illness, while those who had been on long-term prescribed medication have less dramatic improvements. Each have treated thousands of schizophrenic patients. Using their methods, I have also seen extraordinary recoveries, often complete.

Now let's take a look at the various biochemical imbalances that can be the true culprits in a diagnosis of schizophrenia.

Problems with Essential Fats

One of the hottest areas of research in schizophrenia is brain fats. We build our brain from specialized essential fats. Of course, this isn't a static process. We are always building membranes, then breaking them down, and building new ones. The breaking down, or stripping of essential fats from brain membranes, is done by an enzyme called phospholipase A2 (PLA2). This is often overactive in schizophrenia, and this leads to a greater need for these fats, which are quickly lost from the brain. This explains earlier findings that schizophrenic patients have much lower levels of fatty acids in the frontal cortex of the brain.[34][35]

This also explains another anomaly. If a person swallows niacin, or vitamin B_3, they get a blushing reaction and go bright red for a few minutes. The same thing happens if you paint a patch of niacin on the skin. But not so in many schizophrenic patients.[36][37] Craig Hudson and colleagues at Stratford General Hospital in Ontario, Canada, have discovered that the blushing reaction is caused by the very same fats that the PLA2 enzyme strips out.[38] They've developed a niacin skin test to determine which patients will respond best to treatment with essential fats.

So, what's the evidence that increasing a person's intakes of essential fats makes a difference?

The World Health Organization conducted a survey of the incidence and outcome of schizophrenia in eight countries in Africa, Asia, Europe, and the Americas. They found that while the incidence was surprisingly similar in all countries, the outcomes were very different. In some countries, schizophrenia seemed to be a relatively mild and self-limiting disease, whereas in others it was a severe and lifelong condition. Of all the factors considered that might explain this, by far the strongest correlation was with the fat content of the diet. Those countries with a high intake of essential fats from fish and vegetables, as opposed to meat, had much less severe outcomes.[39]

Dr. Iain Glen from the mental health department of Aberdeen University found that 80 percent of schizophrenics are EFA deficient. He gave fifty patients EFA supplements and reported a dramatic response.[40] A larger placebo-controlled, crossover, ten-month study of the effects of EFA supplementation in schizophrenics, including supplements of zinc, B_6, B_3, and vitamin C with omega-6 fats, also produced significant improvements in schizophrenic symptoms.[41]

But not all results are positive. A trial using only omega-3 fats versus placebo found no significant improvement in mental health.[42]

To date, the evidence strongly suggests that some people diagnosed with schizophrenia do need, and respond well to, increased amounts of both omega-6 fats, such as evening primrose oil or borage oil, and omega-3 fats, together with the "cofactor" nutrients (zinc, B_6, B_3, and vitamin C) that help convert them into vital brain fats. The question is, who is likely to respond?

There are three promising tests: One is a blood test testing essential fat levels in red blood cells. The other is the niacin skin flush test, and the third is an ingenious "breath test" which measures the release of the gas ethane, a breakdown product of that enzyme PLA2, stripping out the brain's essential fats. The more ethane released in the breath, the more essential fats you need. These tests can be used to determine if a person is more likely to respond to essential fat therapy.

Too Many Oxidants, Not Enough Antioxidants

There's another part to the essential fat story. These fats are also prone to destruction in the brain, and in the diet, by oxidants (see Chapter 8). Indeed, there is evidence of more oxidation in the frontal cortex of those with schizophrenia. Therefore, as well as increasing the intake of essential fats, it makes sense to give a person a diet (and lifestyle) that minimizes oxidants from fried or burned food and maximizes intake of antioxidant nutrients such as vitamins A, C, and E. These alone have been shown to help. Vitamin C is also an antistress vitamin and may counter too much adrenaline, which is often found in those diagnosed with schizophrenia.

Vitamin C deficiency is also far more common than realized in mentally ill people, often because they don't look after themselves properly and eat poorly. Pronounced vitamin C deficiency can make you crazy, as reported by Professor Derri Shtasel from the department of psychiatry at the University of Pennsylvania School of Medicine in Philadelphia. She describes a case of a woman who was confused and hearing voices, as well as having physical symptoms. She was tested for vitamin C status and found to be very deficient. After being given vitamin C she had fewer hallucinations, her speech improved, and she became more motivated and sociable.[43] Vitamin C has been shown to reduce the symptoms of schizophrenia in research trials,[44] and a number of studies have shown that people diagnosed with mental illness may have much greater requirements for this vitamin—often ten times higher—and are frequently deficient.[45]

The Niacin Connection

One of the classic vitamin deficiency diseases is pellagra. At the turn of this century there were said to be 25,000 cases annually in the United States, focused in the southern states where corn, lacking in tryptophan, was a staple food. The amino acid tryptophan can be converted into niacin. A lack of dietary tryptophan and a lack of niacin can trigger pellagra. The classic symptoms of this condition are the "3 Ds"—dermatitis, diarrhea, and dementia. A more extensive list of symptoms might include headaches, sleep disturbance, hallucinations, thought disorder, anxiety, and depression.

Officially it doesn't really exist any more in the Western world, due to improved nutrition and the fortification of foods with niacin. Yet I come across people that fit this description every year. For instance, a girl diagnosed with schizophrenia came to see me. I always ask what other symptoms a person remembers at the time they started to feel mentally unwell. She remembered loose bowels and eczema—classic symptoms of pellagra. At the time, her doctors and psychiatrists obviously didn't make the connection. I doubt that many doctors or specialists even hold the possibility of nutrient deficiency on their checklist of causes of so-called schizophrenia. She proved B_3 deficient after blood tests and made great improvement when she began taking niacin, plus other nutrients.

Two other cases illustrate another important point. In this case, two male teenagers, both diagnosed as schizophrenic and hospitalized, didn't have the associated symptoms of diarrhea and dermatitis. Both responded so well to 1,000–2,000 mg of niacin (100 times the RDA) that within days they both became lucid, were discharged, and have continued to improve, requiring less or no medication. From their diets one wouldn't suspect they had been chronically deficient in vitamin B_3, yet their body chemistry responded to 100 times the amount needed by most. Some practitioners call this "vitamin dependency," but we are all vitamin dependent. It's just that some people need more, perhaps for genetic reasons, than others.

The use of "megadoses" of niacin was first tried by Drs. Humphrey Osmond and Abram Hoffer in 1951. So impressed were they with the results in acute schizophrenics that, in 1953, they ran the first double-blind therapeutic trials in the history of psychiatry. Their first two trials showed significant improvement giving at least 3 g (3,000 mg) a day, compared to placebos. They also found that chronic schizophrenics, not first-time sufferers but long-term inpatients, showed little improvement. The results of six double-blind controlled trials showed that the natural recovery rate was doubled. Later they found that even chronic patients, treated for several years with niacin in combination with other nutrients, showed a 60 percent recovery rate.

Why Niacin Therapy Fell Out of Favor

Over the next twenty years more than a dozen trials tested the effects of niacin therapy, often with negative results, so niacin therapy fell out of favor. The main reason other researchers have often failed to corroborate Hoffer's claims for megavitamin treatment is that the regimen he had proven successful wasn't properly followed in subsequent trials—for example, they used the wrong substances or a dosage that was much too low, or used it for too brief a period, or they discontinued tranquilizer medications too quickly.[46]

In 1973, an American Psychiatric Association task force report examined Hoffer's theory by reviewing a number of studies including Hoffer and Osmond's, the subsequent trials, and also some that failed to differentiate between acute and chronic patients. For example, Dr. Richard Wittenborn, consultant to the American Psychiatric Association, said this in a study of eighty-six schizophrenic patients: "Despite the reassuring clinical observations of Hoffer and others, the present findings challenge claims of general efficacy for a two-year regimen of niacin supplementation in the treatment of schizophrenia." [47]

However, Wittenborn had included both acute (recently diagnosed) and chronic (long-term) patients in his study. When he separated these subgroups, as Hoffer suggested, and looked at his findings again, his results did indeed support Hoffer and Osmond's claims for the benefits of niacin therapy. In a second paper he concluded that acute patients "may respond well with high dosage niacin as supplementary to other medication and treatment," observing that, "persons whose premorbid history suggests a participatory lifestyle tend to return to a participatory pattern of living after a year or more of high niacin supplementation. No such trend was indicated for the control patients." While five out of nine acute patients undergoing conventional treatment experienced a reduction in schizophrenic symptoms after two years, this positive outcome was seen in eight of the nine patients who also received niacin supplementation. While this may seem only a moderate improvement, the overall score for important social markers (happiness, friends, a job, hobbies, and so on) worsened in the group that received conventional treatment only and improved significantly in the niacin group.[48]

Wittenborn sent a copy of this second paper to Dr. Hoffer with an apology for his previous publication. Hoffer reports that "when Wittenborn's first report came out, it was treated as gospel by our critics. The second report was totally ignored."

Since then, Dr. Hoffer has published ten-year follow-ups on schizophrenics treated with niacin, compared to those not treated with niacin. In the niacin patients there were substantially fewer admissions, days in the hospital, and suicides. He continues to treat acute schizophrenics with niacin, plus other nutrients, including vitamin C, folic acid, and essential fats, and reports a 90 percent cure rate in acute schizophrenics who follow his nutritional program.

Here's a typical case from Dr. Hoffer.

> In October 1990 a twenty-four-year-old woman arrived in my office. Six months earlier she had begun to hallucinate and become paranoid. During three weeks in hospital she began taking a tranquilizer. For several months after a premature discharge, she almost starved until a retired physician took her into her home to feed her. When I saw her, she still suffered visual hallucinations, but no longer heard voices. I started her on 3 g of niacin and 3 g of vitamin C, daily. Three days later she was much better. By February 1991 she was well. By February 1995 she no longer needed drugs. She is still well and lives with her sister.

Now in his eighties and still actively practicing in Vancouver, Canada, Dr. Hoffer has recorded 4,000 cases and published double-blind trials. He is convinced that his approach is a major breakthrough in the treatment of mental illness.

Five Reasons Why Niacin Works

Just how niacin works is still a bit of a mystery. Knowing that people with schizophrenia had hallucinations, Dr. Hoffer's explanation is that niacin stops the brain from producing adrenochrome from adrenaline, a chemical known to induce hallucinations. Working together with vitamin B_{12} and folic acid, niacin helps keep adrenaline and noradrenaline levels in balance, and prevents the abnormal production of adrenochrome in the brain. These nutrients are "methyl" donors and acceptors, and act intelligently in the brain to keep everything in check (see Figure 25). Once again, some people may simply need more to stay healthy.

Niacin, together with vitamin B_{12} and folic acid, also helps to raise abnormally low histamine levels, an imbalance that is associated with hallucinations. (This happens because it stops histamine from being "demethylated" and hence put out of action. This is why people with high histamine levels occasionally get worse on high doses of folic acid, which may further increase histamine levels.)

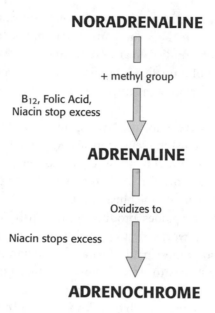

NORADRENALINE

+ methyl group

B$_{12}$, Folic Acid,
Niacin stop excess

ADRENALINE

Oxidizes to

Niacin stops excess

ADRENOCHROME

Fig 25   How niacin, B$_{12}$, and folic acid keep your brain healthy

Niacin, through its flushing action, also helps to detoxify copper and other toxic elements that are associated with mental illness, and improves oxygen supply to the brain. Niacin is also needed for the brain to make use of essential fats. The "happy" neurotransmitter serotonin also needs niacin. Serotonin is made from the amino acid tryptophan, but only in the presence of enough niacin. So there are many possible ways this vitamin could affect brain function.

Hoffer has also found that patients who test positive for pyroluria (see below) are more likely to respond well to increased intakes of niacin. So large doses of niacin are most likely to be effective for acute, not chronic, schizophrenics who are pyroluric and have some of the classic low histamine symptoms of hallucinations, anxiety, and thought disorder.

A Safe and Effective Dose

The amount of niacin that's needed is around 1–6 g a day. A minimum therapeutic level is 1 g a day. These levels are in the order of 100 times the RDA. Levels of niacin much higher than these, particularly in sustained-release tablets, can be liver toxic. Out of perhaps 100,000 people taking megadoses of niacin at levels of several grams over the past forty years, there have been two deaths due to liver failure. In a third case, jaundice resulted from a slow-release preparation. When the same patient was placed back on standard niacin, he no longer got jaundice. In any event, anything over 1 g is best taken under the supervision of a qualified practitioner. If you become nauseated, that is an indication to stop supplementation and resume three days later, with a lower amount.

Niacin comes in different forms. Niacin (formerly known as nicotinic acid) causes a harmless blushing sensation, accompanied with an increase in skin temperature and slight itching. This effect can be quite severe and lasts for up to thirty minutes. However, if 500 mg or 1,000 mg of niacin are taken twice a day at regular intervals, the blushing stops.

Some supplement companies produce a "no-flush" niacin by binding niacin with inositol. This works, so it's probably the best form, but it is more expensive. Niacin also comes in the form of niacinamide, which doesn't cause blushing either. It has to be said, however, that both of these forms appear to be slightly less effective than niacin. This may be because the blushing effect of niacin improves blood flow, and hence nutrient supply to the brain.

Combined Niacin, Folic Acid, and B_{12} Work Best

The best results are achieved, not by supplementing only niacin, but by combining niacin with folic acid and B_{12}. Both folic acid and vitamin B_{12} are often deficient in people diagnosed with schizophrenia—[49] and both have been proven to help reduce the symptoms—but only at high doses.

Research at Kings College Hospital psychiatry department in London has found high doses of folic acid to be highly effective in schizophrenic patients.[50] They used 15 mg a day, which is seventy-five times the RDA! Folic acid is not toxic at this level. I generally recommend starting with 5 mg a day and increasing up to 10 mg, then 15 mg if no improvement occurs within two months.

Vitamin B_{12}, which like folic acid is involved in methylation, has also been shown to help schizophrenic patients.[51] B_{12} is difficult to absorb, especially in large amounts, and some doctors have reported good results giving weekly, or twice-weekly, injections of 1mg of vitamin B_{12}. Some supplements provide sublingual vitamin B_{12}, which is absorbed in the mouth. It's hard to absorb much this way, but does avoid the most common reason for B_{12} deficiency—a lack of "intrinsic factor" in the gut needed for B_{12} absorption. Sublingual liquid B_{12} supplements providing 50 mcg daily may be able to help normalize a B_{12} deficiency. Weekly B_{12} shots, at least to start with, tend to produce a much more rapid improvement.

Are You Pyroluric? The Zinc Link

Possibly one of the most significant "undiscovered" discoveries in the nutritional treatment of mental illness is that many mentally ill people are deficient in vitamin B_6 and zinc. But this deficiency is no ordinary deficiency: You can't correct it by simply eating more foods that are rich in zinc and B_6. It is connected with the abnormal production of a group of chemicals called "pyrroles." A person with a high level of pyrroles in the urine needs more B_6 and zinc than usual, since they rob the body of these essential nutrients, increasing a person's requirements to stay healthy. More than 50 percent of people diagnosed with schizophrenia have "pyroluria."

The test for pyroluria is remarkably simple and very inexpensive. When you add a chemical known as Erhlich's reagant to urine, it will turn mauve if there are kryptopyrroles present. Dubbed "mauve factor" in the 1960s, this was found in 11 percent of normal people, 24 percent of disturbed children, 42 percent of psychiatric patients, and 52 percent of schizophrenics.[52] Dr. Carl Pfeiffer and Dr. Arthur Sohler at Princeton's Brain Bio Center worked out that these abnormal chemicals would bind to B_6 and zinc, inducing deficiency. With this knowledge, effective therapy was at hand. Since 1971, thanks to Dr. Pfeiffer's pioneering work, thousands of pyroluric patients have been successfully treated with B_6 and zinc, both at the Brain Bio Center and more recently at the Institute for Optimum Nutrition in London.

Here's a case in point from Dr. Pfeiffer.

> Since she was eleven, Sara's life had been a nightmare of mental and physical suffering. Her history included chronic insomnia, episodic loss of reality, attempted suicide by hanging, amnesia, partial seizures, nausea, vomiting, and loss of periods. Her knees were so painful (x-rays showed poor cartilages) and her mind so disperceptive that she walked slowly with her feet wide apart, like a peasant following a hand plough drawn by tired oxen. Psychiatrists at three different hospitals gave her various labels—"schizophrenia," "paranoid schizophrenia," and "schizophrenia with convulsive disorder." At times her left side went into spasms with foot clawed and fist doubled up. Both arm and leg had a wild flaying motion. Restraints were needed at these times. Psychotherapy was ineffective, and most tranquilizers accentuated the muscle symptoms.
>
> Then Sara tested positive for pyroluria and was given B_6 and zinc. Her urinary kryptopyrrole level was at times as high as 1,000 mcg%, the normal range being less than 15. She was diagnosed as B_6 and zinc deficient and treatment was started. Over three months her knees became normal, the depression subsided along with the seizures, her periods returned, the

nausea vanished, and so did the abdominal pain. She has had no recurrence of her grave illness, has finished college, and now works in New York. She takes zinc and B$_6$ daily. When under stress of any kind, she increases her intake of vitamin B$_6$.

The Signs and Symptoms of Pyroluria

Pyroluria is often a stress-related condition, with symptoms usually beginning in the teenage years after a stressful event such as exams or the split-up of a relationship. Those with pyroluria often become reclusive and socially withdrawn, depending on the family and avoiding any stressful situations.

Pyrolurics often have weak immune systems and may suffer from frequent ear infections as a child, colds, fevers, and chills. Other symptoms include fatigue, nervous exhaustion, insomnia, poor memory, hyperactivity, seizures, poor learning ability, confusion, an inability to think clearly, depression, and mood swings. In girls there can be irregular periods and in boys relative impotence. The pyroluric patient can have bad breath and a strange body odor, a poor tolerance of alcohol or drugs, may wake up with nausea, and have cold hands and feet and abdominal pain.

A lack of dream recall is very common. It is normal to remember dreams, and many people, whether or not they have mental health problems, report better dream recall once they start supplementing optimal amounts of vitamin B$_6$ and zinc. Other telltale signs include pale skin, white marks on the nails, and, in extreme cases, poor hair growth and loss of hair color. Often a person with pyroluria also has skin problems such as acne or eczema.

Not all these symptoms are present in all pyrolurics, but if you are experiencing a number of them, it is well worth testing for. As we've seen, the simple urine test measures the level of kryptopyrroles in the urine, which should not be above 15 mg% (different laboratories use different measurement methods so be guided by their "normal" ranges). You can also check the probability of pyroluria, based on symptoms, using the online questionnaire at www.mentalhealthproject.com.

David was another case in point.

David was diagnosed as having schizophrenia at twenty, having suffered from acute depression, paranoia, and extreme mental confusion. He was also seeing and hearing things. He was put on the drug Stelazine, which calmed him down, but he felt disoriented and couldn't go back to college or relate with friends and family in a normal way. He was living a reclusive life, with his family. He came to see me at the Institute for Optimum Nutrition. He tested positive for pyroluria and zinc deficiency, as well as having blood sugar problems. Within days of adding B$_6$ and zinc supplements, changing his diet, and avoiding sugar, coffee, and alcohol, he became symptom-free. He was able to stop taking Stelazine and, within months, got a place at the university to continue his education.

Mark Vonnegut, the son of American novelist Kurt Vonnegut, is another example of someone who had a rapid recovery after been diagnosed with pyroluria at the Brain Bio Center. At the time Mark was stricken with insomnia, which led to "crazes" while in college, and he had no dream recall. He showed the usual rapid improvement when given daily zinc and enough B$_6$, and he started dreaming again. After recovering from pyroluria, Mark wrote *Eden Express*. His book must be read to learn the difficulties that the patient encounters in a mental hospital.

Only Zinc Deficiency?

Many of these symptoms are now recognized as classic signs of zinc deficiency, but this possibility is rarely tested for or corrected with zinc supplements. It amounts to a tremendous oversight within psychiatry: Zinc is, after all, probably the most commonly deficient mineral. The average intake in Britain is 7.6 mg a day, while the RDA is 15 mg, so almost half the population gets less than half the RDA of zinc. Seeds, nuts, meat, fish, and whole foods are all rich in it.

There's more to the story, however. People with pyroluria often come from families with a history of mental health problems. Dr. Pfeiffer also noted that it was more common in all-girl families. Although nothing is proven at this stage, it is likely that pyroluria is a genetic predisposition that makes an individual need more vitamin B$_6$ and zinc to feel well. Like so many imbalances discussed in this book, it illustrates how we are all biochemically unique and need to discover our own optimum nutrition to stay healthy and mentally well.

For people with pyroluria, this means both eating a healthy diet and supplementing relatively large amounts of zinc, starting with 25 mg and going up to 50 mg a day, as well as vitamin B$_6$, starting at 100 mg and going up to 500 mg. Those with pyroluria seem to do better on relatively low-protein diets, or, at least, not high-protein diets. Some pyroluric patients react badly to high-protein foods such as meat. This may be because you need adequate amounts of B$_6$ and zinc to digest, absorb, and use protein.

Allergic to Wheat or Milk?

Many people with mental health problems are sensitive to gluten, especially wheat gluten, which can bring on all sorts of symptoms of mental illness. This has been known since the 1950s, when Dr. Lauretta Bender noted that schizophrenic children were extraordinarily subject to celiac disease (severe gluten allergy).[53] By 1966 she had recorded twenty such cases among around 2,000 schizophrenic children. In 1961 Drs. Graff and Handford published data showing that four out of thirty-seven adult male schizophrenics admitted to the University of Pennsylvania Hospital in Philadelphia had a history of celiac disease in childhood.[54]

These early observations greatly interested Dr. Curtis Dohan at the University of Pennsylvania. He suspected that the two were linked and decided to test his theory by randomly placing all men admitted to a locked psychiatric ward in a Veterans Administration Hospital in Coatsville, Pennsylvania, either on a diet containing no milk or cereals, or on one that was relatively high in cereals. (Milk was eliminated from the diet because some people do not benefit when only glutens are removed.) All other treatment continued as normal. Midway through the experiment, 62 percent of the group on no milk and cereals were released to a "full privileges" ward. Only 36 percent of those patients receiving a diet including cereal were able to leave the locked ward. When the wheat gluten was secretly placed back into the diet, the improved patients once again relapsed.[55]

These results have since been confirmed by other double-blind, placebo-controlled trials. In one, published in the *Journal of Biological Psychiatry*, thirty patients suffering from anxiety, depression, confusion, or difficulty in concentration were tested, using a placebo-controlled trial, as to whether individual food allergies could really produce mental symptoms in these individuals. The results showed that allergies alone, not placebos, were able to produce the following symptoms: severe depression, nervousness, feeling of anger without a particular object, loss of motivation, and severe mental blankness. The foods/chemicals that produced most severe mental reactions were wheat, milk, cane sugar, tobacco smoke, and eggs.[56]

In the 1980s, when more accurate methods for allergy testing became available, the American allergy expert Dr. William Philpott followed up Dr. Dohan's theory by testing fifty-three patients diagnosed with schizophrenia. Sixty-four percent reacted adversely to wheat, 50 percent to cow's milk, 75 percent to tobacco and 30 percent to petrochemical hydrocarbons. The emotional symptoms caused by allergic intolerance ranged from dizziness, blurred vision, anxiety, depression, tension, hyperactivity, and speech difficulties to gross psychotic symptoms. At the same time, the individuals also experienced various adverse physical symptoms such as headaches, feeling of unsteadiness, weakness, palpitations, and muscle pains.[57]

Why Some Can't Stomach It

A class of peptides made in the body called endorphins and enkephalins are extremely potent painkilling substances. They perform this task by locking onto receptors in the brain to abolish the perception of pain. These receptors are heavily clustered in the frontal lobes and the lower limbic regions of the brain, where abnormalities have been found in those with schizophrenia. The wheat protein gluten mimics endorphins and enkephalins and is capable of reacting with the brain's endorphin receptors in either a stimulatory or suppressive way, very similar to certain drugs that have been known to produce psychosislike symptoms in patients. Casein proteins in dairy products are also thought to have amino acid sequences similar to those in enkephalins, and so may also be capable of interacting with brain receptors. The term "exorphins" (a contraction of "external endorphins") has been coined to describe these substances in relation to their pharmacological effects.[58]

Historical and cultural correlations would support the view that gluten has some kind of pathological effect on certain individuals with schizophrenia. Schizophrenia was extremely rare in southern Pacific nations prior to the introduction of cereal grains, though levels there are now similar to levels in Europe.

There is now more than enough evidence to investigate the possibility of food and chemical sensitivities in people diagnosed with schizophrenia. At the very least, a trial period of two weeks without wheat or milk products is well worth exploring.

To find out more about the best tests for allergies and how to follow an elimination diet, see Chapter 11.

And What Else?

Histamine imbalances are another biochemical twist in the tale of schizophrenia. In Chapter 22 we explored "histadelia," how very high histamine levels can lead to compulsive and obsessive behavior, and pits of depression. In Chapter 16 we explored how very low levels of histamine are associated with feelings of anxiety, paranoia, and hallucinations.

Beyond histamine, where do we go? In this chapter we explored only seven of many promising avenues that can induce severe symptoms of mental illness associated with a diagnosis of schizophrenia. Like so many complex diseases, from chronic fatigue syndrome to autism, there is also evidence of immune system weaknesses, of links with viral infections,[59] of evidence of gut-related problems, liver detoxification problems,[60] and even links with difficult births and Caesareans.[61] A newcomer to this field of science will be understandably confused and wonder where to begin.

I have two answers. The first is at the beginning of this book. By working through Parts 1 and 2, and making the changes to your diet and lifestyle, this gives you the best possible chance to give your brain and body a tune-up. My second answer is to see a clinical nutritionist, preferably trained at the Institute for Optimum Nutrition, who is qualified to help you unravel the many strands that can lead to mental illness.

In my view, people diagnosed with schizophrenia are like "canaries in a coal mine" (if you recall, the hapless birds were lowered into mines to check if the air was safe to breathe). More sensitive than the rest of us to the insults of modern living and eating, to the suboptimal nutrition we almost all are victims of, those diagnosed with schizophrenia need all the help they can get through a personalized program of optimum nutrition. With this, and the right level of personal and social support, many can be released from the hellish symptoms of schizophrenia and the chemical straitjacket of the major tranquilizers to lead a happy and productive life.

The starting point to tackling a diagnosis of schizophrenia is to:

- Balance your blood sugar.

- Check for, and correct, essential fat imbalances.

- Up your intake of antioxidants and especially vitamin C to 3 g a day.

- Consider high-dose niacin, B_{12}, and folic acid supplements.

- Get checked for pyroluria and, if so, supplement zinc and B_6.

- Check yourself for wheat and other allergies.

- Check your histamine status. If low, try high-dose niacin, B_{12}, and folic acid. If high, don't take large amounts of folic acid or B_{12}.

PART 6

Mental Health in the Young

Are children today having a "kid life crisis"? Mental health problems are very much on the increase in children—from autism to learning difficulties, hyperactivity, and depression. A major reason for these increases is often suboptimum nutrition. Here you'll find out how to maximize your child's potential and help him or her be and stay mentally and emotionally healthy.

Chapter 26

LEARNING DIFFICULTIES, DYSLEXIA, AND DYSPRAXIA

Nowadays children with learning and behavioral problems tend to get put into one of a number of boxes. Are they dyslexic, having problems with words and writing? Are they dyspraxic, having problems with coordination? Do they have "attention deficit hyperactivity disorder" (ADHD), the official term for what used to be known as hyperactivity, with poor attention span, concentration, and hyperactive behavior?

Rightly or wrongly, the treatment depends on the box. If your child is diagnosed as having ADHD, the drug Ritalin will most likely be offered, but not if the diagnosis is dyslexia. But does ADHD actually exist? A top group of child psychiatrists and psychologists, convened by the National Institutes of Health in the United States in 1988, failed to find any substantial evidence that there is a disease called ADHD.[1] ADHD is purely a descriptive label given to children with a variety of behavioral and learning difficulties, and the diagnosis tells us nothing about the cause or treatment. In other words, almost every child is different, showing his or her own unique pattern of difficulties in learning, coordination, and behavior, and as you will see, with optimum nutrition many of these difficulties often go away without recourse to drugs.

In truth, there are substantial clinical overlaps between learning difficulties, dyslexia, dyspraxia, and ADHD. While a minority of children are purely dyslexic, more often the same individual will show features of two, three, or all of these conditions in differing degrees of severity. Around half the dyslexic population is likely to be dyspraxic, and vice versa, and the mutual overlap between ADHD and dyslexia/dyspraxia is also around 50 percent.[2]

Unfortunately, there is usually no such overlap in diagnosis or treatment. ADHD lies in the realm of psychiatry, with stimulant medication the most likely course of action (see Chapter 27). Current evidence suggests that up to 20 percent of the population may be affected to some degree by one or more of these conditions, and the associated difficulties usually persist into adulthood, causing serious problems not only for those affected but for society as a whole.

Dyslexia is characterized by specific problems in learning to read and write due to sutble probelms in visaul percetpion (just testing you!). Problems with arithmetic and reading musical notation are also common, as are poor working memory, difficulties with the sounds of words, and a poor sense of direction. Dyslexia affects around 5 percent of the population in a severe form, though many more when milder forms are also included. If you suspect your child might be dyslexic, many schools have special needs

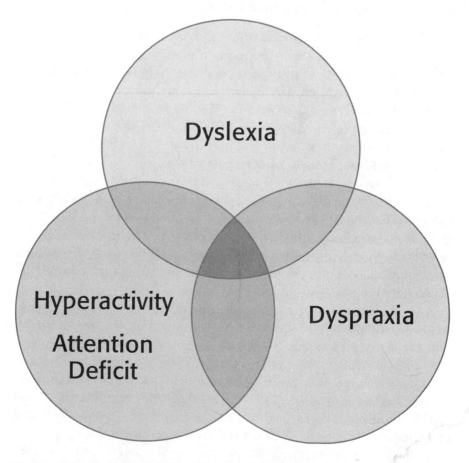

Fig 26 Dyslexia, dyspraxia, and attention deficit hyperactivity disorder overlap.

teachers who can test them for dyslexia. If your child's school doesn't, contact the Dyslexia Institute (see Useful Addresses, page 363), who can put you in touch with an educational psychologist who can carry out this test. This can help your child in a number of ways: first, by being aware he or she has a difficulty, by working with a special needs teacher to help minimize that difficulty, and by the special privileges in time for exams and using computers at school, that are routinely offered to those with dyslexia.

Dyspraxia is less well known, but its prevalence is similar to that of dyslexia. It is characterized by clumsiness and difficulties in carrying out complex, sequenced actions. Poor coordination results in difficulties with acts such as catching a ball, tying shoelaces or doing buttons, but more seriously results in extremely poor handwriting and difficulties with organization, attention, and concentration.

Where Nutrition Comes Into Learning

The link between optimum nutrition and later intelligence starts very early—during pregnancy and then in the very early stages of life. Dr. Alan Lucas's sixteen-year study at the Medical Research Council shows just how critical optimum nutrition is in the early years. In this study, more than 400 premature babies were fed either a standard or an enriched milk formula containing extra protein, vitamins, and minerals. At eighteen months, those fed standard milk "were doing significantly less well" then the others, and at eight years old had IQs up to fourteen points lower![3]

A large number of studies using nutritional supplements have shown dramatic improvements in IQ and mental performance later in childhood too, especially among children with dyslexia and other learning difficulties, even Down's syndrome (discussed in Chapter 29). The many studies discussed in Chapter 12 provide ample evidence that supplementation of nutrients can result in significant improvements in mental abilities, especially in children with learning difficulties.

As early as the 1960s researchers had observed that increased vitamin status was associated with increased intelligence.[4] Similarly, researchers at MIT found that the less refined foods children eat the cleverer they are, with diets high in refined carbohydrates—such as sugar, commercial breakfast cereals, white bread, and sweets—lowering their IQ by up to twenty-five points.[5] Stephen Schoenthaler of California State University later confirmed that the main effect of diets high in sugar and refined carbohydrates is that they lower the levels of nutrients in the diet.[6]

To further investigate the effects of poor nutrient intake on intelligence and learning abilities, Schoenthaler and his colleagues gave 245 schoolchildren aged six to twelve years a daily multivitamin/mineral containing just 50 percent of the RDAs or a placebo for three months. The supplements were designed to raise nutrient intakes just to the equivalent of a "well-balanced diet," and confirmed that vitamin-mineral supplementation can significantly raise the nonverbal intelligence of some schoolchildren by up to sixteen points if they are too poorly nourished before supplementation for optimal brain function.[7]

Investigating what this means for children with learning difficulties, Dr. Richard Carlton and colleagues at the Stony Brook University Medical School, New York, provided nutritional supplements on an individualized basis to nineteen learning-disabled children. All of them showed significant academic and behavioral improvements within a few weeks or months, and some children gained three to five years in reading comprehension in the first year of treatment. Most important, all the children in special education classes became able to attended mainstream schooling, and their grades rose significantly.[8]

In another study, this time with thirty-two children with learning and behavioral difficulties, Dr. Michael Colgan supplemented half of the children according to their individual nutritional needs and reduced sugars and refined foods in their diet. The other children were given a standard multivitamin/mineral supplement daily, though no dietary changes were made. All the children attended a remedial reading course designed to improve reading age by one year, and over twenty-two weeks teachers carefully monitored the reading age, IQ, and behavior of the children. Those taking the multi showed an average increase in IQ of 8.4 points, and in reading age of 1.1 years. However, the group on individually tailored supplements and less sugar and refined carbohydrates had an improvement in IQ of 17.9 points and their reading age went up by 1.8 years, suggesting that subtle nutritional variables exert a substantial influence on learning and behavior.[9]

If your child is having problems with schoolwork, it's well worth seeing a clinical nutritionist who can tune up his or her nutrition to maximize intellectual performance.

One theory as to how certain nutrients help improve intelligence is their antioxidant activity in the protection of essential fats needed for optimal brain function (see Chapter 8), though another is that they aid in the metabolism of energy, not just to the body but also to the brain. A key nutrient used as fuel for the brain, the amino-acid L-glutamine, has been shown to significantly improve the IQ of intellectually impaired children, compared to controls.[10] Glutamine is also important for the health and integrity of the digestive system, an important consideration in autism, a related condition discussed in Chapter 28.

Fats Are Essential for Brain Development

We discussed the importance of essential fats for proper brain function in Chapter 4. Children with dyslexia, dyspraxia, and learning difficulties are very often deficient in these essential fats and/or the nutrients needed to properly utilize them, and the benefits of increasing the intake of these fats have been clearly documented in many studies.[11]

A study of ninety-seven dyslexic children by Dr. Alex Richardson and colleagues at Hammersmith Hospital, London, revealed that fatty acid deficiency clearly contributes to the severity of dyslexic problems. Those children with the worst fatty acid deficiencies showed significantly poorer reading and lower general ability than the nondeficient children.[12]

How do you know if your child is deficient in essential fatty acids? You could start with the checklist in Chapter 4. A key indicator is dry skin or eczema, and in a study of sixty children at the Royal London Hospital, Dr. Christine Absolon and colleagues found twice the rate of psychological disturbance in children with eczema compared with those without.[13]

So the many visible symptoms of essential fatty acid deficiency—rough dry patches on the skin, cracked lips, dull or dry hair, soft or brittle nails, and excessive thirst—can be important indicators as to an underlying cause of learning difficulties, concentration problems, visual difficulties, mood swings, disturbed sleep patterns, and in some cases behavioral problems. This is because the related conditions of dyslexia, dyspraxia, learning difficulties, and ADHD all involve poor nerve cell communications in the brain, and fatty acids crucially influence how your brain cells talk to each other.[14]

To test the value of supplementing essential fatty acids in dyspraxia, Dr. Jacqueline Stordy of the University of Surrey gave essential fat supplements (containing DHA, EPA, AA, and DGLA) to fifteen children whose performance on standardized measures of motor and coordination skills placed them in the bottom 1 percent of the population. After twelve weeks of supplementation they all showed significant improvements in manual dexterity, ball skills, balance, and in parental ratings of their dyspraxic symptoms.[15]

Stordy also assessed the benefit of EFA supplementation in dyslexia and found that after just four weeks of supplementation with the omega-3 fatty acids EPA and DHA, night vision and dark adaptation (usually very poor in dyslexics) had completely normalized.[16]

Brain Pollution

Another possible explanation for improvements in intelligence resulting from improved nutrient intakes is that they help detoxify toxic metals like lead, which are known to have detrimental effects on intelligence.[17]

A number of studies have proved the connection between high lead levels and low intelligence. One researcher, Dr. Herbert Needleman, who has tested thousands of children, has not yet found a single child with high lead who has an IQ above 125.[18] Normally 5 percent of the population fall above this measurement. In Britain, lead levels in an estimated 50 percent of all children were high enough in the 1980s to actually impair intelligence. Since the advent of lead-free gas, blood lead levels are fortunately dropping.

Copper is another toxic element that has been reported to be high in dyslexic children.[19] Since zinc and vitamin C are both antagonists of copper, this is another possible explanation for their reported benefits.

In summary, I recommend the following for anyone who is dealing with learning difficulties, dyslexia, or dyspraxia:

- Ensure an optimal intake of nutrients from your diet as well as a good-quality multivitamin/mineral supplement.

- Minimize your intake of sugar and refined or processed foods that provide ample calories but few nutrients and prevent you from eating more nutrient-rich foods.

- Ensure an optimal intake of essential fats from seeds, their cold-pressed oils, and oily fish, plus sufficient antioxidants, especially vitamin E, to protect them from damage.

- Minimize your intake of fried food, processed food, and saturated fat from meat and dairy.

- Have a hair mineral analysis to check for any heavy metal toxicities (see Useful Addresses on page 365).

These are a good start. But also check out the additional factors outlined in the next two chapters, and the guidelines at the end of each.

Chapter 27

THE ATTENTION
DEFICIT DISASTER

Some children just can't sit still. With a short attention span and volatile moods, they get into fights and disrupt the class at school. These are classic signs of an ever-increasing syndrome known as attention deficit hyperactivity disorder, sometimes abbreviated to ADHD or hyperactivity. These children have a hard time at school and at home, performing badly, getting into trouble, and are often shunted from school to school. Untreated, the hyperactive six-year-old might grow up to be come a delinquent teen-ager, often going off the rails with drugs and alcohol. Now affecting an esti-mated one in ten boys in the United States, ADHD is often blamed on poor parenting or schooling. But there are other potential causative factors: heredity, smoking, drinking or drug use during pregnancy, oxygen depriva-tion at birth, prenatal trauma, and environmental pollution.

The good news is that more often than not, children with ADHD have one or more nutritional imbalances that, once identified and corrected, can dramatically improve their energy, focus, concentration, and behavior.

The Rise of Ritalin

Sadly, many hyperactive children are not evaluated for chemical, nutritional, and allergic factors, nor are they treated nutritionally. Instead, they are quickly put on drugs such as Ritalin, which as we saw in Chapter 21 is a habit-forming amphetamine with many properties similar to those of cocaine. Using brain-imaging techniques, Dr. Nora Volkow of the Brookhaven National Laboratory in Upton, New York, has shown that Ritalin is actually more potent than cocaine, and the only reason Ritalin has not produced an army of addicted schoolchildren is that it takes about an hour for it in pill form to affect the brain, while smoked or injected cocaine works in seconds.[20] Despite these facts, Ritalin prescriptions are more and more common. In the United States, 8 million children are now on Ritalin—that's 10 percent of all boys between the ages of six and fourteen.

It's thought that the calming effect of stimulants like Ritalin on hyperactive children is because there is not enough of the neurotransmitter noradrenaline in the part of the brain that is supposed to filter out unimportant stimuli. Dr. Joan Baizer at the University of Buffalo has shown that Ritalin, previously thought to have only short-term effects, initiates changes in brain structure and function that remain long after the therapeutic effects have dissipated.[21]

This is not good news when you consider the United States Drug Enforcement Agency's list of Ritalin's side effects. On top of increased blood pressure, heart rate, respiration, and temperature, people taking Ritalin can experience appetite suppression, stomach pains, weight loss, growth retardation, facial tics, muscle twitching, euphoria, nervousness, irritability, agitation, insomnia, psychotic episodes, violent behavior, paranoid delusions, hallucinations, bizarre behaviors, heart arrhythmias and palpitations, psychological dependence, and even death.[22]

Ritalin also doesn't work. The National Institutes of Health concluded that there is no evidence of any long-term improvement in scholastic performance on Ritalin.[23] What's more, a child given Ritalin or other stimulant drugs is more likely to become addicted to smoking and abuse other stimulant substances later in life, such as cocaine. The long and short of it is, don't let your child be prescribed these drugs.[24]

The use of stimulant drugs to control children's behavior has risen dramatically in the last decade. Ritalin is now given to up to 20 percent of children in some American schools, and researchers looking at its effectiveness have found that it can worsen the behavior of more children than it helps.

In contrast, nutritional treatment has proven very helpful for many hyperactive children and has few, if any, side effects. Given the substantial overlap between learning difficulties, dyslexia, dyspraxia, and ADHD, I will begin by reiterating the vital importance of optimal nutrient and essential fatty acid intakes and checking for brain pollutants, as discussed in the last chapter, before considering other potential factors in this distressing condition for children, parents, and teachers alike.

Is Your Child Hyperactive?

It can be difficult to draw the line between the behavior of a child that is within the normal limits of high energy and abnormally active behavior. Do these characteristics apply?

- [ ] Overactive
- [ ] Fidgets
- [ ] Can't sit still at meals
- [ ] Talks too much
- [ ] Clumsy
- [ ] Unpredictable
- [ ] Doesn't respond to discipline
- [ ] Speech problem
- [ ] Doesn't listen to whole story
- [ ] Hard to get to bed
- [ ] Reckless
- [ ] Impatient
- [ ] Accident prone
- [ ] Destructive

- [ ] Doesn't finish projects
- [ ] Wears out toys, furniture, etc.
- [ ] Doesn't stay with games
- [ ] Doesn't follow directions
- [ ] Fights with other children
- [ ] Teases
- [ ] Gets into things
- [ ] Temper tantrums
- [ ] Defiant
- [ ] Irritable
- [ ] Unpopular with peers
- [ ] Lies
- [ ] Bed wetter

Score 2 if a symptom is severe, 1 if moderate, and 0 if not present. A score below 12 is normal. Higher scores indicate your child may benefit from the following nutritional strategies.

Eat to Calm Down

As we've now seen abundantly, studies have shown that academic performance improves and behavioral problems diminish significantly when children are given nutritional supplements. Although it is unlikely, on the basis of the studies to date, that ADHD is purely a nutrient deficiency disease, some children are deficient and do respond very well.

In one study by Dr. Abram Hoffer, a pioneer in orthomolecular medicine, large amounts of vitamin C (3 g) and B$_3$ (niacinamide 1.5 g or more) significantly improved the behavior of 32 out of 33 children with ADHD.[25] Some children may be zinc or magnesium deficient, both of which can produce symptoms associated with ADHD. The symptoms of magnesium deficiency, for example, are excessive fidgeting, anxious restlessness, coordination problems, and learning difficulties despite having a normal IQ. Polish researchers examining the magnesium status of 116 children with ADHD found that magnesium deficiency occurred far more frequently than in healthy children (95 percent of children with ADHD were deficient), and they also noted a correlation between levels of magnesium and severity of symptoms. Supplementation of 200 milligrams (mg) of magnesium for six months improved their magnesium status (determined by hair analysis) and significantly reduced their hyperactivity, which worsened in the control group that did not receive magnesium supplementation.[26]

Given that a possible effect of Ritalin is to correct a noradrenaline deficiency in the part of the brain that is supposed to filter out unimportant stimuli, it is interesting to note that magnesium plays a key role in promoting production of noradrenaline. Dr. Lendon Smith reports that around 80 percent of children are able to stop taking Ritalin after as little as three weeks once they start supplementing 500 mg of magnesium daily. Other nutrients also involved in the production of noradrenaline include manganese, iron, copper, zinc, vitamin C, and vitamin B_6,[27] and many of these nutrients are also involved in the proper metabolism of essential fats (see below).

Vitamin B_6 and Magnesium

Despite the tremendous results reported for nutritional approaches, Ritalin is far more commonly prescribed than nutritional supplements. Dr. Bernard Rimland assessed the relative effectiveness of different nutrient strategies compared to drugs such as Ritalin, and found that supplementing B_6 and magnesium was ten times more effective than Ritalin!

In fact, the best drug was Mellaril, not Ritalin. However, neither of these drugs were as effective as vitamin B_6 and magnesium or the brain nutrient DMAE, prescribed as Deanol in the United States, which was also twice as effective as Ritalin (see pages 97–98).

Dr. Neil Ward of the University of Surrey has found one way that children become deficient in these important nutrients. In a study of 530 hyperactive children, he found that a significantly higher percentage of children with ADHD had taken several courses of antibiotics in early childhood than those children without ADHD.[28] Further investigations revealed that children who had had three or more antibiotic courses before the age of three tested for significantly lower levels of zinc, calcium, chromium, and selenium.[29]

Vitamins vs. Drugs—Which Work Best?

Dr. Bernard Rimland studied the effect of the nutrient approach to ADHD on 191 children. Dr. Humphrey Osmond decided to compare this to the reported results with drugs. He reported the total number taking each drug, the number helped, the number worsened, and the "relative efficacy ratio." This is the number helped divided by the number worsened. So if twice as many are helped as worsened, the ratio is 2. If the same numbers of people are helped as worsened then the ratio is 1. The results showed that as many ADHD sufferers are worsened by medication as are helped. In stark contrast 18 times as many sufferers are helped than harmed with a nutritional approach, with 66 percent responding positively.

Medication	Total	No. Helped	No. Worsened	Relative Efficacy Ratio
Dexedrine	172	44	80	0.55
Ritalin	66	22	27	0.81
Mysoline	10	4	4	1.00
Valium	106	31	31	1.00
Dilantin	204	57	43	1.33
Benadril	151	34	25	1.36
Stelazine	120	40	28	1.43
Deanol	73	17	10	1.70
Mellari	277	101	55	1.84
All drugs	1591	440	425	1.04
Vitamins	191	127	7	18.14

Even without supplements, significant improvements in behavior can result from dietary changes that increase nutrient intakes. Dr. Stephen Schoenthaler of the Department of Social and Criminal Justice at California State University has conducted extensive investigations into the relationship between poor diet, nutrient status, and bad behavior. In his many placebo-controlled studies conducted over eighteen months in Alabama, Florida, and Virginia, involving over a thousand long-term young offenders, improving their diets improved their behavior by between 40 and 60 percent. Blood tests for vitamins and minerals showed that around one-third of the juveniles involved had low levels of one or more vitamins and minerals before the trial, and those whose levels had become normal by the end of the study demonstrated a massive improvement in behavior of between 70 and 90 percent.[30]

Essential Fatty Acids

Many children with ADHD have known symptoms of essential fatty acid deficiency such as excessive thirst, dry skin, eczema, and asthma. It is also interesting that males, who have a much higher EFA requirement than females, are more commonly affected: Four out of five ADHD sufferers are boys. Researchers have theorized that ADHD children may be deficient in essential fatty acids not just because they have inadequate dietary intake (though this is not uncommon), but rather because their need is higher, they absorb them poorly, or they don't convert them well into prostaglandins that help the brain communicate.[31]

It is of interest then that EFA conversion to prostaglandins can be inhibited by most of the foods that cause symptoms in children with ADHD such as wheat, dairy products, and foods containing salicylates. Conversion is also hindered by deficiencies of the various vitamins and minerals needed for the enzymes that power the conversions, including vitamin B_3 (niacin), B_6, C, biotin, zinc, and magnesium. Zinc deficiency is common in ADHD sufferers.

Research carried out at Purdue University in the United States confirmed that children with ADHD had an inadequate dietary intake of the nutrients required for EFA conversion to prostaglandins and subsequently had lower levels of the fatty acids EPA, DHA, and AA (all produced in the body from EFAs) than children without ADHD.[32] Supplementation with all these preconverted fatty acids and with GLA reduced ADHD symptoms such as anxiety, attention difficulties, and general behavior problems.[33 34 35]

Research at Oxford University has proven the value of these essential fats in a "double-blind" trial involving forty-one children aged eight to twelve years who had ADHD symptoms and specific learning difficulties. Those children receiving extra essential fats in supplements were both behaving and learning better within twelve weeks.[36]

Stephen's story, courtesy of the Hyperactive Childrens Support Group, is a case in point.

> Stephen, aged six, had a history of hyperactivity, with severely disturbed sleep and disruptive behavior at home and at school. Threatened with expulsion from school because of his impossible behavior, his parents were given two weeks to improve matters. They contacted the Hyperactive Chil-

drens Support Group and evening primrose oil was suggested. A dose of 1.5g was rubbed into the skin morning and evening. The school was unaware of this, but after five days the teacher telephoned the mother to say that never in thirty years of teaching had she seen such a dramatic change in a child's behavior. After three weeks the evening primrose oil was stopped, and one week later the school again complained. The oil was then introduced with good effect.

Many children do not eat rich sources of omega-3 EFAs and could benefit from eating more oily fish (salmon, sardines, fresh tuna, mackerel) and seeds such as flax, hemp, sunflower, and pumpkin or their cold-pressed oils. It is also important to replace foods that are known to hinder the conversion of EFAs to prostaglandins while supplementing the nutrients needed for the conversion, discussed above.

Other Culprits Behind ADHD

Toxic Nasties

Looking beyond low levels of essential nutrients, excess antinutrients can also induce ADHD symptoms. Just as in learning difficulties (discussed above), top of the list is lead, which produces symptoms of aggression, poor impulse control, and short attention span. Another is excess copper, which is found in some children with ADHD. Studies have also revealed a link between high aluminium and hyperactivity. Many toxic elements deplete the body of essential nutrients, for example zinc, and may contribute to nutritional deficiencies. A hair mineral analysis to rule out heavy metal intoxication is therefore an important component of an overall nutritional approach.

Just an Allergy?

Of all the avenues so far researched, though, the link between hyperactivity and allergy is the most established and worthy of pursuit in any child showing signs of this syndrome.

Manufacturers now use an extraordinary number of artificial additives in food, and we can each end up eating as much as 5 kg (11 pounds) of additives every year. Some children clearly aren't coping well with this chemical onslaught. A preliminary study by Dr. Joseph Bellanti of Georgetown University in Washington DC found that children with ADHD are seven times more likely to have food allergies than other children. According to his research, 56 percent of ADHD children aged seven to ten tested positive for food allergies, compared to less than 8 percent of controls. A separate investigation by the Hyperactive Childrens Support Group found that 89 percent of children with ADHD reacted to food colorings, 72 percent to flavorings, 60 percent to MSG, 45 percent to all synthetic additives, 50 percent to cow's milk, 60 percent to chocolate, and 40 percent to oranges.[37]

The yellow food coloring tartrazine (E102) is the best known of many chemical additives linked to allergic reactions and ADHD. In a double-blind, placebo-controlled study, Dr. Neil Ward found emotional and behavioral changes in every child who consumed tartrazine, observing that the additive decreased blood levels of zinc by increasing the amount of zinc excreted in the urine.[38] Four out of the ten children in the study had severe reactions, three developing eczema or asthma within forty-five minutes of ingestion.

Other substances often found to induce behavioral changes are wheat, dairy, corn, yeast, soy, citrus, chocolate, peanuts, and eggs.[39] Associated symptoms that are strongly linked to allergy include nasal problems and excessive mucus, ear infections, facial swelling and discoloration around the eyes, tonsillitis, digestive problems, bad breath, eczema, asthma, headaches, and bedwetting. It's relatively simple to identify foods that may be causing or aggravating symptoms by excluding them for two weeks before a carefully observed reintroduction. Testing in this way is not always conclusive, so it may be worth considering a proper allergy test using the IgG ELISA method. Such a test can identify foods that an individual reacts to from a single blood sample, though they do cost $250 to $500, depending on the number of foods tested and the chosen laboratory (see Useful Addresses, page 361, and Chapter 11). While most intolerances are IgG mediated, some are IgE mediated so it's best to have both an IgE and an IgG test.

Up to 90 percent of hyperactive children benefit from eliminating foods that contain artificial colors, flavors, and preservatives, processed and manufactured foods, and "culprit" foods identified by either an exclusion diet or blood test.[40] Some have also reported success with the Feingold diet, removing not only all artificial additives but also foods that naturally contain compounds called salicylates. Although there have been few double-blind studies on the Feingold diet, researchers at the Univesity of Sydney, Australia, found that of eighty-six children with ADHD, 75 percent of them reacted adversely to a double-blind challenge with salicylates.[41] Foods rich in salicylates include prunes, raisins, raspberries, almonds, apricots, canned cherries, blackcurrants, oranges, strawberries, grapes, tomato sauce, plums, cucumbers, and Granny Smith apples. As the list is very long and contains many otherwise nutritious foods, this should be considered only as a secondary course of action, and must be carefully planned and monitored by a nutritionist to ensure adequate nutritional intake.

Understanding how a low-salicylate diet helps children with ADHD offers us an alternative. Salicylates inhibit the conversion and utilization of essential fatty acids, which we know from the discussion above are essential for proper brain function and are also often low in children with ADHD. So instead of avoiding the inhibitor (salicylates), it may be sufficient to increase the supply of EFAs, which has indeed been shown to help.

Sugar Problems

A diet high in refined carbohydrates is not good for anyone, and many parents believe that eating sweets promotes hyperactivity and aggression in their children. In contrast, some recent research has suggested that sugar itself is not to blame for hyperactivity, and can even have a calming effect on certain individuals. Yet dietary studies do consistently reveal that hyperactive children eat more sugar than other children,[42] and reducing dietary sugar has been found to halve disciplinary actions in young offenders.[43] It seems then that reactions to sugar are not due to allergy as such, but a craving brought on by low blood sugar levels.

Other research has confirmed that the problem is not sugar itself but the forms it comes in, the absence of a well-balanced diet overall, and abnormal glucose metabolism. A study of 265 hyperactive children found that more than three-quarters displayed abnormal glucose tolerance.[44] As the main fuel for the brain and body, when blood glucose levels fluctuate wildly all day on a roller-coaster ride of refined carbohydrates, stimulants, sweets, chocolate, fizzy drinks, juices, and little or no fiber to slow the glucose absorption, it is not surprising that levels of activity, concentration, focus, and behavior will also fluctuate wildly, as is seen in children with ADHD. The calming effect sometimes observed after sugar consumption may well be the initial normalization of blood sugar from a hypoglycemic state during which the brain and cognitive functions controlling behavior were starved of fuel.

The advice then is to remove from the diet all forms of refined sugar and any foods that contain it, and replace them with whole foods and complex carbohydrates (brown rice and other whole grains, oats, lentils, beans, quinoa, and vegetables), which should be eaten throughout the day. Carbohydrates should always be balanced with protein (half as much protein as carbohydrates at every meal and snack) to improve glucose tolerance. Two easy examples are eating nuts with fruit, or fish with rice. Supplementing 200 mcg of chromium also helps stabilize blood sugar.

Bipolar Children

Some children diagnosed with ADHD have "bipolar disorder," formerly called manic depression. They may oscillate from states of mania and hyperactivity to crying spells and depression. The trouble is that bipolar disorder simply isn't diagnosed in childhood. In fact, it used to be thought that the condition didn't start before the age of twenty, but this is a myth. Bipolar disorder can and does occur in infancy, but the majority of these children get wrongly classified as having ADHD. Drs. Janet Wozniak and Joseph Biederman from Harvard Medical School found that 94 percent of children with mania met the criteria for a diagnosis of ADHD.

This is bad news because the last thing a bipolar child needs is stimulant drugs such as Ritalin. Dr. Demitri Papalos, associate professor of psychiatry at Albert Einstein College of Medicine in New York City, studied the effects of stimulant drugs on seventy-three children diagnosed as bipolar and found that forth-seven of these children were thrown into states of mania or psychosis by stimulant medication.[45] His excellent book, The Bipolar Child, coauthored with his wife Janice Papalos, helps to differentiate between those suffering from bipolar disorder (see Chapter 23) and ADHD. These are the differences they've observed:

- Children with bipolar disorder essentially have a mood disorder and go from the extreme highs of mania, tantrums, and anger into extreme lows. Some may go through four cycles in the year, while for others these cycles can happen in a week. This rapid cycling is rarely seen in adults.

- Bipolar children also have different kinds of angry outbursts. While most children will calm down in twenty to thirty minutes, bipolar children can rage on for hours, often with destructive, even sadistic, aggressiveness. They can also display disorganized thinking, language, and body positions during an angry outburst.

- Bipolar children have bouts of depression, which is not a usual pattern of ADHD. They often show giftedness, perhaps in verbal or artistic skills, often early in life. Their misbehavior is often more intentional, while the classic ADHD child often misbehaves through their own inattention. A bipolar child can, for example, be the bully in the playground.

The nutritional approach outlined at the end of this chapter is much more likely to be helpful, together with those outlined in Chapter 23. Ritalin, and other stimulant drugs, can be an absolute disaster.

Reward Deficiency Syndrome

Some children with ADHD disturbances suffer from "reward deficiency syndrome," [46] characterized by a constant need for stimulation. This is thought to occur because they either don't produce enough of the motivating neurotransmitter dopamine (from which adrenaline and noradrenaline are made) or don't respond strongly enough to their own dopamine. Drugs like cocaine and Ritalin both increase dopamine production and dopamine sensitivity, at least in the short term. For these children, Ritalin can seem a miraculous cure. But in the long term, they cause "down-regulation" so you need even more stimulation. This is probably why children given Ritalin are more likely to abuse other dopamine-promoting drugs and are more likely to become dependent on such drugs later in life. [47]

For these children, the stimulating brain nutrient DMAE (sold as Deanol in the United States) is highly effective. Researcher and psychiatrist Dr. Charles Grant discovered that in addition to increasing acetylcholine, in higher doses DMAE can actually block the acetylcholine receptor. This allows more dopamine to be released, thereby stimulating the brain. This action could explain DMAE's proven success with reward deficiency syndrome and ADHD. Unlike Ritalin, DMAE doesn't increase the need for external stimulation and doesn't have all the undesirable side effects.

The optimum nutrition approach to ADHD involves a combination of all the above factors, and practitioners have reported significant improvements in at least two-thirds of children. This is substantially better than any drugs currently prescribed for ADHD. Ritalin, the most frequently prescribed, helps about a third of children and makes a third worse.

In summary, I recommend that anyone with ADHD:

- Follow the guidelines at the end of Chapter 26 regarding nutrients, sugar, essential fats, and heavy metals.

- Eliminate chemical food additives and check other potential allergens such as wheat, dairy, chocolate, oranges, and eggs.

- Supplement DMAE.

One last note. ADHD is a complex condition requiring supervision and treatment by a qualified practitioner who can devise the correct nutritional strategy for your child. Individual assessment of supplement requirements is essential and should always be accompanied by a healthy diet. A minimum of three to six months is required before you see any substantial results, but a general slowing of the hyperactivity and increased concentration can happen within weeks. As the children start to feel better and behave better, the positive feedback they receive from their parents and teachers can encourage them to commit to the program and considerable improvements can quickly follow. Gut problems, allergies, and poor liver detoxification are also worthy of consideration in ADHD cases, and are discussed in the next related chapter on autism.

Chapter 28

ANSWERS FOR AUTISM

Few conditions are as mysterious as autism. All of the overlapping conditions in the previous two chapters—dyslexia, dyspraxia, and ADHD—are often present in autism, but there are other symptoms that lead to a diagnosis of autism. These include difficulties with speech, abnormalities of posture or gesture, impaired understanding of the feelings of others, sensory and visual disperceptions, fears and anxieties, and behavioral abnormalities such as compulsive/obsessive behavior and ritualistic movements.

The U.S. State Department of Developmental Services has found that the incidence of autism more than tripled between 1987 and 1999.[48] The figures for the United Kingdom range from three to ten times more cases in the last decade. While autism used to occur primarily "from birth," or at least was detected within the first six months, over the past ten years there has been a dramatic increase in "late onset" autism, most frequently diagnosed in the second year of life, in both the United States and United Kingdom. According to the National Autistic Society, the incidence may now be higher than 1 in every 100 children. This strongly suggests that something new is triggering this epidemic. Possible culprits include diet, vaccinations, and gut problems, which are also very much on the increase in children.

Unraveling Autism

As with all conditions like this, there is the question as to whether it is "inherited" or caused by something in the diet or environment. Autism is

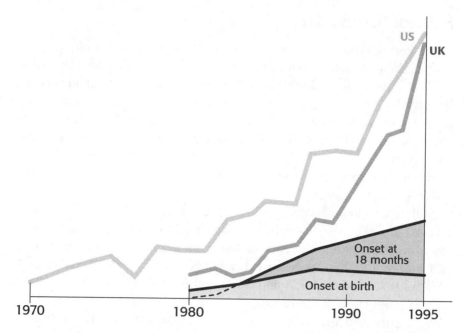

Fig 27   Autism is on the increase in the United States and the United
Kingdom; and change in relation to onset of autism

four times as common in boys as girls. Parents and siblings of autistic
children are far more likely to suffer from milk or gluten allergy, have
digestive disorders such as irritable bowel syndrome, have high cholesterol,
night blindness or light sensitivity, thyroid problems, and cancer. Being
breast-fed also increases the risk. At first glance, one might suspect that
autistic children may inherit certain imbalances. However, an alternative
explanation might be that other family members eat the same food and may
be lacking the same nutrients.

Given the overlaps with dyslexia, dyspraxia, and ADHD, all of the factors discussed in the previous two chapters are equally relevant when considering the causes of autism. Specifically, you'll need to look at balancing
blood sugar, checking for brain-polluting heavy metals, excluding food
additives, correcting possible nutrient deficiencies, and ensuring an optimal intake of essential fatty acids. There is growing evidence that these
approaches can really make a big difference to the autistic child. In fact, it is
probably better to consider all these conditions as part of the "autistic spectrum" of diseases, with dyslexia and mild hyperactivity at one extreme and
autism at the other.

Nutrient Deficiencies

We've known since the 1970s that nutrients can make a big difference to autistic children, thanks to the pioneering research by Dr. Bernard Rimland of the Institute for Child Behavior Research in San Diego, California. He showed that vitamin B_6, C, and magnesium supplements significantly improved symptoms in autistic children. In one of his early studies back in 1978, twelve out of sixteen autistic children improved, then regressed when the vitamins were swapped for placebos.[49] In the decades following Dr. Rimland's pioneering study, many other researchers have also reported positive results with this approach.[50]

Still others have, however, failed to confirm positive outcomes with certain nutrients. For example, a French study of sixty autistic children found significant improvements resulted from a combination of vitamin B_6 and magnesium, but not when either nutrient was supplemented alone.[51] This study shows how important it is to get the balance of these nutrients right. It's likely to be different for each child.

B_6 in particular may help in part because many children with autism or learning difficulties have a condition known as pyroluria (see Chapter 25, page 213), a condition in which, for genetic reasons, high levels of compounds called pyroles are excreted in the urine and cause a deficiency of zinc and vitamin B_6. In children who have facial swelling and a history of frequent colds and middle ear infections, pyroluria should be suspected, and can be tested with a simple urine test (see References and Resources).

A Lack of the Right Fats

We've already discussed how essential fatty acids are essential for brain function, and deficiencies are common in autism sufferers.[52] Research by Dr. Gordon Bell at Stirling University has shown that some autistic children have an enzymatic defect that removes essential fatty acids from brain cell membranes more quickly than it should. Consequently, supplementing the omega-3 fatty acid EPA, which can slow the activity of this enzyme, has clinically improved behavior, mood, imagination, spontaneous speech, sleep patterns, and focus of autistic children.[53 54]

Visual Problems and Vitamin A Deficiency

Pediatrician Mary Megson from Richmond, Virginia, believes that many autistic children are lacking in vitamin A. Otherwise known as retinol, vitamin A is essential for vision. It is also vital for building healthy cells in the gut and in the brain. There is no real doubt that something funny is going on in the digestive tracts of autistic children. Could this be related to vitamin A deficiency, she wondered?

The best sources of vitamin A are breast milk, organ meats, milk fat, fish, and cod liver oil, none of which are prevalent in our diets. Instead, we have formula milk, fortified food, and multivitamins, many of which contain altered forms of retinol such as retinyl palmitate, which doesn't work as well as the fish or animal derived retinol. What would happen, wondered Dr. Megson, if these children weren't getting enough natural vitamin A?[55] Not only would this affect the integrity of the digestive tract, potentially leading to allergies, but it would also affect the development of their brains and disturb their vision. Both brain differences and visual defects have been detected in autistic children. The visual defects, she deduced, were an important clue because lack of vitamin A would mean poor black and white vision, a symptom often seen in the relatives of autistic kids.

If you can't see black and white, what you lose is shadow. Without shadow you'd lose the ability to perceive three-dimensionality, and as a consequence, you couldn't make sense of people's expressions so well. This might explain why autistic children tend not to look straight at you. They look to the side. Long thought to be a sign of poor socialization, it may in fact be the best way they can see people's expressions because there are more black and white light receptors at the edge of the visual field than in the middle! Your whole visual world would become fragmented snapshots.

Of course, the proof is in the pudding. Dr. Megson has reported rapid and dramatic improvements in autism simply by giving cod liver oil containing natural, unadulterated vitamin A. Often she has seen results within a week of starting cod liver oil![56] Here are some of the comments her patients have made after cod liver supplementation. "Now I know where my fingers are." "Now I can see my arms at the same time I see my fingers!" "My box is getting bigger every day. Now I can see emotion on the faces on TV."

The Allergy Link

In addition to these likely deficiencies, the most significant contributing factor in autism appears to be undesirable foods and chemicals that often reach the brain via the bloodstream because of faulty digestion and absorption. Much of the impetus for recognizing the importance of dietary intervention has come from parents who've noticed vast improvements in their children when changing their diets. Certain offending foods and substances appear to adversely influence a large number of children, including:

- Wheat and other gluten-containing grains

- Milk and other dairy products containing casein

- Citrus fruits

- Chocolate

- Artificial food colorings

- Paracetamol

- Salicylates (see Chapter 27, page 233)

- Nightshade family foods (potatoes, tomatoes, aubergines)

The strongest direct evidence of foods linked to autism involves wheat and dairy, and the specific proteins they contain—namely gluten and casein. These are difficult to digest and, especially if introduced too early in life, may result in an allergy. Fragments of these proteins, called peptides, can mimic chemicals in the brain called endorphins, so they're often referred to as "exorphins." These exorphin peptides have damaging opioidlike effects in the brain, leading to the many symptoms we describe as autism. Researchers at the Autism Research Unit at Sunderland University have found increased levels of these peptides in the blood and urine of children with autism.[57]

What's Going on in the Gut

To understand how these common foods can be so harmful to sensitive individuals, we need to look at how they get into the body via the gut. Opioid peptides are derived from the incomplete digestion of proteins, particularly food containing gluten and casein. One such peptide, IAG, derived from gluten in wheat, is detected in 80 percent of autistic patients,[58] while another, Gliadoprhin-7, has been found in very large amounts in 54 percent of autistic children, but only in very small amounts in just 32 percent of non-autistic children.[59] So the first problem is the poor digestion of proteins. Earlier in this chapter we learned how zinc and vitamin B_6 can help autistic children, and here it is worth noting that these two nutrients are essential for proper stomach acid production and therefore protein digestion. But even then, these partially digested protein fragments shouldn't enter the bloodstream. So how do they? Vitamin A deficiency is certainly one culprit, but there may be more.

A large proportion of parents with autistic children report that their children received repeated or prolonged courses of antibiotic drugs for ear or other respiratory infections during the first year of life, prior to the diagnosis of autism. Broad-spectrum antibiotics kill good as well as bad bacteria in the gut, weakening the intestinal membranes. This can lead to what is known as leaky gut syndrome, in which large molecules that shouldn't be absorbed through the gut membrane do get through.[60] Dr. Andrew Wakefield of London's Royal Free hospital, in a study of 60 autistic children with gastrointestinal symptoms, found much greater incidences of intestinal lesions than in nonautistic children with similar digestive problems. Over 90 percent of autistic children showed clinical evidence of chronic inflammation of the small and large intestine as a result of infection, at levels greater than six times that found in nonautistic children with inflammatory bowel disease.[61]

So restoring a healthy gut in autistic children is very important. Supplementing digestive enzymes and probiotics is known to produce positive clinical results in autistic children, as these nutrients help heal the digestive tract and restore normal absorption.[62] Improving the healthy balance of bacteria in the digestive tract, which can be helped by taking probiotic supplements, may also help by digesting exorphins in the gut before they can be inappropriately absorbed.[63] The amino acid L-glutamine is especially important in restoring the integrity of the digestive tract. Drinking 5g dissolved in water just before bedtime can help heal the gut.

Cutting Out Wheat and Dairy

Clearly though, removing suspect foods from the diet is key, and there are many anecdotal reports of dramatic improvements from parents who remove casein and gluten from their autistic children's diet.[64] It can take some time for the harmful peptides to be removed from the blood and brain, so results can be slow to emerge. Dr. Robert Cade, professor of medicine and physiology at the University of Florida, has observed that as the levels of peptides in the blood decrease, the symptoms of autism decrease. "If they can be reduced to normal range," he says, "most patients either improve dramatically or become completely normal." (See the graph on page 244.) But you need to rigidly adhere to a gluten/casein-free diet to accomplish this.[65]

The Autism Research Unit at Sunderland University recommends a gradual withdrawal of foods, waiting three weeks after the removal of casein (dairy) before removing gluten (wheat, oats, barley, rye) from the diet. Keep a food diary and note behaviors and symptoms alongside. This can help to identify other problematic foods, which commonly include citrus fruits, chocolate, artificial food colorings, salicylates, eggs, tomatoes, avocados, aubergine, red peppers, soy, and corn.[66] Because you need to ensure that

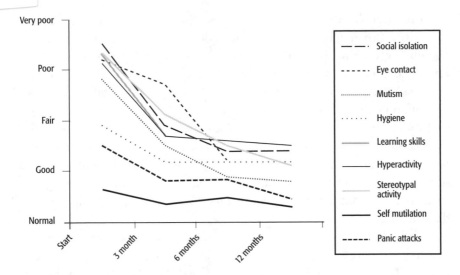

Fig 28 Symptom improvement observed in seventy autistic children while on a gluten/casein-free diet over twelve months

these foods are replaced rather than just removed, as well as being fully aware of all those foods that contain gluten and/or casein (see below), this is best done under the guidance of a nutritional practitioner (see Useful Addresses, page 366).

Grains containing gluten include wheat, oats, barley, and rye. This makes unsuitable most bread, biscuits, cakes, pasta, breakfast cereals, bulgur, couscous, pizza, pita bread, wraps, chapattis, naans, egg noodles, pastry, bagels, crumpets, pot noodles, pies, sausages, ready meals, and processed foods. Check ingredients lists carefully and avoid flour, rusk, malted flakes, and wheat starch. Most alternatives are based on rice or corn, and gluten-free breads, pastas, cereals, biscuits, crackers, cakes, and bars are now readily available in health food shops and some supermarkets.

Casein is in all dairy products, including cow's milk, butter, cheese, yogurt, ice-cream and milk chocolate. Sometimes goat's or sheep's milk are better tolerated, though a better alternative is to make use of the many soy alternatives now available, including milk, cheese, yogurt and ice cream. If soy is suspected, alternatives made from rice are also now available.

A Need to Detox

Another way peptides can harm the autistic child involves the liver. This organ's job is to detoxify harmful chemicals and break down hormones and neurotransmitters to avoid excesses, keeping the brain's chemistry in check. Through a process called sulphation, the liver inactivates excessive amounts of many neurotransmitters in the brain that modulate mood and behavior, so keeping the brain in balance. Thus any reduction in sulphation can upset the brain. Ninety-five percent of autistic children have low sulphate levels, compared to 15 percent of controls, which can result in the inadequate inactivation of these neurotransmitters. Not only that: Reduced sulphation also affects the mucin proteins that line the gastrointestinal tract, increasing gut permeability and inflammatory bowel disease. This is where peptides, known to be high in autistic children, come in, in their turn reducing sulphate production. It's a vicious circle.

Sulphate production is also dependent on the enzyme sulphite oxidase, levels of which are often low in autistic children, as indicated by high levels of sulphite in their urine. Sulphite oxidase is dependent on adequate levels of the mineral molybdenum, so supplementing this can be helpful. About 20 percent of autistic children respond well to such supplements.[67] Also potentially helpful is a highly usable form of sulphur called MSM (short for methylsulfonylmethane).

Autistic children often have dysbiosis—that is, the presence of undesirable microorganisms in the gut, whether bacteria, yeasts, fungi, or parasites. Treatment with antifungal drugs such as Nystatin can produce remarkable improvements, but children often get worse before they get better. This is because fungi such as candida produce all sorts of toxins as they die off. Other less aggressive antifungal agents, including caprylic acid from coconut, charcoal, and the yeast *Saccharomyces boulardi* can be equally effective, causing less severe reactions.

The Metallothionein Connection

The idea that autistic children have a problem detoxifying led Dr. William Walsh at the Pfeiffer Treatment Center in Naperville, Illinois, to look for differences in trace and toxic elements in autistic versus nonautistic children. He found that autistic children, almost invariably, have a high blood copper/zinc ratio and high levels of copper.[68] This discovery led to the theory that a type of protein called metallothionein could be defective in autistic children, leading to an inability to rid the body of toxic metals such as copper, mercury, cadmium, and so on (see Chapter 10). The could happen either because the child has a genetic defect that leads to less metallothionein, or due to early overexposure to such toxic metals, possibly coupled with zinc deficiency. This is because metallothionein contains zinc, which it releases to latch on to an undesirable element such as copper or mercury. In any event, the child ends up overloaded with toxic metals that are well known to induce many of the symptoms associated with autism.

Of course, as eloquent as this theory sounds, does it work? The answer is a resounding yes. By giving autistic children specific nutrients that help detoxify the body and get the metallothionein working properly, the Pfeiffer Treatment Center has reported consistent remarkable recoveries. Some of these cases are reported on www.hriptc.org.

The MMR Vaccine Debate

The official line is that there's no good evidence of a danger of the MMR vaccine causing autism in children. There's some truth to this, in that Dr. Andrew Wakefield's research at the Royal Free Hospital,[69] while important, is the first hint of a problem, but it may be too early to jump to conclusions. Of course, the last thing the medical profession wants is a whole lot of children not being vaccinated, since that increases the risk of epidemics. Wakefield says, "Although MMR cannot by any means be described as a cause of autism, a child genetically predisposed to asthma, eczema, food allergy, or intolerance, perhaps with possible disruption of the gut flora or with a fungal overgrowth, deficient in vitamins, minerals, and essential fatty acids, may be at risk from MMR. For them MMR could be described as the straw that broke the camel's back, tipping the balance of normal childhood development into a retrogressive state."[70]

For most children, the MMR vaccine is unlikely to be a problem, but having said this, no one really knows the full consequences of giving a child three immune attacks—mumps, measles, and rubella—all at the same time. Getting all three illnesses at once simply doesn't occur in nature, so there's a logical argument for single vaccines if a parent so chooses, especially for children with weakened immune systems. Perhaps for these children, with nutrient deficiencies, lacking in essential fatty acids, susceptible to food allergies, infections and/or gut problems, these triple vaccines are the last straw.

So just what is the evidence against MMR? First, studies have shown a high incidence of autism in children whose mothers had received live virus vaccines (particularly the MMR or rubella vaccine) immediately prior to conception during pregnancy or immediately following birth.[71] Second, there are two classifications of autism: the first where autistic traits are noted from birth and the second where symptoms are noted at eighteen months plus. Autism onset at eighteen months was uncommon until the mid-1980s, when the MMR vaccine came into wide use. After that the incidence shot up.[72]

According to Dr. Bernard Rimland, the problem may not be the vaccine itself but a preservative used in multi-dose vials of many childhood vaccines until very recently. Thimerosal, a preservative containing high levels of mercury, was used in many vaccines up until 2001. Before this, each vaccine injection exposed the child to levels of toxic mercury in excess of the United States federal government's own safety guidelines, and a child receiving all his shots could have received a total of 187.5 mcg of mercury—enough to give them heavy metal poisoning.[73] Mercury is known to inhibit the enzyme that digests gluten and casein, possibly increasing a child's susceptibility to wheat and milk allergy.

There's another fact that makes the link between autism and MMR stronger. Many autistic children are found to have measles antibodies in the gut. It's a bit like having a chronic infection. It seems that this triple vaccine makes measles persist. The antidote for measles is vitamin A. This is one of the most important infection fighters for this virus. Although it is too early to conclude, it is entirely possible that late-onset autism may be triggered by multiple vaccinations, allergies, toxic overload, or nutritional deficiencies, and especially combinations of any of these, that send a child's gut and brain into distress.

Tackling Autism Naturally

The optimum nutrition approach to autism involves healing the digestive tract, avoiding sources of casein and gluten plus any other identified allergens, eating healthy foods, and supplementing nutrients that help support digestion, absorption, liver detoxification, the immune system, and the brain.

This approach, although hard work, is much more effective than conventional drugs. One survey of 8,700 parents, asked to rate the effectiveness of drugs and other interventions, reported that Ritalin was the most commonly prescribed. Only 26 percent of the parents reported an improvement, while 46 percent said their child got worse on Ritalin. The most efficient drug in this survey, Nystatin, which is an antifungal drug, still only helped 49 percent of children taking it, according to their parents.[74] Worth considering is secretin. This is a human digestive enzyme, patented as a drug, that seems to trigger improvements in brain function in many autistic children. See www.autism.com/ari for details on this approach.

With this optimum nutrition approach tremendous improvements can result, as the case of Habbo illustrates:

> Habbo was diagnosed as autistic at the age of four. He had serious speech and language problems, was severely behind in social and emotional development, and attended special education for children with developmental delay. He had shown some improvement with the use of special multivitamins, minerals, and DMG (dimethyl glycine) prior to visiting the clinic, attached to the European Laboratory of Nutrients. He was then given comprehensive biochemical testing for deficiencies and imbalances. The clinic found low levels of five vitamins (A, beta-carotene, B_3, B_5 and biotin) and three minerals (magnesium, zinc, and selenium). He also had low levels of omega-3 fats and GLA, an omega-6 fat, and the amino acids taurine and carnitine. His digestion was poor, and he had abnormal gut flora and indications of a yeast infection. Food allergy testing showed clear sensitivity to milk products and some other foods.
>
> He was given a special diet free from milk and casein, a personalized supplement program, and later some Nystatin, which is an antifungal drug. He also started a program of Applied Behavior Analysis, working with a therapist.
>
> He improved steadily and was able to attend his local elementary school from the age of six.
>
> According to the Autism Research Institute's evaluation list, his improvements were:

Speech/language	from 36 to 89 percent
Sociability	from 13 to 68 percent
Sensory/cognitive awareness	from 22 to 97 percent
Health/physical behavior	from 64 to 96 percent

(Where 100 percent means nonautistic behavior)

> At the time of his fifth birthday, Habbo had absolutely no interest in presents or visitors. One year after the evaluation, just before his eighth birthday, he made a list of eight presents he would like to have, including a computer. His parents told him the evening before to wake them at 7:30 A.M. on his birthday, and that's exactly what he did. During the day he couldn't wait for his friends to arrive and celebrate the special day.

(Case kindly supplied by Emar Vogelaar from the European Laboratory of Nutrients in Holland.)

Given the promising research on the many factors discussed in this part of the book so far, the following nutritional strategy, in addition to the recommendations at the end of Chapters 26 and 27, is a very real alternative to drug-based approaches:

- **Eliminate wheat and dairy from the diet completely, replacing with now readily available alternatives, while also checking the possibility of other food sensitivities under the guidance of a nutritional practitioner.**

- **Supplement cod liver oil, vitamin B$_6$, magnesium, zinc, vitamin C, molybdenum, L-glutamine (before bed), and high-strength probiotics (minimum 4 billion microorganisms) daily.**

- **Check for pyroluria and if present, ensure the supplement regimen includes zinc and vitamin B$_6$.**

- **When considering the MMR vaccination, if your child has a weak immune system or you suspect nutrient deficiencies, low essential fatty acids, susceptibility to food allergies, infections, and/or gut problems, consider giving him or her single vaccines if they are available. Alternatively, address all of these issues with a clinical nutritionist prior to your child receiving the triple vaccine.**

As the recommended amounts of the supplements listed above depend on the age of your child, it is certainly best to see a clinical nutritionist who can work out your child's ideal nutritional strategy.

Chapter 29

———

THE WAY UP FROM
DOWN'S SYNDROME

M any of the antenatal tests offered to pregnant women are investigating whether the baby has Down's syndrome. The condition causes so much concern in prospective parents that, in the United States, at least 90 percent of pregnancies with a Down's baby are terminated.

The typical description of the syndrome makes bleak reading. Though many people born with Down's syndrome live for forty to sixty years, that is still at least fifteen years short of the United States average of about seventy-five. About four in ten will have heart problems, and half of them will require surgery. Thyroid problems are also common. They have developmental delays in walking, saying their first words, and so forth, and they have learning disabilities. On top of that they have an increased risk of Alzheimer's disease, starting as early as the age of thirty. They often have difficulties in seeing and hearing. They also have a number of minor problems including dry skin and more coughs and colds.

A person with Down's syndrome is born with forty-seven chromosomes instead of the normal forty-six. Chromosomes carry the genetic information that makes us who we are. In most people, twenty-three of them come from each parent. People with Down's have an extra twenty-first chromosome (or part of it) from either parent. Each chromosome contains the information to make a particular set of proteins. The extra chromosome leads to the overproduction of the proteins coded for on chromosome 21. The syndrome is clearly genetic. But just because a condition has its roots in genetics does not mean the condition cannot be treated by changing the chemical environment in which the genes bathe. In the vast majority of cases, something can be done to prevent, stop, or even reserve a genetic disorder by changing the environment in which the gene operates. This means finding out what is optimum nutrition for the condition: There is a way up from Down's.

Megavitamin Therapy

Treating Down's syndrome through nutrition all began with Dr. Henry Turkel's pioneering work in Michigan in the 1930s, using treatments including large amounts of antioxidants (to protect against damage caused by highly reactive oxidants—see Chapter 8), enzymes, and other nutrients. By the 1960s he was getting remarkable results with severely retarded children, as the case of Wendy testifies.

> Wendy was four years old but her mental age was twenty-one months. She achieved an IQ of forty-four and was classified as retarded. When she began megavitamin therapy, her attention span went from ten seconds to fifteen seconds to ten minutes. Within three months she began speaking in complete sentences. After six months of treatment her IQ score had jumped to seventy-two. By the age of eight her IQ score was eight-five, classifying her as no longer retarded, with low-average ability—a 40-point shift in four years.[75]

Wendy's remarkable transformation, which led to her no longer being classified as educationally subnormal, was verified by an independent psychologist. When researcher Dr. Ruth Harrell heard of Turkel's amazing results, she decided to explore the ideas that many mentally retarded children might have been born with increased needs for certain vitamins and minerals. In her first study she took twenty-two mentally retarded children and divided them into two groups. One received vitamin and mineral supplements, while the other received placebos. After four months, the IQ in the group taking the supplements had increased by between 5 and 9.6 points, while those on placebos showed no change. For the next four months, both groups of children were given the supplements, and the average improvement rose to 10.2 points. Of those children with Down's syndrome taking the supplements, three of the four gained between ten and twenty-five units in IQ and also underwent positive facial and skeletal changes![76]

The results seemed too good to be true. After all, Down's syndrome is a genetic disease, so how could vitamin supplements increase the intelligence of six of the children so dramatically? This sort of improvement in intelligence would put most of our educationally subnormal children back in mainstream education! These findings have since been confirmed by three researchers—and contradicted by three more.[77]

Why the apparent contradiction? Researcher Dr. Alex Schauss believes he may have found the confounding variable: It appears that only those children taking thyroid treatment, commonly needed by those with Down's syndrome, plus the supplements, improved. Neither supplements nor thyroid treatment on their own are expected to help improve intelligence in children with Down's syndrome. Also, you need the right kind of supplements, and this is likely to vary from child to child.

Pinning Down the Right Nutrients

The Trisomy 21 Research Foundation was founded to do just that—research and identify what optimum nutrition was for Down's babies. ("Trisomy 21" is another name for Down's syndrome.) Their approach does not involve large quantities of individual nutrients but rather targets nutrients to deal with the particular biochemical difficulties that people with Down's syndrome have.

A popular misconception is that Down's babies are born with abnormal brains. However, at birth their brain appears to be normal. Within the first four to six months most of the damage that might be done to the brain is done. Nutritional therapy can help prevent the damage. Much is now known about what the effect of the extra chromosome is. One of the biggest problems is that it leads to the overproduction of a key enzyme known as superoxide dimutase (SOD).

SOD is a critical part of a chain of enzyme reactions that protects us from oxidants, so extra SOD may seem an advantage. But it isn't, because it's only part of the oxidant hit squad. Its role is to produce hydrogen peroxide (H_2O_2), a dangerous substance that is usually then disarmed by the next two enzymes in the pathway. However, these two enzymes are not found on chromosome 21. So only part of the hydrogen peroxide produced in Down's people is disarmed. The rest begins to damage the brain and body.

It now appears that the extent of that damage can be reduced by an optimal intake of nutrients that help to disarm the hydrogen peroxide and boost the body's antioxidant defenses. There are a number of nutrients that will assist, including the protective antioxidants of vitamins C and E, lipoic acid, selenium, and bioflavanoids. Essential fats are also important since these are destroyed by oxidation.

Problems with SAMe and Tryptophan

Another problem caused by Down's syndrome is the disruption of a key brain chemical pathway involving the amino acid s-adenosyl methionine (SAMe). This causes a number of biochemical problems including the conversion of folic acid, which is vital to brain and nerve function, into an unusable form. This difficulty can be minimized by providing extra folic acid and vitamins B_6 and B_{12}. One investigation showed that it is possible to correct SAMe-related problems in Down's cells in a test tube by using chemical variants of folic acid and vitamin B_{12}.[78] Many parents have reported improvements after supplementation with methyl donors (DMAE, choline, DMG, and TMG) and methylation catalysts (folic acid, B_6, and B_{12}). SAMe itself has also been used to treat children with attention-deficit disorders, as has MSM, a highly absorbable form of sulphur, an essential mineral that is needed by the body to make SAMe. These are explained in Chapter 7.

Down's people also suffer from the overproduction of collagen, disruptions of their hormones, deficiency in key growth factors, accumulation of toxic ammonia, and deficiency in the amino acid tryptophan (needed for the production of the key neurotransmitter serotonin). These problems are addressed by a large variety of nutrients in the NuTriVene formula recommended by the Trisomy 21 Research Foundation, which contains not only vitamins and minerals but also specific amino acids and some other nutrients.

Dr. Lawrence Leichtman, a geneticist and pediatrician, is founder member of the American College of Medical Genetics and a member of the Scientific Advisory Committee of the Trisomy 21 Research Foundation. To date he has treated over 700 patients at his Genetics and Disabilities Diagnostic Care Center in Virginia Beach, Virginia. In a trial observing Down's children for three years, 113 of whom (aged one month to twelve years) were using the NuTriVene-D formula, and 32 of whom (aged four months to twelve years) were on multivitamins, both groups showed benefit, but those on NuTriVene-D had the best improvements. Their growth rate went up. They had fewer infections, and their white blood cell counts and levels of immunogloblin A, which are an indication of immune strength, improved. There were also clear improvements in speech, coordination, and learning abilities.[79] Madison, daughter of Dixie Lawrence, director of an adoption agency in Louisiana, is a case in point.

> Madison was given the TNI formula [a specific supplement program] and, at around thirty-three months old, was started on Piracetam with choline and vitamin B_5. Five days later she potty-trained herself. On the fifth or sixth day she started saying the odd word and this soon developed into brief sentences. She developed an imagination, unheard of in Down's children of that age. She plays ball with a strong and accurate arm.

To date, the results are promising, but proper double-blind trials testing this formula have yet to be carried out. One such trial, giving nineteen children large amounts of vitamins and minerals over three months, did not find any benefit.[80]

Piracetam and Choline

Piracetam is not part of the NuTriVene-D formula, but many parents give their Down's children both, sometimes together with choline. Piracetam is an intelligence booster and general stimulant (see Chapter 37). Its effects and safety are so impressive that it prompted the creation of a new category of pharmaceuticals called "nootropics," designed to boost intelligence.

There has been considerable media interest, not all positive, in the use of piracetam in Down's children in the United States. One double-blind study giving Down's children piracetam or a placebo, carried out by Nancy Lobaugh and colleagues of Sunnybook and Women's College Health Centre of the University of Toronto, claimed that piracetam therapy did not enhance cognition or behavior but was associated with adverse effects.[81]

The study has, however, been criticized, not for its design but for the interpretation of the results. Dr. Stephen Black of Bishop's University, Quebec, states that a number of positive effects were overlooked. Of seventy-two outcomes measured, including attention, memory perceptual abilities, executive function, and fine motor skills, forty-six produced results that were better in those on piracetam compared with those on the placebo. Eleven out of eighteen parents reported that they had noticed cognitive improvement in children taking piracetam, compared to two out of eighteen parents of children taking the placebo, despite being unaware whether their child had been on piracetam when they made their comment. Teachers also reported that children had significantly "fewer total problems" when taking piracetam. The well-publicized negative effects were apparently spontaneous comments by the parents rather than questionnaire responses. Black suggests that there has been bias in the reporting of the study, and concluded, "A more justifiable conclusion would have been that while dramatic effects were not observed, and there were adverse effects with certain children, small gains in cognition and behavior were also evident." [82]

Getting Help With Optimum Nutrition

There are currently two multinutrient supplements specifically designed for those with Down's syndrome on the market: NuTriVene-D and MSB Plus Version 4. Both products are very similar, differing mainly in dosage size.

They include a daily supplement, a daily enzyme, and a nighttime formula. The daily supplement consists of vitamins, minerals, amino acids, and other essential nutrients. The digestive enzyme compensates for deficiencies in Down's children and their associated malabsorption problems. The night-time formula is designed to provide essential nutrients for increased growth (night time is the main period of growth for a child) and to ease common sleep disorders found in Down's children. It is also possible to have a custom-made version based on blood and urine analysis of the patient.

Any supplement program for the treatment of Down's syndrome must be undertaken with professional guidance, monitoring, and support, and must be followed alongside a healthy diet. Do not compile your own program using over-the-counter vitamin and mineral supplements because certain nutrients can accelerate the degeneration process, and these are often included in general multivitamin and mineral supplements. To find help in the United States, contact the Trisomy 21 Research Foundation (see Useful Addresses, page 362).

In summary, the aim of optimum nutrition is to give a person with Down's syndrome the best possible biochemical support, given his or her genetic uniqueness. This needs to be done with professional guidance. As one mystic says, "Down's syndrome children are those who have given so much, who have served so completely in a pre-vious life, that they come back in this life to be looked after. Who knows if this is true, but like the rest of us, they too deserve optimum nutrition."

Chapter 30

DIET, CRIME, AND DELINQUENCY

Anne was notorious for her antiauthoritarian attitudes and violence. She had lived in care since the age of ten and had a history of assault and burglary, and bouts of severe depression and solvent abuse. Analyses showed abnormal glucose tolerance, zinc, magnesium, and B-vitamin deficiencies. Her energy level was very low in the morning, and she'd often have drops in energy during the day, leaving her depressed and edgy. Within three weeks on a low-sugar diet plus supplements, she had freed herself of drugs, was no longer depressed, had improved energy, and described how she had never felt so relaxed.

Crime and incidences of violent behavior are going up all over the world. Why? Could changes in diet be playing a part? When someone commits a crime what do you do? Punish him or her, remove him or her from society to prevent further crime, or try to understand the causes of deviant behavior in order to socially rehabilitate the offender? In the world of rehabilitation, one factor that is almost completely overlooked is nutrition.

Bernard Gesch came across Anne's case in the course of his work. A former probation officer, he is now director of the United Kingdom-based charity Natural Justice, which investigates the root cause of crime. Gesch believes that the criminal justice system falsely places all the emphasis on social issues, ignoring physical factors such as nutrition. "There are many chemicals around us that are known to affect behavior. Our environment is increasingly polluted. Our food supply has fundamentally changed. In the

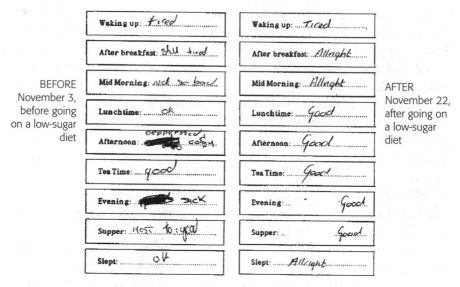

Fig 29 Handwriting and mood: before and after sugar

Reproduced with the kind permission of Natural Justice.

same way that we don't notice aging, how would we notice the effects of gradual changes to our diet and environment?" Yet the effects are there.

The fact is that all thoughts and consequently behavior are processed through the brain and nervous system, which are totally dependent on nutrition. Approximately half of all the glucose in the blood goes to power the brain, which is also dependent on a second-by-second supply of micronutrients—vitamins, minerals, and essential fatty acids. Antinutrients such as lead and cadmium fundamentally affect brain function. "What we're trying to do," says Gesch "is introduce something new into the criminal justice system: that is, the existence of the human brain." His research, and that of others, has identified biochemical factors that influence behavior: exposure to neurotoxins, nutrient deficiencies, paradoxical reactions to given substances, and reactive hypoglycemia.

What's Behind the Crimes?

Sugar Blues

In a remarkable pilot project known as SCASO (South Cumbria Alternative Sentencing Options), young offenders were required, as part of their sentences, to undergo "nutritional rehabilitation." The participants underwent a series of tests for vitamin and mineral levels, toxic minerals, blood sugar balance, as well as dietary assessment. "The most common problems were glucose intolerance and zinc deficiency. Every single person we tested had abnormal glucose tolerance on a five-hour glucose tolerance test," says Gesch.[83] The importance of glucose control in relation to behavior is a consistent finding in the criminal population. In Finland Dr. Matti Virkkunen investigated sixty-nine habitual offenders for glucose balance. Every single one had reactive hypoglycemia. A later study confirmed higher insulin activity during glucose tolerance tests among habitually violent offenders.[84]

In the United States, Professor Stephen Schoenthaler, head of the Department of Sociology and Criminal Justice at California State University, has reported a 21 percent reduction in antisocial behavior, a 25 percent reduction in assaults, a 75 percent reduction in the use of restraints, and a 100 percent reduction in suicides when 3,000 inmates were placed on an experimental diet that reduced refined and sugary foods.[85] These results were confirmed in a double-blind study involving 1,382 detained juvenile offenders placed on a reduced sugar diet. There was a 44 percent reduction in antisocial behavior with most significant reductions among the serious offenders.[86]

A rebound low, otherwise known as reactive hypoglycemia, occurring after a rapid increase in blood sugar levels from consuming sugar, sweets, or stimulants, is associated with extreme tiredness, depression, aggression, and attempted suicide. In other words, if you feel bad, you're much more likely to behave badly. According to Gesch, "Of the forty to fifty people we worked with on SCASO we could create an effect within a week or two." His team taught the young offenders how to prepare simple and nutritious meals and develop an interest in food.

Heavy Metals

One of the most insidious effects on behavior is that of unseen pollution. A worldwide consensus of research has shown that high lead levels correspond to low intellectual performance and antisocial behavior. The correlation between high lead and increased antisocial or delinquent behavior was found in an observational study of 1,000 children by R. Freeman and coworkers in New South Wales,[87] by Herbert Needleman and coworkers in the United States who found antisocial behavior correlated to high dentine lead levels in 2,146 children,[88] and by G. Thomson and coworkers, Department of Education, University of Edinburgh, who found deviant behavior correlated with high blood lead levels.[89] Professor Richard Pihl from the Department of Psychology, McGill University, Montreal, Quebec, Canada, found a correlation between high hair lead and cadmium in violent inmates compared to nonviolent inmates.[90] Other researchers have confirmed an association between high lead and cadmium and deviant behavior.

The levels of neurotoxins like lead, cadmium, copper, and mercury needed to produce an effect on behavior is around 1 percent of the level needed to produce physical symptoms. This indicates how sensitive that part of the brain involved with socialization is to environmental and nutritional changes.

Nutritional Deficiencies

Zinc is an antagonist of heavy metals, and supplementing it has had favorable effects on behavior. Dr. Alex Schauss found significantly higher levels of lead, cadmium, and copper in violent, antisocial adults compared to nonoffenders.[91] The effect of zinc on brain function is consistent with previous studies that have linked zinc deficiency to hyperactivity and learning and eating disorders.

Needless to say, nutritional deficiency is rife among young offenders. Professor Stephen Schoenthaler found evidence of widespread folic acid, thiamine (vitamin B_1), and vitamin C deficiencies. Even adding orange juice to the diets of detainees, which contains each of these nutrients, produced a staggering 47 percent reduction in antisocial behavior among juvenile offenders.[92]

Deficiencies in calcium, magnesium, zinc, selenium, and essential fatty acids have also been shown to correlate with increases in violence. The simple addition of a multivitamin and mineral supplement containing RDA levels of nutrients has been shown to have extremely positive effects on behavior in prison populations in the United States, according to extensive research by Professor Schoenthaler. In a recent study he compared the behavior of young offenders in the three months prior to and during supplementation, versus those given a placebo, and showed an overall reduction in recorded offenses of 40 percent, with the subjects on supplements producing 22 percent fewer assaults on staff, and a 21 percent reduction in violent and nonviolent antisocial behavior when compared with the subjects on placebo. Blood tests for vitamins and minerals showed that around one-third of the juveniles had low levels of one or more vitamins and minerals before the trial. Those whose levels had become normal by the end of the study demonstrated a massive improvement in behavior of between 70 and 90 percent.[93]

Recently, deficiencies in essential fats have started to be considered as a real contributor to deviant behavior. Changes in modern diets have certainly reduced our intake of these essential fats and, if deficient during pregnancy, could have long-lasting effects on mental development and behavior (see Chapter 4). Recent research from Dr. Tomohito Hamazaki of Toyama University in Japan suggests that omega-3 fats help control anger and hostility. He reasoned that, under conditions of stress, from an evolutionary point of view, a certain level of aggression could have survival value, but too much aggression would have the opposite effect.

So, he decided to see what would happen to students, under the stress of exams, if given omega-3 fats, specifically 1.5 grams of DHA, or a placebo. He measured hostility at the start of the study and again, three months later, just before the exams. He measured hostility by showing the participants potentially emotionally charged cartoons with speech bubbles for the characters. The students then filled in the bubbles. The second measure, just before the exams, showed a big increase, a 59 percent jump in hostile reactions in those taking the placebo but no change at all in the students taking the omega-3 fats![94] Omega-3 fats, it seems, help you to keep your head when all around you are losing theirs.

Antisocial Foods

The fourth factor proving to be significant is that of paradoxical reactions to foods. Menzies found that, in a study of twenty-five children with tension fatigue syndrome, all had disturbed sleep, 84 percent had abnormal EEG (brain wave patterns), and 72 percent had digestive problems. All consumed a diet unusually high in refined foods and chemical additives.[95]

Severe allergic reactions can produce Jekyll-and-Hyde changes in behavior as has been well reported in hyperactive children with chemical or food intolerances[96] and juvenile offenders.[97] The same can be true for adults, as illustrated by this extraordinary case report by Dr. Alex Schauss.

> A president of a large American Company, with no previous history of arrest, goes for a drink at his local bar. For some reason he decides to have a glass of red wine, a drink he's never had before. Ten minutes later he pulls out a revolver and guns down a man walking past him. He shoots anyone trying to help this man and ends up injuring twenty-two people. Miraculously, none are killed, but many have serious wounds to their thighs, arms, and torsos. A few hours later, in the local police station, he asks for a psychiatrist. When the psychiatrist arrives, the man asks, "Why am I here?"
>
> Fortunately this man was able to afford the best psychiatrist, neurologists, and doctors. But none could find out what triggered this atrocious action. He could not even remember committing the crime, and was deeply horrified at having done so. Tests eventually showed he had a very imbalanced immune system and the common allergic symptoms of rhinitis and headaches.

The businessman was then tested for two months (by injection, sub-lingual drops, and ingestion) for sensitivity to various substances, including red wine—the likely offender. But, without anyone else's knowledge, he was simply being given placebos—non-reactive "dummy" substances. Then, again without anyone else's knowledge, he was given exactly the same wine he had drunk that fateful evening. Within ten minutes he became increasingly violent and aggressive, grabbing the nurse present and tearing things apart in the laboratory. He was literally going through a Jekyll-and-Hyde-like metamorphosis: The psychiatrists present classified him as acutely paranoid schizophrenic.

Twelve years before this incident, the man had moved to a very expensive block of apartments in which a type of natural gas was used for heating and cooking. In the following years, most people left their apartments because of the health-damaging effects of the gas, even though they had no chance of getting their money back. Birds had been known to die because of exposure to the gas. This man had spent seven years in the apartment. It is likely the gas considerably weakened his immune system, contributing to his aggressive reaction, which was probably to an "amine" in the wine.

Of the few studies so far conducted, all show dramatic reductions in re-offending rates among offenders maintained on low-sugar, high-nutrient diets. Although much harder to identify (and eliminate), it is certainly possible that the introduction of 3,500 new chemicals into the food supply could be contributing to deviant behavior. Suspect foods include wheat and milk, overconsumption of which has been reported in delinquent behavior.

According to Gesch, whose SCASO project encouraged whole foods and no refined sugar, "Seventy-five percent of our referrals were for violent offenses, many of whom were multiple offenders. Of those kept on the combined social and nutritional regimen, none reoffended with a violent offense by the end of the eighteen-month pilot study."[98] The nutritional supplements used in the treament only cost between $7 and $17 a month, compared to the average cost of over $3,000 a month to keep someone in prison.

Crime: Nourishment or Punishment?

Of course, many offenders are suffering from undiagnosed or untreated mental illness such as manic depression or schizophrenia. Any of the most common biochemical imbalances (see Chapter 20), including pyroluria, neurotransmitter imbalances, and hormonal imbalances, can lead to aggressive and delinquent behavior.

One of the most promising treatments is the role of tryptophan in correcting serotonin deficiency, which leads to depression and, in some, aggressive and violent behavior.[99] Antidepressant drugs that block the reuptake of serotonin can also lead to aggressive behavior in some people (see Chapter 21), which shows the importance of this neurotransmitter in relation to antisocial behavior. So many of these biochemical imbalances could be nutritionally treated, if only they were checked for.

However, the focus within the criminal justice system is culpability, not testing for and correcting biochemical imbalances. If behavior is thought of purely as a psychological/social phenomenon, then the blame rests on the individual and his or her relationship with society. Hence the current strategy of punishment: removal from society and social rehabilitation. If brain function, and all the factors that affect brain function, are put into the equation, then issues around nutrition and environmental pollution have to be considered.

This will necessitate the establishment of diagnostic centers at each prison and hospital. Education is so often the key, and the establishment of prison nutrition clubs to promote awareness of good nutrition among patients, prisoners, and security personnel, backed up by the availability of food charts and literature, would do much to improve the awareness that's currently so sadly lacking. Perhaps even more pressing is the need for a research institute dealing with psychopathic, violent, or antisocial behavior.

After years of fund-raising and campaigning, Natural Justice persuaded the Home Office to allow the first United Kingdom double-blind trial on young offenders in a maximum security prison in Aylesbury, England, giving them either a multi-nutrient containing vitamins, minerals, and essential fatty acids, or a placebo. The results, published in the *British Journal of Psychiatry*, showed a staggering 35 percent decrease in acts of aggression after only two weeks.[100] Since prison diets are, if anything, better than those most young offenders eat, this shows just how important optimum nutrition is for reducing violent and deviant behavior. When the trial was over and the supplements were stopped, there was a 40 percent increase in offenses in the prison.

Chapter 31

BEATING ADDICTIONS

Chris, a heroin addict, was taken off heroin and given prescriptions for methadone, temazepam, diazepam, and Valium, to which he became addicted. He then tried a nutrition-based detox program, which includes a "purification phase" involving large amounts of niacin and other nutrients, plus daily saunas. "It's the easiest detox I've ever done. Having gone through the purification I understand why, after previous detoxes, I was still craving. In the beginning of the sauna program I would get flashbacks, but after two weeks I was feeling full of energy, and happy, which has stayed with me since I finished. I'm keeping on the vitamins. I've closed that chapter of my life without a doubt."

In the words of one of the first pioneers of the optimum nutrition approach, Dr. Roger Williams, "No one who follows good nutrition practice will ever become alcoholic." Addiction, whether it be to alcohol, tranquilizers, cigarettes, or heroin, is less likely to occur in those who are well nourished, for a number of reasons. First, the use of stimulants, like caffeine, nicotine, or cocaine, is more attractive if you are constantly tired. Secondly, the use of relaxants such as alcohol or tranquilizers is more attractive if you suffer from anxiety. The more your brain chemistry is out of balance, the more out of balance it will become if you expose yourself to potentially addictive substances.

Of course, addiction is not only chemical. Psychological factors, as well as the drug abuse itself, are usually present in those who become addicted.

Obviously, such psychological factors that predispose a person to addiction will need to be dealt with alongside nutritional intervention. However, whatever the cause, once a person is addicted, this has chemical and physiological effects. You can't just remove the addictive substance without inducing withdrawal symptoms, sometimes severe enough to cause death.

One in Four People Are Addicted

Addiction affects every one of us. The use of addictive substances, from caffeine in tea and coffee, to alcohol and cigarettes, is part of everyday life for most. Take a look at the table below to get an idea of how many people currently suffer from addictions.

Number of people dependent/addicted (percent of United States population)		
Nicotine	55 million	(20 percent)
Caffeine	87 million	(30 percent)
Alcohol	18 million	(6 percent)
Prescription drugs	9 million	(3 percent)
Heroin	0.5 million	(0.2 percent)
Cocaine	3.6 million	(1.2 percent)

Sources: National Institute on Drug Abuse, National Institute of Alcohol Abuse and Alcoholism (NIAAA)

Some of these substances are legal, some illegal. Some are prescribed by your doctor and some are self-prescribed. But all are addictive and harm mind and body to varying degrees.

The classic symptoms of addiction include depression or feelings of doom, nervousness and anxiety, craving for sweets or alcohol, irritability or rages, headaches, weight problems (either way), extreme tiredness or weakness, dizziness or feeling faint, morning nausea, blurred vision, transient muscle aches or joint pain, and insomnia and nightmares. If you have quite a number of these symptoms, it may be time to do something about your addictions.

Why Addiction?

Is it in the Genes?

There is supporting evidence for a genetic factor in some people, predisposing them to addictions. Since the 1990s, evidence has been growing for a genetic link to alcoholism and possibly other addictions. The gene in question, the D2 dopamine receptor gene, encourages the building of receptor sites for the pleasure-giving neurotransmitter dopamine. Some people have a variation of this gene that means less dopamine receptors, hence less pleasure.[101] These individuals are therefore more prone to lower moods and motivation. As a natural consequence, they then seek activities and substances that promote dopamine activity in the brain. Dr. Kenneth Blum, one of the pioneers in this research, calls this "reward deficiency syndrome" (see Chapter 27, page 236).

Such people are especially prone to overuse of stimulants (caffeine, nicotine, and cocaine), as well as alcohol. They are also more likely to seek stimulating activities, from daring sports to gambling.

Many addictive types are also histadelic—genetically pre-programmed to overproduce high levels of histamine. This makes a person more prone to compulsive and obsessive behavior. Once nutrient-depleted, the high-histamine type often becomes seriously, sometimes suicidally depressed. Alcohol abuse can become a way of slowly killing yourself.

Both of these genetic factors run through families, so a history of addiction, depression, suicide, and mental illness of a compulsive/obsessive nature is a good clue, although, of course, behaviors can be inherited in addition to genes.

Empty Calories Lead to Addiction

Genes are only one side of the equation. They don't determine behavior, just predispose it. By providing optimum nutrition for a person with reward deficiency syndrome or histadelia, his or her mood, energy, and general well-being can be so substantially improved that compensations using addictive substances no longer become necessary.

One study with mice shows how poor nutrition also predisposes addiction. The mice in this study were split into two groups: One was given a healthy diet, the other a junk food diet. Both had free access to water or alcohol. The junk food mice soon became alcoholic and died prematurely. The health food mice stayed teetotal and lived to a ripe old age.[102]

As the alcoholic mice became more and more nutrient deficient, they became less interested in food and more interested in alcohol. Alcohol not only stops you from absorbing, it also affects appetite. So bad nutrition not only leads to alcoholism, but alcoholism leads to bad nutrition. It's a vicious downhill spiral. The same link between junk food and addiction has also been recorded in humans.[103]

How Addiction Happens

Before looking at specific types of addiction, and how to break the habit, let's understand more about the chemical nature of addiction itself. Most addictive substances either promote more of a particular neurotransmitter, such as dopamine, or mimic a desirable brain chemical by docking onto its receptor sites.

Caffeine, for example, blocks the breakdown of dopamine and adrenaline, hence elevating circulating levels of these motivating neurotransmitters. Cocaine also blocks the breakdown, giving a more intense dopamine high. Heroin, on the other hand, looks like the brain's own opioids, instantly killing pain and inducing a euphoric state.

The Sugar Link

Most alcoholics and drug addicts have dysglycemia. One way of raising your blood sugar level is to smoke a cigarette, have coffee, eat chocolate, drink alcohol, or take a drug, from cannabis to cocaine. A group of researchers in 1973 decided to test how many of 200 alcoholics had abnormal blood sugar balance with a glucose tolerance test. No less than 97 percent came up positive.[104] The same is true for most other addicts.

Many people have learned to control their blood sugar levels by eating, drinking, and smoking substances that alter their body chemistry. There's also a synergy of these pharmacological agents in food and drink. High coffee consumption can precipitate alcoholism, because the shakiness from coffee can be controlled by alcohol. In animal studies, giving animals caffeine increases consumption of alcohol, confirming a complex interaction between these addictive psychoactive substances.[105]

Allergy or Addiction?

Addictions have a lot in common with "hidden" allergies. Often the allergic substance becomes addictive, and if it isn't consumed, withdrawal symptoms set in which can be relieved by consuming the allergen. This is why people often feel worse on a short fast, until the withdrawal phase is over, and then feel much better.

Addicts also test allergic to their addictive substance. Many people who regularly consume alcohol become allergic to it, or to something in it. For example, many beer drinkers become allergic to brewer's yeast. Drs. William Philpott and Dwight Kalita found that 75 percent of tobacco smokers tested allergic to tobacco on skin tests.[106] I tested this when working in a medical allergy treatment center and failed to find a single smoker who wasn't allergic to tobacco on intradermal testing. This is why, with regular consumption, people often find they don't feel so good after alcohol, cigarettes, cannabis, or whatever has become their drug of choice. Most allergies require a five- to ten-day avoidance before a person becomes symptom-free. A similar length of time is often required for addictions.

Alcohol: The Greatest Antinutrient of Them All

There are costs and benefits attributable to the drinks and leisure industries. On the one hand this sector of business employs over a million people and, in 1996, generated in excess of $17 billion in revenue for the government. On the other hand it has been estimated that 60 percent of parasuicides, 30 percent of divorces, 40 percent of domestic violence, and 20 percent of child abuse cases are associated with alcohol misuse.[107]

Pronounced nutritional deficiency states are well recorded in many drug addictions, but none so obviously as in addiction to alcohol. Alcohol is the greatest antinutrient of all. It is well proven to deplete almost every vitamin (vitamins A, B_1, B_2, B_6, folic acid, B_{12}, C, D, and E), mineral (calcium, magnesium, potassium, zinc, and selenium), amino acid (tryptophan, taurine, glutathione, and so on), essential fat (omega-3 and 6), as well as disturbing blood sugar control.[108] Just reading the mountains of research on how alcohol destroys nutrients in the body is sobering!

Many of the symptoms and problems of alcohol abuse arise directly from these nutritional deficiencies. For example, tryptophan depletion leads to depression, while B-vitamin deficiencies make you anxious, unable to concentrate, and even crazy. B_6 deficiency may account for some of the perceptual distortions that occur in both alcohol intoxication and withdrawal.

Even without alcohol these deficiencies can bring on mental illness, as illustrated by the story of one sixty-one-year-old woman from New Zealand, diagnosed with schizophrenia.[109] She refused medication for four months, had the delusion she was dying from cancer, and neglected her nutrition. She was admitted to hospital and went into a coma. She was given thiamine, vitamin B_1, and responded in three hours.

As well as inducing deficiencies, alcohol reduces appetite and impairs absorption. When there is organic damage such as pancreatitis, cirrhosis, or hepatitis, appetite is further impaired, creating even more deficiencies. So, the first step in treating addiction is to prepare the person for withdrawal by correcting these deficiencies. Giving all essential nutrients in optimal amounts dramatically reduces craving for alcohol. In animal studies, rats given vitamin B_1 cut their drinking by a staggering 80 percent.[110] Those given the amino acid glutamine cut their drinking by 34 percent.[111] The amino acid taurine, at 3 g a day, reduces withdrawal symptoms.[112] There are also many nutrients that protect the liver from damage from alcohol. These include taurine, choline, glutamine, glutathione, and many others.

How to Quit

Coming off Booze without Side Effects

It is no surprise to find that a number of researchers report that megadoses of a cocktail of nutrients, given orally as supplements or intravenously, can virtually eliminate symptoms of withdrawal. Even the basics—that's a whole food diet plus a multivitamin—kept 81 percent of alcoholics off booze six months after withdrawal, compared to 38 percent left to their own devices.[113]

Large amounts of specific nutrients can help. In 1974 Dr. Russel Smith in the United States gave 507 hardcore alcoholics 3–5 g of niacin/vitamin C a day for a year.[114] At the end of the year 71 percent were sober. Drs. Hoffer and Osmond have reported on the combined use of niacin, B_6, and vitamin C.[115] They reported a 75 percent success rate after a year, compared to 30 percent success from counseling alone.

However, the best results are achieved by providing high amounts of all the key nutrients, especially B vitamins, vitamin C, glutamine, taurine, tryptophan, and essential fats. The extraordinary and sad fact is that most alcohol recovery units don't do this, so people both have to go through the agony of withdrawal without optimal nutrition support, and have a much greater chance of going back on the booze. For an up-to-date list of addiction treatment centres I recommend the website www.mentalhealthproject.com.

Heroin Withdrawal Made Easier

Drs. Alfred Libby and Irwin Stone pioneered a detoxifying treatment for drug addicts using megadoses of vitamin C.[116] In one study involving thirty heroin addicts, they gave 30–85 g a day and achieved a 100 percent success rate. Others have reported similar positive results using vitamin C combined with niacin.

Both heroin addiction and alcoholism increases acid levels in the body, causing a depletion of calcium and potassium. In 1973 Dr. Blackman decided to test what would happen if he neutralized this acidity. He gave nineteen heroin addicts sodium bicarbonate, potassium bicarbonate, and calcium carbonate every half hour for two hours, followed by a two-hour break, repeating the cycle until withdrawal was over. All volunteers said the withdrawal symptoms were either completely eliminated or considerably reduced. Sixteen out of nineteen reported no severe withdrawal symptoms. Of the others, symptoms lasted for no more than four hours.

Once again, giving heroin addicts high levels of a cocktail of vitamins, minerals, amino acids, and essential fats can dramatically reduce symptoms of withdrawal and increase chances of staying clean.

Quitting Cigarettes

One of the most common and socially acceptable addictions is to nicotine in tobacco. The same principles apply here as with other addictions. An alkaline diet, with plenty of fruit and vegetables, or the use of alkaline salts certainly helps reduce craving, as do megadoses of vitamin C and niacin, among other nutrients. Most smokers are hypoglycemic, so a diet with slow-releasing carbohydrates, no sugar, tea, and coffee is essential. Extra chromium, B_6 and zinc also help to stabilize blood sugar. These nutritional factors, plus counseling to deal with the psychological and behavioral factors, plus gradual reduction of nicotine intake, are highly effective for those who wish to quit. Exactly how to do all this is explained in my book *How to Beat Stress and Fatigue* and on the website www.mentalhealthproject.com under "How to Quit Smoking."

Kicking Addiction to Prescription Drugs

The sad truth is that many prescription drugs used to treat mental health problems are addictive. The most commonly prescribed antidepressant drugs, originally marketed as completely safe "happy" pills, were originally touted to benefit even those who didn't think they were depressed. Yet recently the United States authorities found that when people try to come off these drugs, even with a gradual reduction, at least 2 in every 100 people suffered abnormal dreams or pains resembling electric shocks, and 7 in every 100 experienced dizziness. They are now insisting that these drugs carry a new warning requiring doctors to monitor patients for any side effects that may indicate a physical dependency.

Most concerning of all is tranquilizer addiction. There are an estimated 1.5 million people addicted to tranquilizers in Britain. Coming off them is not only difficult, but without the right support it can be very dangerous, even fatal in some instances. The longer people are on these dangerous drugs, the more forgetful, drowsy, and withdrawn they become. If they try to stop, they become anxious and can't sleep. They may experience tremors, tremendous irritability, headaches, even seizures. That's why it's vital to come off tranquilizers gradually, with support, and with the support of natural relaxants such as kava and valerian. The names of good organizations and information on how to do this are found on the website www.mentalhealthproject.com under "Coming Off Tranquillisers."

Are You a Stimulant Addict?

The most widespread addiction of all is to stimulants—tea, coffee, caffeinated drinks, sugar, chocolate, and cigarettes. To be in tip-top mental health, you need to address this issue too. The odd cup of tea or coffee is no big deal, but if you "need" these substances every day, or every hour, you are in trouble! Any trip through a mental health ward will show you that most people with mental health problems are stimulant addicts. Whether legal or illegal drugs, the see-saw between tranquilizers or alcohol and stimulants keeps your brain out of balance. Chapter 9 explains how to quit stimulants and what to eat and drink instead.

Why Withdrawal and Detoxification Are Different

Optimum nutrition during the first week of drug withdrawal can make all the difference, as the studies above have shown. Very large amounts of vitamin C, B vitamins, glutamine, and other amino acids should be given four times a day, under supervision. Calcium and magnesium are especially important because they can virtually eliminate the terrible cramping and nerve pain associated with opiate withdrawal. During this time 24-hour counseling support is essential.

One consistent and yet widely ignored finding is that withdrawal from a drug doesn't mean the person is decontaminated. Most drugs take months to completely leave the system, as residues are stored in body cells. Hence, high-level nutritional support in the months following withdrawal is vital for long-term success, until the addict is truly "clean."

One particularly effective method of speeding up drug detoxification is the combined use of niacin, saunas, and water. Niacin helps eliminate toxins from cells. It is best taken thirty minutes before entering a sauna, on an empty stomach. The sauna needs to be set at 80°F. The participant then stays in the sauna for an hour, coming out if need be, while keeping very hydrated by drinking water. Some people experience some level of "flashbacks", so such an approach needs to be done under supervision. This needs to be done every day until the person feels significantly better, which can take from five to twenty-five days depending on the former level of intoxication.

So some highly successful strategies for dealing with addiction have been tested and proven to work. Sadly, very few addiction treatment centers apply these strategies and consequently have poor success rates. Many ignore biochemical aspects of addiction and simply involve withdrawal and counseling. A radical rethink on the treatment of addiction is badly needed.

In summary, if you are dealing with addiction:

- Get professional help and guidance.

- Deal with psychological issues with a psychotherapist.

- Increase your intake of nutrients, including a high-strength B complex plus niacin 500 mg, pantothenic acid (B$_5$) 500 mg, vitamin B$_6$ 100 mg, folic acid 1 mg, vitamin C 3–10 g a day spread throughout the day.

- Take L-glutamine powder, 5 g A.M. and P.M., plus enough essential fats including GLA , EPA, and DHA, and minerals including calcium, magnesium, potassium, and zinc.

- Eat an extremely healthy diet that supports your brain (see Part 1).

- Come off slowly, replacing your addictive drug with natural relaxants/stimulants as appropriate.

Chapter 32

OVERCOMING EATING DISORDERS

One of the greatest shortcomings of human logic is the unquestioned belief that psychological problems, whether involving behavior or intelligence, are influenced only by psychological factors, and that physical problems are influenced only by physical factors. This presupposes that mind and body are separate, that the energy of mind and of body are two different things. Ask a chemist, an anatomist, and a psychologist to define where the mind starts and the body ends and they will find that the two are intimately interconnected. The same is especially true of anorexia nervosa and bulimia because they are behavioral disorders involving eating, a physiological event.

Anorexia was first identified by Dr. William Gull in 1874. This is his treatment: "The patient should be fed at regular intervals and surrounded by persons who could have moral control over them, relations and friends being generally the worst attendants." Today, treatment is often essentially the same, summed up as "drug them, feed them, and let them get on with their lives" in an article in the *Guardian* describing treatment in "leading hospitals." The "modern" approach includes "behavior therapy," that is, rewards and privileges, and drugs to induce compliance. The drugs include psychotropic drugs such as chlorpromazine, sedatives, and antidepressants. The diet is high carbohydrate, sometimes as much as 5,000 kcals, with little regard to quality.

Bulimia is binge eating followed by self-induced vomiting and is probably a more common condition nowadays. Some anorexics are bulimic. Some bulimics are not anorexic. It is still a food/weight, compulsive/obsessive disorder, and is classified as follows:

- Recurrent episodes of binge eating (rapid consumption of large amounts of food in a discrete period of time).

- A feeling of lack of control over eating behavior during the binges.

- The person regularly engages in self-induced vomiting, use of laxatives, diuretics, strict dieting, fasting, or exercise in order to prevent weight gain.

- A minimum average of two binge eating sessions a week.

- Persistent over-concern with body shape and weight.

The Zinc Link

The idea that nutrition, or malnutrition, could play a part in the development and treatment of this condition did not really emerge until the 1980s, when scientists began to realize just how similar the symptoms and risk factors of anorexia and zinc deficiency were (see table below). As early as 1973 two zinc researchers, K. Hambidge and A. Silverman, concluded that "whenever there is appetite loss in children, zinc deficiency should be suspected."[117] In 1979, Rita Bakan, a Canadian health researcher, noticed that the symptoms of anorexia and zinc deficiency were similar in a number of

Anorexia	Zinc
Symptoms	
Weight loss	Weight loss
Loss of appetite	Loss of appetite
Amenorrhea	Amenorrhea
Impotence in males	Impotence in males
Nausea	Nausea
Skin lesions	Skin lesions
Malabsorption	Malabsorption
Disperceptions	Disperceptions
Depression	Depression
Anxiety	Anxiety
Risk factors	
Female under 25	Female under 25
Stress	Stress
Puberty	Puberty

respects and proposed that clinical trials be undertaken to test its effectiveness in treatment.[118] Meanwhile, David Horrobin, most renowned for his research into evening primrose oil, proposed that "anorexia nervosa is due to a combined deficiency of zinc and EFAs."[119] More recently, strong evidence has come to light that those with anorexia and bulimia may be more prone to tryptophan deficiency. Tryptophan is the building block for serotonin, the brain's "happy" neurotransmitter, that also helps control appetite.

Zinc Hypothesis Confirmed

In 1980, when the zinc link had been reported, the first trial started at the University of Kentucky. The researchers discovered that ten out of thirteen patients admitted with anorexia and eight out of fourteen patients with bulimia were zinc deficient on admission. After vigorous feeding they became even more zinc deficient. Since zinc is required to digest and utilize protein, from which body tissue is made, they recommended that extra zinc, above that required to correct deficiency, should be given as the anorexic starts to eat and gain weight.[120]

In 1984 the penny dropped with two important research findings and the first case of an anorexic treated with zinc. The first study, since confirmed, showed that animals deprived of zinc very rapidly developed anorexic behavior and loss of appetite, and that if these animals were force-fed a zinc-deficient diet to gain weight, they became seriously ill.[121] The second study showed that zinc deficiency damages the intestinal wall and therefore the absorption of nutrients including zinc, potentially leading to a vicious spiral of deficiency.[122]

Then, in 1984, Professor Derek Bryce-Smith, now patron of the Institute for Optimum Nutrition, reported the first case of anorexia treated with zinc. The patient was a thirteen-year-old girl, tearful and depressed, weighing 37 kg (81.4 lbs). She was referred to a consultant psychiatrist, but, despite counselling, three months later her weight was 31.5 kg (69.3 lbs). Within two months of zinc supplementation at a level of 45 mg per day, her weight returned to 44.5 kg (97.9 lbs), she was cheerful again, and tests for zinc deficiency were normal.[123]

Meanwhile, the first double-blind trial with fifteen anorexics was being carried out at the University of California. In 1987 the researchers reported, "Zinc supplementation was followed by a decrease in depression and anxiety. Our data suggest that individuals with anorexia nervosa may be at risk for zinc deficiency and may respond favorably after zinc supplementation."[124] By 1990, many researchers had found that over half of anorexic patients showed clear biochemical evidence of zinc deficiency.[125] In 1994 Dr. Carl

Birmingham and colleagues carried out a double-blind, controlled trial giving 100 mg of zinc gluconate or a placebo to thirty-five women with anorexia. They concluded that "the rate of increase in body mass of the zinc supplemented group was twice that of the placebo group, and this difference was statistically significan."[126] Sadly, many treatment centers still fail to supplement those suffering from anorexia with zinc.

Zinc: The Chicken or the Egg?

The evidence linking zinc and anorexia is now beyond question. In fact, a recent review of all the research concludes, "There is evidence that suggests zinc deficiency may be intimately involved with anorexia in humans: if not as an initiating cause, then as an accelerating or exacerbating factor that may deepen the pathology of anorexia."[127] The fact that high levels of zinc supplementation help to treat anorexia does not mean the cause of anorexia is zinc deficiency. Psychological issues may, and probably do, bring about change in the eating habits of susceptible people.

By avoiding eating, a young girl can repress the signs of growing up. Menstruation stops, breast size decreases, and the body stays small. Starvation induces a kind of "high" by stimulating changes in important brain chemicals, which may help to block out difficult feelings and issues that are too hard to face. Many anorexics also choose to become vegetarian, and most vegetarian diets are lower in zinc, essential fats, and protein, according to a study at the Health Sciences Department of the British Columbia Institute of Technology in Burnaby, Canada, which analyzed the diets of vegetarian anorexics, versus nonvegetarian patients.[128]

Whether vegetarian or not, once the route of not eating is chosen and becomes established, zinc deficiency is almost inevitable, both due to poor intake and poor absorption. With it comes a further loss of appetite and even more depression, disperceptions, and the inability to cope with the stresses that face many adolescents, especially girls, growing up in the twenty-first century.

The optimum nutrition approach to help someone with anorexia or bulimia is best carried alongside work with a skilled psychotherapist. The nutritional approach emphasizes quality of food rather than quantity, including supplements to ensure vitamin and mineral sufficiency, and of course 45mg of elemental zinc per day, halving this level once weight gain is achieved and maintained.

Low Tryptophan: The Appetite Controller

Loss of weight and loss of muscle tissue is an indication of protein deficiency.

This can be the result of either insufficient intake, or inadequate digestion, absorption, or metabolism. The amino acids valine, isoleucine, and tryptophan have been found to be low in people with anorexia. Supplementing valine and isoleucine helps to build muscle, while tryptophan is the building block of serotonin, a neurotransmitter that controls both mood and appetite.

Recent research has found striking differences in blood levels of tryptophan in anorexic patients.[129] Also, both starvation and excessive exercise have been shown to influence the availability of tryptophan in the blood of anorexic patients.[130] To date, the evidence is pointing toward a problem with how people with eating disorders respond to low tryptophan. In fact, the conversion of tryptophan into serotonin is both zinc and B_6 dependent. These three nutrients may all be needed for proper appetite control, as well as a balanced, happy mood.

The interplay between body and mind, or nutrients and behavior, is well illustrated by recent research at Oxford University's psychiatry department by Dr. Philip Cowen and colleagues which found, not surprisingly, that women on calorie-restricted diets develop lower levels of tryptophan and serotonin. However, recovered bulimics, when put on a diet free of tryptophan, rapidly become more depressed and overly concerned about their weight and shape, as well as more fearful of their loss of control over their eating.[131] In a similar trial that deprived both women with bulimia and healthy "controls" of tryptophan for one day, the bulimic women became more depressed and had a much greater desire to binge than the controls.[132]

All this research strongly suggests that those prone to anorexia or bulimia have a special need for tryptophan, and probably zinc and B_6, and that when deprived of these nutrients they are more likely to develop unhealthy reactions, including loss of appetite control.

While supplementing tryptophan, or 5-hydroxytryptophan (5-HTP), plus zinc and B_6, is the most direct way to address these imbalances in people with eating disorders, in the long run the goal must be to change the diet. Often, especially in those with anorexia, supplements, including concentrated fish oils, are more acceptable at first because unlike food they contain virtually no calories. However, as a person's nutrition improves, so his or her anxieties and compulsiveness become better and he or she can see the logic for making dietary changes.

The ideal diet should include easily assimilable foods containing good-quality protein such as quinoa, fish, soy, and spirulina or blue-green algae. Other good foods are ground seeds, lentils, beans, fruits, and vegetables.

Fish and seeds are especially important because they contain essential fats. Since most people with eating disorders go out of their way to avoid fat, their diets are frequently low in these essential nutrients. Also, essential fats are vital for the body to both make serotonin and to receive the serotonin signals that cross between one neuron and another.

The optimum nutrition approach, therefore, involves ensuring all these nutrients are provided in optimal amounts.

What's Your Binge Food?

In the case of bulimia, what a person binges on is very revealing, either of food sensitivities or blood sugar problems. The most common binge foods are sweet foods, wheat foods, or dairy foods. Both wheat and dairy products contain exorphins, chemicals that mimic (and can therefore block) pleasure-giving endorphins in the brain, and again, may influence behavior. Sweetened foods, of course, satisfy a low blood sugar condition, and the cure is to eat foods that keep your blood sugar level even. I have often asked people with bulimia to binge as much as they like for the next two weeks, but not on these foods. Often they report that their desire to binge at all is dramatically reduced. Once again, these foods, in certain people, may provoke a change in mood and behavior that sets them off on a slippery slope.

Don't think, however, that if a person is deficient, or has a biochemical uniqueness that makes them more prone to react strongly to the lack of a nutrient like zinc or tryptophan, that this excludes psychological problems as part of "the cause." Many people with anorexia are the bearers of a secret, a trauma, or a problem that needs to be resolved, and can be with the help and support of a psychotherapist.

In summary, I recommend the following for anyone who is dealing with an eating disorder:

- See a clinical nutritionist who can assess what you are deficient in and advise you accordingly.

- Their advice will probably include 30–50 mg of zinc, 100 mg of B_6, 200 mg of 5-HTP, plus essential fats, either in capsules or in seeds and fish.

- See a psychotherapist with experience of helping people with eating disorders making a full recovery.

Chapter 33

FITS, CONVULSIONS, AND EPILEPSY

Epilepsy is a mysterious condition, characterized by occasional fits, technically called convulsions. It affects almost half a million people in Britain. The convulsions, which last for seconds or minutes, are thought to be caused by a temporary upset in the brain's chemistry, causing neurons to fire off faster than usual and in bursts.

Convulsions can be brought on by neurological problems such as a brain injury, a stroke, an infection, and less frequently, a tumor. High levels of stress and panic attacks can also trigger a convulsion. So too can heart disease, especially irregular heartbeats, and blood sugar problems. Whatever the triggers, convulsions indicate that the brain is out of balance. An obvious place to start is to ensure an optimal intake of the brain's best friends—nutrients. The optimum nutrition approach can be highly effective, as Francis's story illustrates.

> While teaching classes in Oxford, Francis had a bad car accident. This left him with severe headaches, poor memory and concentration, severe depression, but most of all, epilepsy. So bad was his epilepsy that he complained of what he called "epileptic storms," sometimes daily. During the night he would often have five or six fits, despite being on antiepilepsy drugs. His memory had so deteriorated he could no longer teach, and being epileptic, he found it hard to get work. Naturally he became depressed.
>
> After years under medical supervision he decided to try some alternatives and was referred to me. He promised to avoid tea, coffee, and

sugar, and we discussed how to eat a balanced diet, with plenty of fruit, vegetables, and whole grains—the "optimum" diet.

I wanted to give him every chance to change and included high levels of supplements giving him B_3, B_5, and B_6, choline, calcium, zinc, magnesium and manganese, as well as other nutrients. Magnesium and manganese have both been shown to help epilepsy, while B_5 and choline have a specific effect on memory.

When he came back after one month, he had made tremendous changes to his diet and had reaped the rewards of his efforts. "I am amazed at how well I feel," he commented and went on to tell me how he hadn't had a single muscle tremor or panic attack. Three months later, he had still only had one epileptic "storm." His brain is working better, his depression completely gone, and he can sleep straight through the night without any fits or muscle tremors.*

Differences in the nutritional status of those with convulsions or epilepsy and those without has been demonstrated by many researchers. The key nutrients that have frequently been shown to be deficient are folic acid, the minerals manganese and magnesium, and essential fats.

Finding What Helps

B Vitamins

Folic acid, a vitamin that is often low in those with mental health problems, is depleted by convulsions. This suggests that it is somehow involved.[133] Ironically, anticonvulsant drugs such as phenytoin, primidone, and phenobarbital further deplete folic acid. Combining a drug such as phenytoin with folic acid works better than giving the drug alone. In one study, epileptics were given the drug with either folic acid or a placebo, and after a year, only those on folic acid reported substantially less fits.[134] However, folic acid could be a double-edged sword. Some uncontrolled studies suggest that folate supplementation may create epileptic fits in a minority of people. Several controlled studies, however, have failed to confirm this observation, suggesting that this effect must be very rare.[135] With the guidance of your doctor, folic acid supplementation is well worth trying, although don't expect immediate results. Also worth supplementing is vitamin B_6.

Unlike folic acid, high doses of vitamin B_6 can produce almost immediate

* Case supplied by Christopher Scarfe.

results. The first research to identify a role for B$_6$ in the treatment of epilespy in children took place in Japan in the 1980s. More than half the children with "infantile spasms" responded very well to B$_6$ supplementation, although the doses used were very high and caused side effects in some of them.[136]

In a more recent study at the University of Heidelberg in Germany, seventeen children were given high doses of vitamin B$_6$ (300 mg/kg/day orally). Five out of the seventeen had immediate relief within two weeks, while after four weeks all patients were more or less free of seizures. No serious adverse reactions were noted. Side effects were mainly gastrointestinal symptoms and were reversible after reduction of the dosage.[137]

Magnesium, Manganese, and Zinc

The mineral manganese is completely essential for proper brain function and, to date, four studies have shown a correlation between low levels and the presence of epilepsy, suggesting that as many as one in three children with epilepsy have low manganese levels.[138] [139] [140] Supplementing manganese helped to reduce fits. In one study published in the *Journal of the American Medical Association*, one child who was found to have half the normal blood manganese levels didn't respond to any medication, but upon supplementing manganese had fewer seizures and improved speech and learning. [141] Dr. Carl Pfeiffer was the first to report the successful treatment of epilepsy with manganese.[142] At the Institute for Optimum Nutrition we have frequently found that patients with convulsions or fits are manganese deficient and have no or fewer fits once supplementation is started.

Magnesium is another mineral well worth checking. Magnesium is also vital for proper nerve and brain function, and, once again, a number of researchers have found low levels in patients with epilepsy and reported fewer fits on supplementation.[143] [144] In animals, magnesium injections have also been shown to instantly suppress convulsions.[145]

If a child is found to have low blood levels of magnesium, as many as 75 percent respond, with fewer fits, according to research from Romania.[146] Supplementing this mineral is especially helpful to those with "temporal lobe" epilepsy. This is especially useful since people with this type of epilepsy rarely respond to conventional anticonvulsant drugs.[147] It is also possible that pregnant women deficient in manganese may be more likely to have children with epilepsy.

It is also well worth testing for zinc. Once again, zinc levels have been found to be lower in children with epilepsy,[148] and anticonvulsant drugs can further deplete this vital mineral. There is also some suggestion that too much copper and not enough zinc may increase the odds of having a seizure.[149] Ideally, we need to take in ten times more zinc than copper. Zinc is also a valuable ally for vitamin B_6, since it helps convert B_6 (pyridoxine) into the active form of the vitamin, called pyridoxal phosphate. It is highly likely that the few children who have had adverse reactions to very high doses of vitamin B_6 may not have done so if given B_6 together with zinc.

In fact, most adverse reactions to vitamins or minerals arise when they are treated like drugs and given at very high doses without other nutrients, thereby completely ignoring the principle of synergy. For this reason I strongly recommend that any person who is experiencing fits, convulsions, or epilepsy see a clinical nutritionist for a thorough nutritional workout.

This should involve both hair and blood analyses for magnesium, manganese, and zinc, as well as folic acid. Levels of magnesium and folic acid are best tested in red blood cells. Depending on the results, a clinical nutritionist can work out what combination of these nutrients, often in high doses, are worth trying, together with basic multivitamin supplementation.

The optimum nutrition approach involving an all-around good diet and supplements program is especially important since other nutrients have also been shown to have positive effects on mental health in those with epilepsy. These include B_1,[150] selenium,[151] and vitamin E.[152]

Absolutely Essential: The Right Fats

Imbalances in essential brain fats is one of the hottest areas of research. It is highly likely, with so many people deficient in essential fats, and especially omega-3 fats, that ensuring an optimal intake and balance of essential fats may help reduce the incidence of fits in epileptics.

The anticonvulsant properties of the two EFAs in a ratio 1:4, omega-3 to omega-6, have been demonstrated in epileptic rats. Three weeks of EFA supplementation resulted in up to 84 percent fewer rats having seizures and up to a 97 percent reduction in the duration of seizures. The experimenters postulated that the anticonvulsant effects of EFAs may be related to the stabilization of neuronal membranes in the brain.[153]

It also works in humans. Reserachers at the Kalanit Institute for the Retarded Child in Israel gave people with epilepsy 3 g of omega-3 fats for six months and found a dramatic reduction in both the number and severity of epileptic seizures.[154]

Amino Acids and Phospholipids

Many of the "brain food" nutrients discussed in Part 1 may also be helpful for those with fits. These include phospholipids such as phosphatidyl choline, and essential fats. Also potentially helpful are the brain's master tuners—SAMe and tri-methyl glycine (TMG). A close relative, di-methyl glycine (DMG), produced remarkable results in one twenty-two-year-old man with long-standing mental retardation, who had been having around seventeen seizures per week despite anticonvulsant medication. Within one week of starting DMG, at 90mg twice daily, his seizures dropped to just three per week. Two attempts to withdraw the DMG caused dramatic increases in seizure frequency.[155]

The amino acid taurine, which helps to calm down the nervous system, may also have a role to play. In animals studies low brain taurine concentrations have been found at the site of maximal seizure activity, and supplementing taurine was found to have a potent, selective, and long-lasting anticonvulsant effect.[156]

However, the most powerful relaxant amino acid has got to be GABA, the brain's peacemaker, because it acts directly as a neurotransmitter. One possible mechanism for explaining why anticonvulsant drugs work is that they block the activity of the excitatory neurotransmitter, glutamic acid, and thereby promote the inhibitory neurotransmitter, GABA. However, I would be cautious about supplementing GABA, and possibly large amounts of taurine, except under medical supervision. This is mainly because animal studies have shown that rats prone to petit mal (absence) seizures sometimes have too much of these amino acids.[157] Another brain-friendly nutrient, DMAE, while potentially helpful, should also be given with caution.

Vinpocetine, an extract of the periwinkle plant (*Vinca minor*), may also help, according to research in Russia.[158] This herbal extract does many useful things in the brain (see Chapter 13). It improves production of cellular energy in brain cells, and it widens blood vessels in the brain, thus improving transport of glucose and oxygen to the brain and their use once they get there. One theory is that epileptic fits may be caused by fluctuations in glucose or oxygen supplies to the brain, which might explain the positive effects of vinpocetine.

Check for Allergies

As with so many types of mental health problems, it's well worth checking for allergies. One epileptic's fits were proven to be induced by certain foods. Without knowing which, they were either given a minute amount of their "trigger" foods or placebos, and only the foods brought on fits.[159] Professor William Rea from Texas, renowned for his special sealed hospital wing that is completely free of all allergens, environmental pollutants, and chemicals, designed specially for those with multiple allergies, has also found some epileptics stop having fits. One of his patients, a twenty-nine-year-old man with a four-year history of grand mal epilepsy as well as double vision, tachy-cardia, dizziness, edema, and spontaneous bruising, none of which had responded to the usual drugs, had complete relief after fasting for six days. When he was reintroduced to certain foods and chemicals, he once more started having fits. For him, peanuts were the worst food.[160] Another power-ful trigger substance for some people with epilepsy is the smell of rosemary oil, found in many essential oil blends.

In summary, if you are prone to fits, convulsions, or epilepsy and haven't been checked out by a clinical nutritionist, there is plenty of room for hope.

- Have your vitamin and mineral levels checked. If low in folic acid, B_6, magnesium, manganese, or zinc, supplementation may well help.

- Make sure you are getting enough essential fats, from seeds, fish, and their oils.

- Other brain-friendly nutrients, including amino acids, choline, DMAE, taurine, and vinpocetine may help, but they are best taken under professional guidance.

PART 7

MENTAL HEALTH IN OLD AGE

Age-related memory decline is not inevitable. Parkinson's disease and Alzheimer's disease can be prevented or even arrested with the right nutrition. This part reports on amazing discoveries in the treatment and prevention of these health problems, backed up by proper science and remarkable recoveries using nutritional therapy.

Chapter 34

Putting the Brakes on Parkinson's Disease

Parkinson's disease isn't just an affliction of old age. In the United States and the United Kingdom there are more than 1.2 million sufferers, ranging from teenagers to the elderly.

Whatever the age of the person with Parkinson's disease, the condition can be very tough to live with. People with this disease first show symptoms of tremor, rigidity, unsteadiness, and slow movement (bradykinesia). The reason for these problems with muscular control and function has been attributed to a deficiency of the neurotransmitter dopamine.

Conventional treatment is based on drug therapy giving L-dopa, the direct precursor of dopamine, which is made from the amino acid phenylalanine, found in dietary protein (see Figure 30).

Other drugs are available which may increase the effectiveness of L-dopa, and there are surgical methods of helping control the tremors. There is also ongoing research in both areas. However helpful, drugs and surgery do run the risk of side effects. As such, so many people with Parkinson's disease opt for drugs only when they cannot function effectively enough without them. With the right nutritional support, this threshold may never be reached.

Thanks to the pioneering work of Dr. Geoffrey Leader and Lucille Leader, a doctor and nutritionist living in London, we now know that the right nutritional intervention can effectively improve the symptoms of Parkinson's disease. Harry's story is a case in point.

Harry was referred by his GP to Dr. Geoffrey Leader and Lucille Leader at their clinic in London (see Useful Addresses on page 367). He made repetitive movements, had tremors (made worse by stress), intractable constipation, very low energy, and was very underweight. The Leaders arranged biochemical tests, which demonstrated that Harry was deficient in nutrients. They also found that he was eating foods that compromised the absorption of his L-dopa medication.

They recommended nutrients to address the deficiencies that were found, dealt successfully with the constipation, and worked out a suitable diet and a schedule for taking the L-dopa in relation to different foods, which

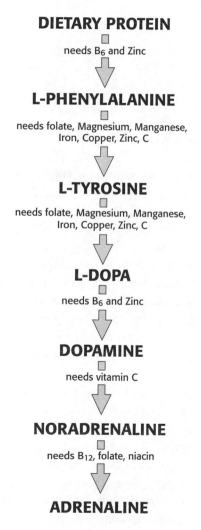

DIETARY PROTEIN

needs B₆ and Zinc

⬇

L-PHENYLALANINE

needs folate, Magnesium, Manganese,
Iron, Copper, Zinc, C

⬇

L-TYROSINE

needs folate, Magnesium, Manganese,
Iron, Copper, Zinc, C

⬇

L-DOPA

needs B₆ and Zinc

⬇

DOPAMINE

needs vitamin C

⬇

NORADRENALINE

needs B₁₂, folate, niacin

⬇

ADRENALINE

Fig 30 How we make dopamine[1]

Adapted with permission from Dr. Geoffrey Leader and Lucille Leader, *Parkinson's Disease—The Way Forward* (see Recommended Reading, page 358).

would maximize the efficacy of Harry's drugs. This enabled him to take smaller doses of L-dopa, which in turn reduced its side effects, which included the distressing dyskinesia. The weight problem was addressed using a specific dietary strategy that was compatible with his drug regimen. They also helped Harry to keep his stress levels low by a special relaxation technique called autogenic training that also helps control the symptoms.

Within a few weeks, Harry was experiencing a feeling of well-being. His bowel function had normalized, his energy had improved, the dyskinesia was a thing of the past, and he was putting on weight. His body movements were more controlled.

Note: The full details of this integrated nutritional strategy are given in the Leader book, *Parkinson's Disease: The Way Forward* (see Recommended Reading on page 358).

Many Roads to Dopamine Deficiency

There is little doubt that dopamine deficiency is the major cause of the symptoms of Parkinson's disease, and most drug therapy aims to improve the body's ability to make dopamine from L-dopa. But, why do some people develop this impaired ability to make this key neurotransmitter? There are many answers to this question.

In some cases the neurons that produce dopamine don't work properly, sometimes because they lack the raw materials or the enzymes that turn the building blocks, amino acids, into neurotransmitters. The neurons can die off or be damaged, for example by oxidants, or by environmental toxins such as pesticides and herbicides. Interestingly, researchers at the University of Miami have found levels of these chemicals to be higher in the brains of Parkinson's sufferers.[2] The incidence of Parkinson's disease is notably higher in rural areas where a lot of crop spraying takes place, and some pesticide combinations have shown a clear geographical correlation with incidences of the disease.[3][4] Deficiency of nutrients such as folic acid can also make these dopamine-producing brain cells more susceptible to damage.[5]

Sometimes there is a problem in how the body detoxifies, a job primarily done by the liver, leaving neurons unprotected.[6] Then there are other factors such as prolonged stress and the likelihood of genetic predispositions.

Geoffrey and Lucille Leader figured that each of these pieces of the jigsaw puzzle could be made a lot better if sufferers followed a targeted optimum nutrition program. They started to test patients with Parkinson's disease and found that literally 100 percent of them had nutritional deficiencies based on tests that measure what is going on within cells. They also found that many people were deficient in stomach acid and digestive enzymes, leading to poor digestion, and had increased intestinal permeability, leading to faulty absorption of nutrients. Intestinal permeability is tested by drinking polyethylene glycol (PEG 400), a substance that shouldn't pass through the gut wall, and then measuring levels of PEG 400 in the urine. Using this test, people with Parkinson's disease may often show an increase in gut permeability or evidence of malabsorption. While there is no conclusive evidence yet that Parkinson's disease is caused by nutrient deficiencies, the Leaders have found that correcting these deficiencies often helps.

Brain Toxins, Oxidants, and the Liver

All this faulty digestion and absorption places extra stress on the liver, the detoxification capital of the body. Since the brain's neurons can't protect themselves from toxins, they depend on the liver. A simple example of this is alcohol—once you drink more than your liver can detoxify, you get drunk, which is what happens when brain cells are exposed to this toxin. In excess, you lose muscular control, and movements, including speech, slow down.

Problems with liver detoxification are often a hallmark of Parkinson's patients. One of the liver's best detox allies is the sulphur-containing amino acids, which have the ability to mop up undesirable toxins in a process called sulphation. Researchers have reported faulty sulphation in patients with Parkinson's disease, which can be helped by supplementing cysteine, methionine, and molybdenum and avoiding wine, coffee, certain cheeses, and chocolate, all known inhibitors of sulphation.[7] Eating foods rich in glucosinolates, such as broccoli, Brussels sprouts, cabbage, cauliflower, and kale, also helps the liver to detoxify.

The greatest toxins of all are oxidants, or "free radicals." Giving antioxidants helps to prevent free-radical damage to brain cells and slows the progression of the disease. In a seven-year pilot study, twenty-one patients with early Parkinson's disease were given 3,000 mg of vitamin C and 3,200 IU of vitamin E daily. The need for drug therapy was delayed up to two to three years compared to those who did not receive the antioxidants.[8]

These nutrients are some but by no means all of the allies that can support liver function, thereby preventing brain damage from toxins. Dr. Jeffrey Bland from Gig Harbor, Washington, an expert in liver detoxification, has also found tremendous improvement by supporting liver function with nutritional supplementation, increasing the effectiveness of drugs, reducing symptoms, and boosting energy levels in those suffering from the early stages of Parkinson's disease in studies.[9]

Personalized Nutrition Works Best

The best results with Parkinson's disease come from a total optimum nutrition approach. This involves both diet and supplements, helping to improve digestion, absorption, liver function, and the cells' ability to work properly and to produce dopamine, thus optimizing cellular metabolism and energy production.

As you can see in Figure 30, the ability to make dopamine efficiently depends on many vitamins and minerals. This includes nutrients such as zinc, magnesium, and the B vitamins, especially B$_6$ and folic acid. Researchers at the National Institute on Aging in the United States found that mice fed a folic acid-deficient diet have a significantly greater risk of developing Parkinson's-like symptoms. One likely reason for this is that without folic acid, the body produces too much homocysteine, a toxic substance that damages brain cells and so hinders dopamine production. Researchers at Boston University have found that a high homocysteine level is a strong, independent risk factor for the development of Alzheimer's disease.[10] In mice fed adequate amounts of folic acid, they were able to repair the damage in dopamine-producing neurons and counteract the adverse effects of homocysteine.[11]

The Leaders have found the best approach involves a tailor-made nutritional program of diet and supplements and have found that this may often reduce symptoms and make drugs more effective, thus optimising dosage. They recommend many supplements based on patients' biochemical individuality, including vitamins, minerals, essential fats, amino acids, antioxidants, phospholipids, and brain-friendly herbs such as ginkgo.

As with so many mental health problems, controlling blood sugar and checking and correcting food allergies or intolerances can make a big difference. The most common allergy-provoking foods are the gluten grains (especially wheat, but also rye, oats, barley, and spelt) and dairy products. Managing stress is also important because we respond to stress by producing the stress hormones noradrenaline and adrenaline, which are made from dopamine (see Figure 30). This is why the symptoms of Parkinson's disease often get worse when the sufferer is stressed.

Working with Medication: What to Eat When

The right diet is very important in such a strategy that tackles every piece of the jigsaw of Parkinson's disease. Movement problems can get worse when dense protein foods containing certain amino acids in high proportion are eaten too close to the times of taking L-dopa medication.[12] This is because

L-dopa competes with the amino acids for absorption at the receptor sites in the intestine and at the blood-brain barrier, so less gets through. To make best use of the L-dopa, protein-rich foods containing the other amino acids should not be eaten at the same time as taking L-dopa medication, according to the following guidelines:

L-dopa medication and diet—what to eat when*

L-dopa is affected by protein-containing foods which contain significant amounts of the following **amino acids**: tyrosine, phenylalanine, valine, leucine, isoleucine, tryptophan, methionine and histidine. Foods that contain these amino acids include eggs, fish, meat, poultry, dairy produce (not butter), beans, green peas, spinach, sago, soy, couscous, bulgar, coconut, avocado, asparagus, and gluten-containing grains (oats, rye, wheat, barley, spelt).

➢ **Take L-dopa medication**
Wait ONE HOUR before eating any of the foods listed above.

➢ After eating any of the foods listed above, wait TWO HOURS, if possible, before taking L-dopa medication again.

---

*This dietary protocol has been developed and proven helpful by Dr. Geoffrey and Lucille Leader and is reproduced with their kind permission.

With older types of the drug L-dopa, vitamin B_6 caused its conversion to dopamine before reaching the brain. This was disastrous. Latterday L-dopa drugs contain a decarboxylase inhibitor, which inhibits premature carboxylation of L-dopa to dopamine. As such, vitamin B_6, which helps turn L-dopa into dopamine, can be used safely together with the Parkinson's drugs Sinemet and Madopar.[13]

The drug selegiline is also often used for Parkinson's disease. In higher doses (above 30 mg), there is a risk of hypertension if a person eats foods rich in another amino acid—tyramine.[14] These include cheddar and other strong cheese, ripe avocado, pepperoni, salami, soy sauce, old liver pâté, overripe bananas, brewer's yeast, broad beans, Chianti, overripe or canned figs, vermouth, Drambuie, yeast extract (marmite, etc.), miso soup, fish (pickled, salted, or smoked), caviar, chocolate (large quantities), or caffeine (large quantities). Some people are more susceptible to this dose-dependent side effect than others, and few react at a dose of 10 mg, which is commonly given to Parkinson's patients.[15]

While being careful to avoid these foods around medication, it is important to get enough protein from foods at other times. Good whole proteins include fish, soy products, and eggs. Many people choose to have their meals containing concentrated protein at night. This is because they do not need as much help with movement control at night as during the day when their L-dopa medication is necessary to see them through all their activities. Some people leave out L-dopa completely after the protein meal. Otherwise it is best to follow the time protocol for taking L-dopa with a protein-rich meal, as above.

It is also important to have a well-balanced diet throughout the day including fruits and vegetables, gluten-free whole grains and plenty of fluids. A common problem in Parkinson's disease is constipation. Having a diet rich in fruits and vegetables and drinking plenty of water throughout the day makes a big difference, as can a few prunes, figs, or dried apricots with each meal, or psyllium husk capsules between meals with water.

In summary, with the appropriate individualized nutritional management there's a good chance you can put the brakes on Parkinson's disease. It may alleviate symptoms and reduce the speed of increasing drug dosages. I recommend the following:

- See a nutrition consultant who can assess you for nutritional deficiencies, digestive problems, and liver function.

- Pursue a tailor-made nutritional strategy, including a specific diet regimen that maximizes the effects of any medication.

- Avoid environmental toxins and eat organic when possible.

- Do all you can to reduce your level of stress.

- Reduce autointoxication from constipation by eating six to eight prunes, figs, or apricots before each meal.

Chapter 35

PREVENTING AGE-RELATED MEMORY DECLINE

We are on the threshold of a new disease. It isn't dementia, senility, or Alzheimer's disease, although for some it marks the beginning of that slippery slope. It's age-related memory and/or mood decline. It affects at least one in four people over the age of sixty and is accepted by most as an inevitable but undesirable consequence of aging.

Imagine this scenario: "Doctor, I'm fifty-five and there's little doubt that my memory isn't as sharp as it used to be. What can you recommend?" You're then asked a sequence of questions that conclude you don't have dementia or Alzheimer's disease, followed by, "It's just what happens later in life." Of course, the drug companies are well aware of this missed opportunity and are pushing for official classification of a disease. "Age-related memory impairment affects many more people than Alzheimer's disease, although, it's certainly true, it is a much less severe condition," says Dr. Paul Williams of Glaxo Pharmaceuticals, adding, "We believe at least 4 million people in the United Kingdom suffer from this." Glaxo has been developing drugs to enhance memory and mental performance. In fact, most major players have already patented and developed "smart drugs," discussed in Chapter 37, that will soon be prescribed in these scenarios. According to the drug companies, memory decline is becoming a massive and widespread problem.

The good news is that there really is something you can do, and the place to start is optimum nutrition.

Boosting the Aging Brain

Vitamin-Fueled Vitality

The misconception that you get everything you need from a well-balanced diet becomes increasingly further from the truth as you age. First, for many people the ability to digest and absorb nutrients decreases. A common finding among older people is that hydrochloric acid production in the stomach declines, immediately affecting the ability to make use of protein, vitamins, and minerals. So too, for most of us at least, does exercise and/or general physical activity, and consequently appetite. Less food means fewer nutrients.

Circulation, at least for many, also becomes worse with age, so fewer nutrients make it from the gut to the brain. An underlying cause of many of the diseases of later life—cancer, heart disease, diabetes, and Alzheimer's disease—is inflammation. Increases in underlying inflammatory processes in the brain, which can ultimately lead to neuronal damage, can leave the brain in dire need of certain nutrients. The famous five are:

- B vitamins

- Antioxidants

- Trace elements

- Essential fats

- Phospholipids

While Part 1 gave you the background to their general importance for brain health, they really come into their own in later life, as overwhelming evidence shows. Many studies have shown that even supplementing a multivitamin containing moderate amounts of vitamins and trace elements can make a noticeable difference. One of the more thorough pieces of research was conducted by Dr. Rakesh Chandra from the Memorial University of Newfoundland in Canada.

Dr. Chandra decided to test whether supplementation with vitamins and trace elements in modest amounts could improve memory and mental performance in healthy, elderly subjects. He gave ninety-six such men and women, all over the age of sixty-five, either a daily supplement of trace elements and vitamins or a placebo for twelve months. Blood-nutrient levels were measured at the beginning and at the end of the study, as was their immediate and long-term memory, abstract thinking, problem-solving ability, and attention. Of the eighty-six people who completed the year, those taking supplements showed a highly significant improvement in all cognitive tests except long-term memory recall. He also found that the lower the blood nutrient levels, the worse the mental performance.[16]

Multivitamins don't just improve your mental performance; they also make you happier. Another double-blind placebo-controlled trial gave elderly people a B-complex supplement, containing 10 mg of B_1, B_2, and B_6. That's about ten times the RDA. Compared to those taking placebos, there was a definite improvement in mood.[17]

Antioxidant Protection

The best vitamins for boosting your mood and memory are the antioxidants, which include A, C, and E, although the minerals selenium and zinc and the semi-essential nutrient coenzyme Q_{10} have antioxidant properties too. These not only protect the brain from oxidation, but also improve the supply of oxygen, the brain's most critical nutrient. So too do B vitamins, especially folic acid and B_{12}, deficiency of which results in anemia and an inability to efficiently transport oxygen to the brain, and vitamins B_1, B_2, and B_3, which help the brain make use of oxygen in generating brain power in every cell.

The more antioxidants you have in your blood, the sharper your mind. That's what researchers at the University of Berne, in Switzerland, found when they tested 442 people, aged 65 to 94 years. Those with the highest levels of vitamin C and beta-carotene in their blood had the best scores on memory tests.[18] Other researchers in the United States have found a similar positive link between vitamin E and memory performance.[19]

The likely explanation for these associations is that antioxidants improve circulation and reduce the risk for heart disease.[20] It is becoming more and more evident that Alzheimer's and heart disease share many of the same risk factors and mechanisms. As arteries become more and more inflamed and damaged, so too does the brain.

Antioxidants not only protect the brain from oxidation; they also reduce inflammation. Inflammation, often characterized by pain, redness, or swelling, but insidiously invisible in the brain, is how the body lets you know something is wrong. When the body exceeds its capacity to detoxify, for example when the liver is overloaded with alcohol, inflammation is the result. Improving liver function by increasing your intake of liver-friendly nutrients such as antioxidants, methylsulfonyl-methane or MSM, glutathione, and cysteine helps lessen the burden on the brain.

In fact, there is a direct link between liver function and cognitive function. Investigating the reason for memory and concentration problems in alcoholics, a study of 280 patients with liver damage at the Johns Hopkins

University School of Medicine in Baltimore found that this cognitive impairment results from liver damage rather than alcohol intake directly, as those with non-alcohol related liver damage had similar reductions in cognitive function.[21]

While most multis give you small amounts of these antioxidants, there's a good case for upping your intake as you get older. As he approached old age, Dr. Linus Pauling upped his intake of vitamin C as high as 10 g. Rats make the equivalent of 3 g a day, while goats make 16 g a day. We humans have lost the ability to make vitamin C, he argued, and suffer the consequences in old age.

I recommend as an optimum amount 3 g of vitamin C when you're forty, 4 g when you're fifty, 5 g when you're sixty, and so on, divided into two daily doses. For vitamin E the magic formula is 100 IUs for every decade. So, if you are sixty years old that's 600 IUs (400 mg) a day.

Go for the Smart Fats

It's also worth upping your intake of essential fats, especially omega-3s. Simply eating three servings of oily fish (herring, salmon, mackerel, or tuna) a week halves your risk of a heart attack. As we are learning, cardiovascular disease and memory decline are intimately connected.

Omega-3 fats are not only extremely powerful anti-inflammatory agents, which is one of the main mechanisms by which brain cells get damaged, they may also be involved in encoding memories. One theory of memories is that they are encoded in lipoproteins, built out of essential fats and phospholipids. Another theory is that memories are encoded through RNA, the messenger molecule in charge of building new cells. Since brain cells are permanently being replaced and rebuilt, memory must be transmittable. If this theory is correct, zinc is important to memory because it is essential for building RNA. Fish is not only a good source of omega-3 fats, it's also rich in both RNA and zinc.

As we'll see in the next chapter, amazing results have been achieved with Alzheimer's patients by supplementing omega-3 fish oils, and there's no reason not to assume that supplements can't sharpen your mind and memory and prevent dementia from ever developing. Once you hit the age of fifty, I recommend 1,000 mg of DHA/EPA a day. Most supplements provide 400–600 mg, so this means two fish oil capsules a day.

Acetylcholine: Memory Key

As we learned in Chapter 5, acetylcholine is the mind and memory neurotransmitter, helping you to learn new information. It is built out of choline, the most usable form of which is CDP choline (also known as citicholine), followed by phosphatidyl choline. These phospholipids also help to make membranes in the brain and therefore protect against declining numbers and efficiency of neurons.

As you get older the number of neurons and synapses you have decreases, which is why both memory and emotion become blunted. However, this doesn't need to happen if you can just get these phospholipids and essential fats into the brain.

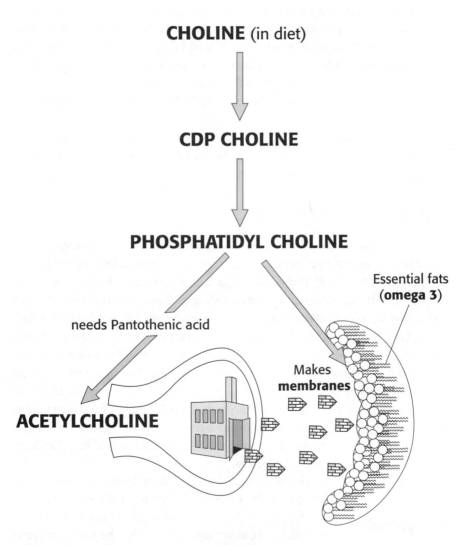

Fig 31   How the brain makes phospholipids

As you can see from the figure above what you want is to get phosphatidyl choline into the brain. While it would be logical to think that supplementing phosphatidyl choline would be the best way to do this, much of this breaks down into choline before it gets into the brain. The same is not true for citicholine. This is the most effective for increasing membrane building in the brain.[22] Since the phospholipids literally soak up essential fats, combining citicholine and phosphatidyl choline, plus essential fats, is like oysters for your brain. These can keep you as sharp as a pencil throughout life. They are also essential nutrients after a stroke.

Another phospholipid, phosphatidyl serine, has well-proven memory-boosting effects. In animal studies phosphatidyl serine was shown to be especially good at reversing age-related memory decline. Research on rats, carried out by the Yakult Central Institute for Microbiological Research, found that sixty days of supplementing phosphatidyl serine could improve some mental function in older rats with age-related memory decline to that of young rats.[23] Human studies have also shown that phosphatidyl serine is effective in reversing memory decline (see Chapter 13).

Other acetylcholine helpers, such as DMAE, pyroglutamate, and pantothenic acid, are well worth supplementing on a daily basis. These are often found together in brain-food formulas.

Ginkgo: Back in Circulation

Another proven brain booster, especially in old age, is the herb ginkgo biloba. While studies on younger people haven't always proven its benefit, studies on older people, especially those with circulation problems, have shown very positive results. A review of ten studies testing ginkgo's effects on people with circulation problems, carried out at the University of Limburg in the Netherlands, found significant improvement in memory, concentration, energy, and mood.[24] A more comprehensive double-blind, placebo-controlled trial carried out in France found remarkable improvement in speed of cognitive processing of sixty- to eighty-year-olds, almost comparable to those of healthy young people, when given 320 mg a day.[25] Ginkgo biloba may also be helpful in elderly depression—it has been shown to increase serotonin receptor sites in elderly but not young rats, suggesting that it may block an age-related loss of serotonin receptors.[26]

Ginkgo contains two phytochemicals called ginkgo flavone glycosides and terpene lactones, which give it its remarkable healing properties. Ginkgo usually comes in capsule form, and you should look for a brand that shows the flavonoid concentration, which determines strength. The recommended flavonoid concentration is 24 percent, of which one would take 30–50 mg up to three times a day. Ginkgo is sometimes also contained in brain-food formulas.

Stay Cool, Use It or Lose It, and Keep Fit

Stress has an enormous impact on our memories, too. A mild dose of stress can actually stimulate memory and mental alertness, but long-term stress is definitely bad news: It puts too much of the hormone cortisol into circulation, and this literally damages the brain. Raised levels of cortisol have been linked to poorer memory and a shrinking of the brain's memory sorting center.

After only two weeks of the raised cortisol levels of stress, the dendrite "arms" of brain cells that reach out to connect with other brain cells start to shrivel up, according to research carried out at Stanford University in California by Robert Sapolsky, professor of neuroscience.[27] The good news is that such damage isn't permanent. Stop the stress and the dendrites grow back. One way to reduce your stress levels is to reduce your intake of sugar and stimulants. The more dependent on stimulants your are, the more your blood sugar levels fluctuate, and the more you are likely to react stressfully to life's inevitable challenges.

With the right nutrition and the right attitude, age-related memory loss doesn't need to happen to you. You can build new brain cells at any age. Research clearly shows that healthy, well-educated elderly people can show no decline in mental function right up to death, and no increased rate of brain shrinkage even after sixty-five. It's a "use it or lose it" situation.

It isn't only your brain you need to exercise. Physical exercise has a direct effect on mental powers, probably by improving circulation. Research published in the *Journal of Internal Medicine* found that regular walking improved memory and reduced signs of dementia.[28] The threshold for this positive effect was about 1,000 steps, or a little over a mile a day.

The steps you need to take to keep all your marbles are, in essence, the same as those needed to maximize your memory and mental alertness earlier in life. So, whether you are twenty or sixty years old, the time to act is now. However, if you are over fifty, it's worth upping the amounts of these brain-friendly nutrients.

In summary, staving off age-related memory decline means:

- Eat oily fish three times a week.

- Eat plenty of antioxidant-rich fruits and vegetables.

- Supplement a high-strength multivitamin and mineral.

- Supplement between 3 and 8 g of vitamin C a day, increasing your intake with age.

- Supplement 100 IU of vitamin E daily for each decade of your age.

- Supplement 2 fish oil capsules giving 1,000 mg of EPA/DHA.

- Supplement phospholipids (phosphatidyl choline, citicholine, and phosphatidyl serine).

- Supplement a brain food formula giving phospholipids, pyroglutamate, DMAE, pantothenic acid, ginkgo biloba, and/or vinpocetine.

- Keep fit.

- Keep learning new things.

- Reduce the stresses in your life.

If you do all this, there is no reason why your memory and mental powers need decline with age. As Leonard Larson, president of the American Medical Association in 1960, said, "There is no diseases of the aged, but simply diseases among the aged."

Chapter 36

Say No to Alzheimer's Disease

Trouble started at work. Just little things: She'd misfile a project, or forget the name of someone in the office. Then she forgot the way to the cafeteria. Her supervisor suggested that perhaps it was time she took retirement. Things started to go downhill from there. Her doctor dismissed her complaints as symptoms of the normal aging process. It wasn't until Joan took a walk one winter afternoon, wearing her best summer dress on a snowy day, that her family finally believed something was seriously wrong.

This case, from neurologist Dr. Jay Lombard and nutritionist Carl Germano, authors of the *Brain Wellness Plan*, is typical. What could be worse than losing your mind, while your body has many years to run? Yet, that is precisely what happens to one in ten people over the age of sixty-five, and one in two people over the age of eighty-five. Currently in Britain half a million people suffer from Alzheimer's disease, costing the National Health Service a staggering $23.5 billion a year.

With an ever-aging population, the prediction is that, by 2030, 20 percent of people over sixty-five will have Alzheimer's disease. The stress it brings, both to the sufferer and their family, is immense. For many people on the slippery slope to Alzheimer's disease, the first signs are depression, irritability, confusion, and forgetfulness.

The good news is that Alzheimer's disease can often be arrested and, in some cases, even possibly reversed by a comprehensive approach using both optimum nutrition and certain "smart" drugs, discussed in the next chapter. Tom Warren is a case in point. Fifteen years ago Tom was diagnosed with

Alzheimer's disease and told by his doctor that he might have just seven years to live, and there wasn't anything he could do. Today Tom is completely cured of his dementia. He has written one book about his recovery, and he's working on another.[29] One of the reason this is possible is that new brain cells are being made all the time, and, under the right conditions, new brain cell growth can be encouraged.[30]

The Roots of Alzheimer's Disease

Alzheimer's is a complex disease without a single cause, but with many contributors. Many researchers are now converging on the idea that it is a degenerative disease that develops largely due to the long-term consequence of faulty nutrition and exposure to antinutrients, much like cardiovascular disease, and that any long-term solution must involve fundamental changes to a person's diet.

The contributory factors may include:

- A genetic predisposition

- Poor nutrition

- Digestive and detoxification problems

- Circulation problems

- Viral infections

- Toxic accumulation in the brain

- Oxidant damage

- Inflammation

- Stress and excess cortisol

Each of these can be prevented, with the exception of the genetic predisposition. Even in this case, having the gene on its own is not enough to cause the disease. The gene in question is called "apolipoprotein E," or ApoE for short. It helps transport cholesterol and build healthy membranes for the brain's neurons. Those who inherit a particular type of this gene, called ApoE4, have more than double the risk of developing Alzheimer's disease. The presence of this defective gene is now being used as a marker to predict risk.

Yet this risk may never manifest as reality unless other circumstances prevail, such as infection and/or faulty nutrition. One of these is infection with the herpes simplex virus, according to research carried out at Manchester's Molecular Neurobiology Laboratory and reported in the *Lancet* in 1997.[31] Their research shows that viruses can damage genes and change the message they deliver to brain cells, causing cellular damage. The question then becomes: What protects your genes? The answer, once again, is optimum nutrition.

Vitamin E for Prevention and Treatment

Both vitamin E and selenium have been shown to stop viruses from changing genetic messages, so it may be that only those deficient in these nutrients who are infected with certain viruses have an increased susceptibility to Alzheimer's disease. This may partly explain why those who supplement vitamin E have a fraction of the risk. A recent study in the United States gave 633 disease-free sixty-five-year-olds large amounts of either vitamin E or vitamin C. By the laws of probability a small number in each group would have been expected to show the signs of Alzheimer's disease five years later. None did.[32] Another study published in the *Journal of the American Medical Association* found that the risk of developing Alzheimer's disease was 67 percent lower in those with a high dietary intake of vitamin E, versus those with a low intake.[33]

Vitamin E not only plays a key role in early prevention in this way, but also in slowing down the progression of the disease. In a landmark study reported in the *New England Journal of Medicine* in 1997, Alzheimer's patients received either 2,000ius of vitamin E, the drug selegiline, or a placebo.[34] Vitamin E was shown to reduce progression most significantly, thus relieving some burden on both patients and their family. Dr. Leon Thal from the University of California, one of the doctors running this study, stated, "The results of this study will be used to change the prescribing practices in the United States and probably many other parts of the world." Now, at least in the United States, the American Psychiatric Association recommends vitamin E supplements for Alzheimer's patients.

Other antioxidants, including vitamin C, beta-carotene, cysteine, lipoic acid, glutathione, anthocyanidins, and coenzyme Q_{10} are also important. These are discussed in Chapter 8 and should be included in any comprehensive nutritional strategy to maximize recovery from Alzheimer's disease.

Alzheimer's Disease Is an Inflammatory Disease

It is highly likely that both cardiovascular and Alzheimer's disease result from the same or a similar disease process. Not only does the presence of cardiovascular disease greatly increase the chances of getting Alzheimer's disease, especially if you have the ApoE4 gene,[35] but many of the same causes, including too many oxidants and not enough antioxidants, apply to both conditions. Once cardiovascular disease is present, blockages in arteries may lead to a poor supply of key nutrients to the brain. Without a good supply of antioxidants, for example, brain cells become more vulnerable to free radical damage.

Cardiovascular disease is intimately linked to both a lack of antioxidants and excess exposure to oxidants, for example from fried food or from smoking cigarettes. Antioxidant nutrients such as vitamin C and E, which are now well proven to help both conditions, not only mop up these brain pollutants, but also reduce inflammation.

The diagnostic proof of Alzheimer's disease, as distinct from other forms of dementia, is the presence of plaques or patches of dead cells and other waste material in the brain. At the core of these plaques has been found a substance called "beta-amyloid." This is an abnormal protein that is also found in the plaques of arterial deposits. Beta-amyloid is a toxic invader that arises when the body is in "emergency mode," resulting in inflammation, as the immune system becomes overreactive. It's a scenario that develops once a person's total environmental overload exceeds his or her genetic capacity to adapt. Looked at in this way, the presence of the ApoE4 gene simply means less adaptive capacity to the insults of modern-day diets and lifestyle, while optimum nutrition means more adaptive capacity by giving your brain and body a less toxic chemical environment. Inflammation, in this model, is the alarm bell.

Indeed, research has shown that taking anti-inflammatory drugs offers some protection from Alzheimer's disease, which is consistent with the hypothesis that the damage that occurs to brain cells is part of an overall inflammatory reaction. It also means that natural anti-inflammatory nutrients may prove to be important in prevention strategies, especially as cortisone-based anti-inflammatory drugs may make matters worse (see below).

Inflammatory reactions invariably mean increased production of oxidants, and hence an increased need for antioxidants such as vitamin A, beta-carotene, and vitamins C and E, all of which have been shown to be low in those with Alzheimer's disease. Also involved in calming down brain inflammation are our old friends, the omega-3 fats, found in salmon, tuna, herring, and mackerel. As well as being anti-inflammatory, they are a vital component of brain cell membranes and help control calcium flow in and out of cells. This factor is important because too much calcium inside brain cells is known to contribute to the production of the toxic beta-amyloid protein.

If inflammation is the key, then the way to prevent and reverse the brain damage that occurs in Alzheimer's patients is to reduce causes of inflammation and increase natural anti-inflammatory nutrients, such as antioxidants and omega-3 fats. Inflammation can be caused by too many oxidants, too much homocysteine, digestive problems leading to poor liver detoxification, and too much stress.

Stress, Cortisol, and Memory Loss

Under prolonged stress, the body produces the adrenal hormone cortisol. In the previous chapter I mentioned the work of Professor Robert Sapolsky of Stanford University. His research has shown that although cortisol is a powerful anti-inflammatory hormone, raised cortisol can damage the brain. In studies with rats he found that two weeks of induced stress causing raised cortisol levels causes dendrites, those connections between brain cells, to shrivel up.[36] He believes that brain cell loss in aging and Alzheimer's disease may be, in part, due to high levels of cortisol and recommends that corticosteroid drugs should not be used in Alzheimer's disease patients for other medical problems like asthma or arthritis.[37] This research also implies that the ability to create a lifestyle that avoids nonstop stress is also important for reducing Alzheimer's risk.

Adrenal exhaustion can also lead to a lack of cortisol, which increases inflammation. It's a question of balance. There is some evidence that DHEA, an adrenal hormone discussed in the next chapter, may be helpful in restoring a normal balance of adrenal hormones in those with Alzheimer's disease with evidence of adrenal burnout.

Digestion and Detoxification

Although vastly underexplored, it is highly likely that digestive problems, leading to poor liver detoxification, leading to an increased toxic load on the brain, is part of the picture that generates inflammation. This is now understood to be part of the picture with Parkinson's disease (see page 289) and is likely to be a significant piece of the jigsaw with Alzheimer's disease. The connection is also more likely because poor nutrition and poor absorption, which are hallmarks of Alzheimer's patients, generally means poor detoxification. Since the brain is unable to deal with many toxins, their presence triggers inflammation, which is the body's natural reaction to an insult.

This also means that the many nutrients that improve digestion, absorption and detoxification may help those with Alzheimer's disease. This includes the amino acids l-glutamine, cysteine, and glutathione.

How's Your Homocysteine?

Homocysteine is an example of a toxin that the brain can't protect itself against. It's made in the body from the normally beneficial amino acid methionine when a person is deficient in either vitamin B_6 or folic acid.

The theory that homocysteine might be behind atherosclerosis and heart disease was first proposed by Dr. Kilmer McCully back in 1969, but never taken seriously. That was, until the European Concerted Action Group, a consortium of doctors and researchers from nineteen medical centers in nine European countries, studied 750 people under the age of sixty with atherosclerosis, compared to 800 people without such cardiovascular disease.[38] They found that having a high level of homocysteine in the blood was as great a risk factor for cardiovascular disease as smoking or having a high blood cholesterol level. Those in the top fifth of homocysteine levels had double the risk of cardiovascular disease. In other words, 20 percent of people had double the risk of cardiovascular disease because of high homocysteine levels.

They also found that those taking vitamin supplements reduced their risk to a third of those not taking supplements. When they compared blood levels of vitamin B_6 and folic acid, they found that there was a direct relationship between increasing homocysteine levels with decreasing levels of folic acid and vitamin B_6, with vitamin B_6 being the strongest association.

What, you might wonder, has all this got to do with Alzheimer's disease? Dr. Matsu Toshifumi and colleagues at Tohoku University, Japan, wondered if homocysteine was also damaging the brain. To check this they conducted brain scans on 153 elderly people and checked them against each individual's homocysteine level. The evidence was clear—the higher the homocysteine, the greater the damage to the brain.[39] They also confirmed that high homocysteine levels were strongly correlated with low folic acid levels. Other researchers have also found that older people with low levels of folic acid have an increased risk of developing Alzheimer's disease,[40] and Dr. David Snowdon at the University of Kentucky has confirmed by autopsies that the lower the levels of serum folic acid, the greater the neurological damage that person suffered.[41]

A recent study in the *New England Journal of Medicine* charted the health of 1,092 elderly people without dementia, measuring their homocysteine levels. Eight years later, 111 were diagnosed with dementia, of which 83 were given the diagnosis of Alzheimer's disease. Those with high blood homocysteine levels (above 14 μmol/l) had nearly double the risk of Alzheimer's disease. This strongly suggests that optimum nutrition should, at the very least, halve your risk of developing Alzheimer's disease in later years by lowering homocysteine.[42]

B Vitamins: Your Brain's Best Friends

Although the homocysteine link is in the early stages of research, it certainly makes sense to ensure an optimal intake of B_6 and folic acid in older people, meaning 100 mg and 1,000 mcg a day, respectively. These B vitamins help the body make proper use of the sulphur-containing and beneficial amino acid methionine, instead of producing toxic homocysteine.

B vitamins do far more for the brain than reduce homocysteine levels. Oxygen, the most critical and dangerous nutrient of them all, depends on vitamin B_{12}, folic acid, niacin, and essential fats to be transported and used by the brain. Vitamin B_1 deficiency has long been known to result in brain damage. One of the most dangerous problems of excessive alcohol consumption is induced B_1 deficiency. The condition is called Wernicke-Korsakof syndrome. The symptoms include anxiety and depression, obsessive thinking, confusion, defective memory (especially of recent events), and time distortion—not so different from Alzheimer's disease.

Vitamin B_3 (niacin) is crucial for oxygen utilization. It is incorporated into the coenzyme NAD (nicotinamide adenosine dinucleotide), and many reactions involving oxygen need NAD. Without it, pellagra and senility can develop. For these reasons, optimal intakes of all the B vitamins is an important part of an Alzheimer's prevention plan.

Aluminum, Mercury, and More

Another brain toxin found in the plaques of Alzheimer's sufferers is aluminum. While plenty of studies have shown this increased accumulation of aluminum, what isn't clear is whether this is a cause or a consequence of the disease. The likelihood is that it's a bit of both and still a significant contributor to memory problems. In a study in the 1980s of 647 Canadian gold miners who had routinely inhaled aluminum since the 1940s (this used to be a common practice, thought to prevent silica poisoning), all tested in the "impaired" range for cognitive function, suggesting a clear link between aluminum and memory loss.[43]

Aluminum is all around us—in aspirin, antacids, antidiarrheal drugs, cake mixes, self-rising flour, processed cheese, baking powder, drinking water, milk, talcum powder, tobacco smoke, drink cans, cooking utensils and pans, air pollution compounds, and aluminum foil. It is poorly absorbed into the body, unless you are zinc deficient, which half of the population is. It also becomes much more absorbable in acidic conditions. So, for example, if you boil tea containing tannic acid, or rhubarb, which contains oxalic acid, in an old aluminum pan, you can leach aluminum from the pan into the food or drink. Your aluminum level is easily tested in a hair mineral analysis. If your level is high, it's important to identify the potential sources in your diet and lifestyle, and reduce them. I have often seen, for example, high levels in those who grill food directly on aluminum foil.

Mercury is another cause for concern. Autopsies of brains from Alzheimer's patients, compared to control patients of the same age, have shown raised levels of mercury.[44] Researchers from the University of Basel, Switzerland, have also found high blood mercury levels, more than double those of the control groups, in Alzheimer's patients, with early-onset Alzheimer's patients having the highest mercury levels of all.[45] Trace amounts of mercury can cause the type of damage to nerves that is characteristic of Alzheimer's disease, according to recent research at the University of Calgary Faculty of Medicine, strongly suggesting that the small amounts we are exposed to, for example from amalgam fillings, may be contributing to memory loss.[46] Although the research on the link of mercury to Alzheimer's disease is in its infancy, it is certainly wise to reduce your exposure to this highly toxic metal. Chapter 10 explains how to test and reduce your toxic load of aluminum, mercury, and other brain pollutants.

Only Connect: Acetylcholine and Memory

Whatever the contributory causes to the brain damage seen in Alzheimer's disease, once the brain damage occurs, there is memory loss. Understanding how that occurs opens up avenues for treatment.

A memory is not held in one, but in several brain cells joined together in a network. The memory itself is thought to be put into storage by the neurotransmitter acetylcholine, and stored by altering the structure of a molecule called RNA within brain cells. The limbic system, which is the "doughnut" on top of the brain stem, then has to decide if the memory is worth keeping. The amygdala, part of the limbic system, decides about more emotional memories, while the hippocampus decides about others. In Alzheimer's patients the hippocampus loses its ability to file memories, resulting in an inability to create new ones. People with Alzheimer's also show marked deficiencies in acetylcholine, no doubt largely because these acetylcholine-producing brain cells have been damaged or destroyed.

Even if a memory is intact, if you don't have enough acetylcholine, you can't connect one part of the memory with others. For example, you know the face but can't remember the name.

Boosting the Memory Molecule

Much like Prozac, which stops the breakdown of the neurotransmitter serotonin (a deficiency of which is connected with depression), current state-of-the-art Alzheimer's drugs block the breakdown of acetylcholine. These drugs cause unpleasant side effects, and the alternative is to supplement the nutrients the brain uses to make acetylcholine in the first place. These are phosphatidyl choline, CDP choline, and pantothenic acid (vitamin B_5).

Studies using piracetam, a drug based on the amino acid pyroglutamate, have demonstrated clear improvement in memory, mood, and cognitive abilities in both animals and humans.[47] One study, published in 1988 by Drs. H. Pilch and W. E. Muller, found that mice given piracetam for two weeks had 30 to 40 percent more acetylcholine receptors than before.[48] This suggests that pyroglutamatelike molecules may also have a regenerative effect on the nervous system. (See the next chapter for more details.) This nutrientlike drug is well worth considering for those with Alzheimer's disease.

The effects of enhancing mental performance through supplementation of "smart nutrients" such as phosphatidyl choline, and citicholine, phosphatidyl serine, pantothenic acid, DMAE, and pyroglutamate are likely to be far greater when taken in combination than individually. These have already been discussed in the last chapter and in Chapters 5 and 13, and are well worth supplementing for those with Alzheimer's disease.

While acetylcholine is the major player as far as memory is concerned, other neurotransmitters are also involved. Some stimulate mental processes, while others calm down information overload. You need a balance. For example, the stimulating neurotransmitter glutamate helps forge links between memories, but too much can literally overexcite neurons to death. This is how MSG (monosodium glutamate) turns up the volume on tastes, but too much can definitely be a bad thing. GABA, a close relative of glutamate, calms down the nervous system. The right balance of these neurotransmitters is important. Supplementing 5 g of glutamine a day, an amino acid from which the brain can build these neurotransmitters, can also help promote memory.

Putting It All Together

The ideal level of nutrients to prevent Alzheimer's disease or help someone with the condition is shown below. It is also well worth considering certain smart drugs and hormones, explained in the next chapter.

Alzheimer's Prevention and Reversal Plan

Nutrients	Prevention Dose	Intervention Dose
Vitamins & Minerals (found in multivitamin and mineral formulas)		
Vitamin A (beta-carotene)	15,000 IUs	15,000–20,000 IUs
Thiamin (vitamin B_1)	50 mg	250 mg
Niacin (vitamin B_3)	100 mg	500–1,000 mg
Pantothenic Aacid (vitamin B_5)	100 mg	300 mg
Vitamin B_6	50 mg	100 mg
Folic acid	400 mcg	1200 mcg
Cyanocobalamin (vitamin B_{12})	10 mcg	100 mcg
Antioxidants (found in antioxidant formulas)		
Vitamin C	2,000 mg	4,000 mg
Vitamin E	400 IUs	1,000 IUs
Zinc	15 mg	30 mg
Selenium	200 mcg	400 mcg
Lipoic Acid	200 mg	200 mg
NAC (n-acetyl-cysteine)	500 mg	1,000 mg
Glutathione	100 mg	300 mg
Coenzyme Q_{10}	30 mg	100 mg
Anthocyanidins	100 mg	300 mg
Phospholipids (found in phospholipid complexes and lecithin)		
Phosphatidyl serine	100 mg	300 mg
Phosphatidyl choline	500 mg	1,000 mg
Citicholine	250 mg	500 mg
Smart Nutrients (often found in "brain food" formulas)		
L-glutamine	1,000 mg	5,000 mg
Ginkgo biloba	150 mg	300 mg
Pyroglutamate	250 mg	750 mg
DMAE	100 mg	500 mg
Essential Fats (found in seed and fish oil supplements)		
GLA (omega-6)	150 mg	300 mg
EPA (omega-3)	600 mg	1,200 mg
DHA (omega-3)	400 mg	800 mg

The moral of this story is that Alzheimer's disease is not inevitable, is almost certainly the long-term consequence of diet and lifestyle, is preventable and, to some extent, reversible with optimum nutrition. The key steps are:

- Eat a diet high in antioxidant nutrients and supplement large amounts of antioxidant nutrients such as vitamins A, C, E, selenium, and zinc, as well as a multivitamin containing B vitamins, especially folic acid.

- Ensure an optimal intake of brain fats, especially omega-3 fats from fish and flax seeds or fish oils and phospholipids.

- Reduce your cortisol load by reducing your level of stress and anxiety.

- Reduce your exposure to aluminum and mercury.

- Supplement acetylcholine-supporting nutrients such as phosphatidyl choline, phosphatidyl serine, DMAE, and pyroglutamate.

Chapter 37

SMART DRUGS AND HORMONES

I'm a purist. I believe in nutrients that are part of our evolutionary design, tried and tested over thousands of years. But what if there were drugs or hormones that were safe and did enhance mental performance, or help restore or retain it? What if there were drugs and hormones that could reverse mental decline above and beyond the positive effects of nutrients? The truth is there are, and, especially in situations of memory decline in old age, they are well worth considering.

What Are Smart Drugs?

Over a hundred "smart drugs" have already been developed, and once age-related memory decline becomes a classified disease, there is no doubt that such drugs will become very widely used in society. Some have also been shown to enhance mental abilities in those without diagnosed memory problems. This raises the important question of whether some of these drugs fit the category of "natural highs" in the sense of improving mental ability without a downside, or whether their use should be restricted to those with cognitive problems.

For the pharmaceuticals industry, the advantage of these drugs is that they are not nutrients but in most cases man-made substances—that is, they can be patented and hence are more profitable. The disadvantage of such man-made chemicals is that they are alien to the human body. They may not produce a "perfect fit" in enzyme systems and while creating the desired effect in the short term, may, in the long term, unbalance the brain's sensitive chemistry. In any case, with many of these new smart drugs, the long-term effects are still unknown, so it is best to proceed with caution.

Smart drugs tend to fall into one of three categories:

- Drugs that block the breakdown of neurotransmitters, thereby keeping more of these information molecules in circulation. These include Deprenyl, Aricept, and Huperzine A.

- Drugs that mimic or improve the action of neurotransmitters. These include piracetam, Hydergine, and Dilantin.

- Hormones that influence brain function. These include DHEA, pregnenolone, progesterone, and melatonin.

These are by no means the only smart drugs and hormones, but they are among the most interesting, well researched, and widely taken, with a track record of relative safety. They therefore have a potential role in restoring an active memory and mind, if not promoting it.

More Mileage from Your Neurotransmitters

Deprenyl, also called selegiline, is part of a group of drugs called monoaminooxidase inhibitors, or MAOIs for short. They work as anti-depressants by preventing neurotransmitters from being broken down. Most of these drugs, however, are MAO-A inhibitors, and as such are associated with potentially dangerous side effects. Deprenyl, on the other hand, does not cause this effect, since it is an MAO-B inhibitor.[49]

Deprenyl is particularly effective at stopping the breakdown of dopamine, a deficiency of which is associated with Parkinson's disease. It is mainly prescribed for both the treatment of Parkinson's and Alzheimer's disease. Some people recommend taking it to prevent these diseases and as a general stimulant to mental functioning, even when no symptoms are present. In animals it has also been shown to extend life span.[50] Deprenyl has a better track record in terms of toxic effects than a number of MAOI drugs, which can have unpleasant side effects.

Research by the National Institutes of Health in the United States has shown that 10 mg of Deprenyl does significantly improve memory, attention span, and learning in people with Alzheimer's disease.[51] To what extent it makes a difference in normal people is a subject of controversy. If you want to experiment, start with 1 or 2 mg and build up to 5 mg. If you experience insomnia, lower the dose. Deprenyl is either available on prescription as Eldepryl, while the liquid form (Deprenyl citrate) can be ordered by mail.

Aricept (donepezil) is a drug widely prescribed for people with Alzheimer's disease. It works by inhibiting the enzyme acetylcholinesterase, which breaks down acetylcholine, hence keeping more of this important memory neuro-transmitter in circulation. There are other drugs that do this such as Cognex (tacrine), but most have very unpleasant side effects. Aricept is perhaps the best drug in this class, but it is neither side effect free nor recommended for those without serious memory problems. A better bet is the plant product *Huperzia serrata.*

Huperzia serrata, a moss used for centuries in China, contains an alkaloid called huperzine A, which is also a powerful and highly selective acetyl-cholinesterase inhibitor, working like the anti-Alzheimer's drug Aricept to keep more acetylcholine in circulation. *Huperzia serrata* has been reported to have fewer side effects than such drugs and may work in a more natural way. It also protects against the toxic effects of glutamate (such as MSG). The recommended daily dose is 200 mcg.

Nootropics: Your Brain's Best Friends?

Piracetam is one of a number of new drugs called "nootropics," which are related to the amino acid pyroglutamate. Over 150 studies have been published on piracetam, which has been shown to have a broad effect on enhancing mental performance. Numerous studies have shown improvements in memory, concentration, coordination, and reaction time.[52] The drug is also being used with reasonable success in the treatment of Alzheimer's disease, although it is more effective in the early stages of memory decline.

One such study tested the effects of piracetam on eighteen people aged fifty and older, with demanding jobs and above-average IQs, who were basically fully functional except that they were having problems retaining and recalling memory. They were extensively tested for cognitive function and assigned to the piracetam or placebo group, without them or the researchers knowing who was on the real thing. On retesting those taking piracetam, they had significantly improved on a number of cognitive tests. These people were then put on the placebo, while those previously on the placebo were given pirac-etam. Again, the piracetam group improved dramatically while those on the placebo did not.[53] Another double-blind placebo trial involved 162 French people aged fifty-five and over with age-related memory decline who had sought help from their doctor. With the group taking piracetam, it proved effective after six weeks.[54] These are just a couple of several convincing studies that have led to piracetam being widely prescribed. Nootropil, one brand of piracetam, has registered sales of over $1 billion in recent years.

So, how does piracetam work? It seems to promote memory retention, improve acetylcholine transmission and reception, reduce the effects of stress, and speed up reaction time. Part of its mode of action is that it improves communication across the corpus callosum, which connects the two hemispheres of the brain, hence improving the link between our analytical and relational thinking processes, most helpful for storing and finding memories.

Piracetam is, by all accounts, very safe and has no side effects at effective doses. It usually comes in 800 mg capsules, and the recommended dose is three to six capsules per day (2,400–4,800 mg). Since positive effects may only occur at higher doses, my recommendation is to start with 4,800 mg for two weeks, then reduce the dose back to 2,400 mg or whatever level continues to be effective. Piracetam is far more effective if given with choline. Piracetam is available on prescription in the United States, or without prescription from overseas.

Hydergine is the most widely used and thoroughly tested prescription drug for improving brain function. It is ergoloid mesylate, an extract of the ergot fungus that grows on rye and was discovered in the 1950s by Albert Hoffman, who is better known for his discovery of that other ergot-based drug, LSD. The way it works is by improving circulation to the brain and protecting against oxidant damage. It also seems to improve the production of neurotransmitters, especially dopamine, noradrenaline, and acetylcholine, and stabilizes the brain's glucose metabolism. In 1994 researchers from the University of California reviewed the results of forty-seven trials testing Hydergine for its effects on reversing memory loss in those with dementia. The majority of these studies proved effective, although it was little help to those with Alzheimer's disease.[55]

There is also some evidence that Hydergine improves memory in healthy people. In a United Kingdom study, twelve volunteers without cognitive problems were given cognitive tests before and after receiving 12 mg of Hydergine for two weeks. The results showed significant improvement in their alertness and cognitive abilities.[56] The usual dose for Hydergine is 9 mg, given as 3 mg three times a day. It appears to be nontoxic although there are rare reports of nausea and headaches that do not occur at lower doses.

Dilantin (phenytoin), which first became popular as an antiseizure drug, has been found to improve concentration, response time, mental performance, and mood. It seems to normalize the electrical activity of the brain and may be especially helpful for those who have difficulty focusing. It was made popular by stockmarket mogul Jack Dreyfus, known as the "lion of Wall Street."

Later in life Dreyfus suffered from crippling anxiety and depression and described his brain as a "bunch of dry twigs." Fearful or angry thoughts set the twigs alight, so to speak, and he couldn't stop these negative thoughts spreading like wildfire. Then he discovered Dilantin, which he described as "gentle rain" keeping his excessive thoughts under control. He went on to fund substantial research that has proven that Dilantin can be very helpful for those people who are unfocused, easily distracted, short-tempered, impulsive, and obsessive. It has now been used for years and is free from side effects, at least at a low dose, is nonaddictive, and doesn't have the sedating effects of tranquilizers. The recommended dose is 100 mg, one to three times a day. It is available on prescription.

A Smarter Hormone

One step closer to nature is the use of "smart hormones." These are naturally occurring hormones that have an effect on performance. In this category are melatonin, pregnenolone and DHEA. In the United States, these natural hormones are sold over the counter to deal with anything from jet lag to life extension. In the United Kingdom and most other countries they are only available on prescription.

DHEA and pregnenolone are naturally occurring hormones, but that certainly doesn't make them harmless. As you can see from Figure 32, they can, if needed, be turned into estrogen and testosterone. Pregnenolone can also be turned into progesterone and adrenal hormones. So they can have a powerful effect on the balance of sex hormones, as well adrenal hormones, which are involved in the stress response. Low levels of estrogen, progesterone, and adrenal hormones are all associated with declining memory.

Both DHEA and pregnenolone levels tend to decrease with age, and the simplistic view is that supplementing them will stop the aging process. The trouble is, having more than you need means the body has to work hard to get rid of the excess. For these hormones, more is not necessarily better. While potentially useful for those with adrenal exhaustion, blood sugar problems, and hormonal imbalances, they are not recommended for supplementation except under the guidance of a health practitioner. Before and after tests should be carried out to determine whether or not there is a deficiency, in which case correcting it is likely to improve mental functioning. The older you are, the more likely you are to have low levels of DHEA and pregnenolone. For this reason, many older people in the United States supplement up to 25 mg of pregnenolone or 15 mg of DHEA a day. More than this is unwise without proper testing. DHEA and pregnenolone should be taken in the morning, before breakfast.

Melatonin became famous as the answer to jet lag. It is a hormone produced by the pineal gland, the master gland of the endocrine system,

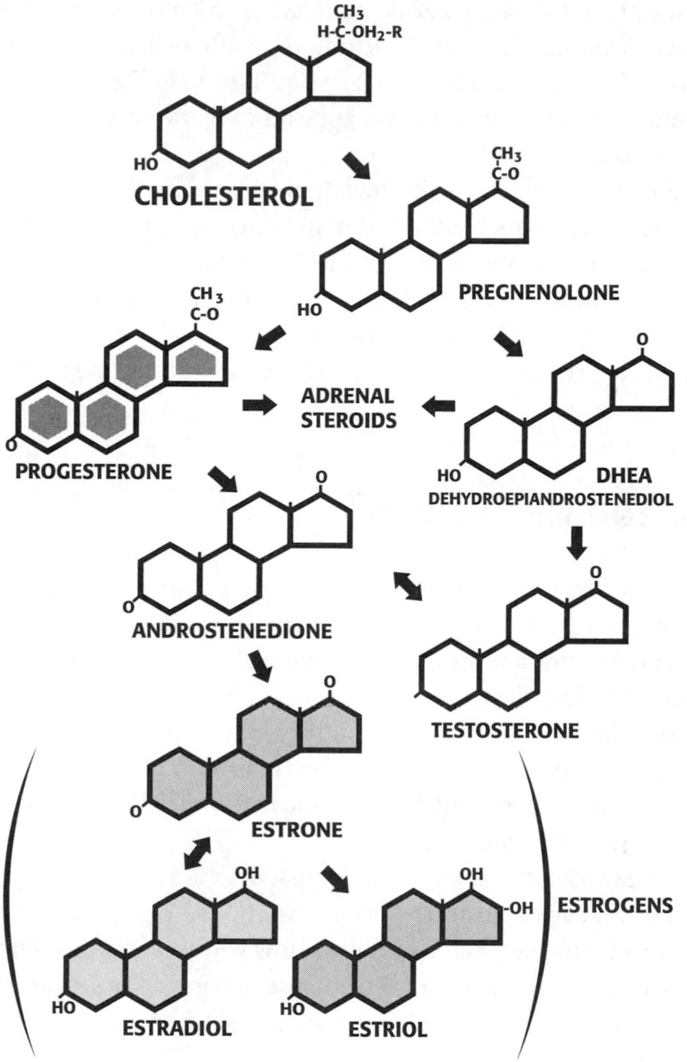

Fig 32   The Hormone Family Tree

which conducts the orchestra of other hormone-producing glands that control blood sugar levels, stress reactions, sex hormones, calcium balance, and other critical processes in the body.

The pineal gland also acts as a biological clock, secreting melatonin during the night. Long-distance traveling upsets this system and can result in jet lag symptoms—fatigue, fuzzy thinking, insomnia, and headaches. By taking melatonin in the evening in the new time zone, many people experience a substantial reduction in these symptoms.[57] More controversial is the recommendation to take melatonin for depression, for memory enhancement, or for extending lifespan. Given at the wrong time of day it can worsen mental functioning, creating the equivalent of jet lag. Taken at night it tends to promote calmness and sleep. However, it appears to work only if you have low levels of melatonin.[58][59]

Of all the smart hormones, it's melatonin I recommend using with the most caution, except possibly for seasonally affected depression (SAD) and short-term use in correcting jet lag. In these situations, 1.5–3 mg in the evening may be worth experimenting with, under the guidance of a health practitioner. Some people supplement 25 mg of melatonin a day, in the evening, and report benefits, but this certainly doesn't suit everybody, and I would urge caution.

But Do You Need Them?

As attractive as smart drugs and hormones might seem, my recommendation is not to take them, at least not in the first instance. In many cases, the combination of mind- and memory-enhancing nutrients as discussed in the last two chapters, does the trick. However, if these steps alone do not produce the effect you are after, and you suffer from the symptoms described below, you may wish to experiment with the following smart drugs and hormones. I recommend you do so with the guidance of your doctor or a suitably qualified health practitioner.

My recommendation under any circumstance is to start with no more than one smart drug or hormone, at the lower dose (with the exception of piracetam), and build up gradually, noting how you respond, and stopping at the dose that produces the best results for you. Then add others as required. Please check with your doctor before taking any smart drug.

Recommendations for Taking Smart Drugs and Hormones

Symptoms	Smart Drug/Hormone	Daily Dose
Poor memory	Piracetam	2,400–4,800 mg
	Hydergine	3–6 mg
	Pregnenolone	25 mg
	DHEA	15 mg
Poor focus, obsessive and excess thoughts	Dilantin	100–300 mg
Lack of brain energy, mental slowdown	Deprynyl	1–10 mg
	Pregnenolone	25 mg
	DHEA	15 mg
Pronounced memory loss, dementia	*Huperzia serrata*	200 mcg
	Hydergine	9 mg
	Piracetam	4,800 mg
	Pregnenolone	25 mg
	DHEA	15 mg
Alzheimer's disease	Deprynyl	10 mg
	Huperzia serrata	200 mcg
	Piracetam	4,800 mg
	Pregnenolone	25 mg
	DHEA	15 mg

PART 8

Action Plan for Mental Health

FINDING HELP

The maxim that ricochets throughout this book is "Treat the cause, not the symptom." Most drug treatments fail to do this. Major tranquilizers may sedate a person to the point where he or she is less of a problem to themselves or others, but they're not addressing the cause. The same can be said for anti-depressants. If you are depressed because your serotonin levels are low, then the causes of this need to be addressed.

Treating the cause, not the symptoms, is easier to say than do, especially in the area of mental health. Often there are many causes. And often there are subtle interplays between psychological problems and physical/chemical problems. A psychological problem can change our behaviour around nourishing ourselves, or misusing mind-altering substances, leading to a chemical imbalance in the brain that makes the psychological problem worse.

I never cease to be amazed at the mind-body link, at what the body says about our minds. The person with backache who needs to stand up for himself. A person with sinus problems who can't breathe, and needs to make space in his or her life for him/herself. A person with digestive problems who is fed up with his or her life and job.

Digging a bit deeper, there's the subject of this book—how our nutrition and biochemical imbalances affect how we think and feel. Depression, anxiety, and memory problems are all linked to what we eat. But, of course, the link isn't obvious. Often it's only after years of faulty nutrition that mental health symptoms emerge.

That's why I strongly recommend that anyone with mental health issues both see a professional nutritionist or doctor specializing in this area, who can assess all the possible underlying physical/chemical causes, and a professional psychotherapist who can delve into underlying psychological issues that may have a bearing on how you think and feel. Rarely can one person be a master of both domains. If you are suffering from a more serious mental health problem, you will also be seeing a doctor or psychiatrist. This is your team to help you get back on the road, firing on all cylinders. And as you've seen here, there are many thousands of people with a vast range of conditions who have managed just that.

Finding a Nutritionist

The good news is that help is widely available throughout Britain and in many other countries. Clinical nutritionists, well qualified to assess these areas of imbalance, are available in most cities and major towns. Since 1984, at the Institute for Optimum Nutrition, we've been training an army of clinical nutritionists who can help you tune up your body and brain so you can experience your full potential. Not all clinical nutritionists or dieticians have experience in the cutting edge of mental health and nutrition, so it's worth asking them if they can help you.

You can find your nearest clinical nutritionist or doctor specializing in this area by visiting www.mentalhealthproject.com. If you don't have access to a computer you can also write to the Mental Health Project, briefly stating your problem, and they will help you find someone suitable (see Useful Addresses, page 360).

Finding a Psychotherapist

Psychotherapists and counselors are also widely available all over the United States. A more extensive level of training is a psychologist, which refers to people with Ph.D., and certified credentials by State Licensing Boards.

There are different types of psychotherapeutic approach. Three often-promising approaches are cognitive-behavior therapy, which helps change the way you think and therefore feel; interpersonal therapy, which works on communication in relationships; and problem-solving therapy, dealing with underlying issues that may be contributing to your issues. Then there's the "transpersonal" approach. This is a conceptual approach to psychological issues that includes the spiritual and therefore considers the deeper "meaning" issues that often underlie chronic depression, anxiety, and schizophrenia. Often, breakdowns are, at one level, spiritual crises and it is good to work with a psychotherapist or counselor who has this level of understanding. See the resources section of the Association for Transpersonal Psychology's website www.atpweb.org.

Most people find therapists through their health-insurance provider, who have lists of certified therapists on their websites. Your doctor may also recommend a therapist. Word of mouth is also important. Ask self-help groups in your area who has experience with your typ4e of problem and gets good ratings from former clients. It is quite normal to have one trial session before committing to a series of appointments. Progress tends to be faster once a person has corrected nutritional imbalances simply because they can think straight and have more energy to change self-defeating patterns of behavior.

Halfway Houses and Hospitals

If you are more seriously in need of help, you may be hospitalized in the short term, then possibly recommended to a number of "halfway houses," often run by local charities.

Hospitals seldom follow the directions of clinical nutritionists. Often, the best strategy for an optimum nutrition program is to have a person's daily supplements packaged into individual sachets and given every day. Sometimes there is resistance to this, which is why your clinical nutritionist must work with your psychiatrist to give you the best possible treatment. What's more, hospital diets usually include wheat, sugar, dairy produce, and large amounts of tea and coffee, none of which are going to aid recovery.

We badly need suitable alternatives to hospitalization. The alternatives may range from halfway houses to treatment in the home under the guidance of a carer and clinical nutritionist. Parents or relatives can also give support in following an optimum nutrition strategy.

Right now there are few options available for halfway houses amenable to administering the optimum nutrition approach. The good news is that there are initiatives in some areas to get such halfway houses set up. The Mental Health Project website (www.mentalhealthproject.com) gives an up-to-date list of what is available.

A halfway house takes years of effort to establish. The usual population of patients at any one time will vary from six to twenty. Plans must be made for proper food, nonallergic housing, daily care and exercise, and discharge of patients. The houses should be organized as a not-for-profit unit and should receive help from government bodies or annual donations from benefactors.

The insurance companies should pay for this care as they do for hospital care, especially since this approach is so much cheaper in the long run, as it helps get people back into the community. Some voluntary help can be used to ease the great financial burden.

I believe the future of mental health care will be best served by having doctors working closely with nutritionists and psychotherapists, with halfway houses offering people a chance to both rebalance their psyche, their body and brain, with healthy eating, exercising, and psychological support. Once achieved, most people can find their way back into the world and lead a meaningful existence.

Chapter 39

THE BRAIN-FRIENDLY DIET
IN A NUTSHELL

The starting point for tuning up your brain is to follow an optimum nutrition diet and take daily supplements. Even if you have no mental health problem as such, this regimen can increase your mental energy, improve your mood, and sharpen your mind. Here are the ten golden rules to follow to make sure your diet is maximizing your mental health:

- Eat whole foods—whole grains, lentils, beans, nuts, seeds, fresh fruit and vegetables—and avoid refined, white, and overcooked foods.

- Eat five or more servings of fruits and vegetables per day. Choose dark green, leafy, and root vegetables such as watercress, carrots, sweet potatoes, broccoli, Brussels sprouts, spinach, green beans, or peppers, raw or lightly cooked. Choose fresh fruit such as apples, pears, berries, melon, or citrus fruit. Have bananas in moderation. Dilute fruit juices, and only eat dried fruits infrequently in small quantities, preferably soaked.

- Eat four or more servings per day of whole grains such as rice, millet, rye, oats, whole wheat, corn, or quinoa as cereal, breads, and pasta.

- Avoid any form of sugar and foods with added sugar.

- Combine protein foods with carbohydrate foods by eating cereals and fruit with nuts or seeds, and ensuring you eat starch foods (potato, bread, pasta, or rice) with fish, lentils, beans, or tofu.

- Eat cold-water carnivorous fish. A serving of herring, mackerel, salmon, or fresh tuna two or three times a week provides a good source of omega-3 fats—or good vegetable protein sources, including beans, lentils, quinoa, tofu (soy), and "seed" vegetables. If eating animal protein, choose lean meat or preferably fish, organic whenever possible.

- Eat eggs—preferably free-range, organic, and high in omega-3s.

- Eat seeds and nuts. The best seeds are flax, hemp, pumpkin, sunflower, and sesame. You get more goodness out of them by grinding them first and sprinkling on cereal, soups, and salads.

- Use cold-pressed seed oils. Choose an oil blend containing flaxseed oil or hemp oil for salad dressings and cold uses, such as drizzling on vegetables, instead of butter.

- Minimize your intake of fried food, processed food, and saturated fat from meat and dairy products.

Chapter 40

BRAIN-FRIENDLY SUPPLEMENTS

The brain uses about a third of all nutrients taken in from food. If you follow the brain-friendly diet described in the last chapter, you will be maximizing your intake of nutrients from your food. In addition, there is great benefit to be had by taking the following supplements on a daily basis to ensure optimum nutrition for your mind.

- Supplement a multivitamin and mineral that gives you at least 25 mg of all the B vitamins, 10 mcg of B_{12}, 100 mcg of folic acid, 200 mg of magnesium, 3 mg of manganese, and 10 mg of zinc.

- Supplement fish oil for omega-3 fats and borage (starflower) or evening primrose oil for omega-6 fats.

- Supplement a brain-food formula providing phosphatidyl choline and phosphatidyl serine, plus other brain-friendly nutrients such as DMAE and pyroglutamate.

- Add a tablespoon of lecithin granules, or a heaping teaspoon of hiPC (phosphatidyl choline) lecithin to your cereal every day.

- Consider supplementing some free-form amino acids, or individual amino acids if you have a related mental health problem.

In addition, you may choose to add the supplemental recommendations in chapters whose content specifically applied to you. Ensure that these recommended amounts of the specified nutrients are included in your daily supplement program. Wherever possible we recommend consultation with a qualified practitioner, who can run the appropriate tests, rather than self-supplementation.

Last Word

This book is about an idea whose time has come. Such ideas tend to go through three stages.

First, the powers that be say it is not true and not important. This denial of the importance of optimum nutrition for the mind was the hallmark of the 1980s, and it only began to be shattered with the advent of our research on vitamins and IQ.

During stage two, they say it's true, but it's not important. That's where we are now. No one in their right mind can deny the overwhelming evidence, presented in this book, that optimizing your nutrient intake can both prevent and reverse mental health problems, as well as improve mental performance and emotional balance.

Finally, they say it's true, and it's important—but it's not new! I can't wait for this day, when children with ADHD are first treated nutritionally and supported psychologically before any stimulant drug is doled out. Or, in fact, the day when schools support children's development with healthy food. I welcome the day when GPs explain the simple diet, supplement, and lifestyle changes that we already know are at least, if not more effective and certainly less dangerous than today's antidepressant drugs. I anticipate the day when those diagnosed with schizophrenia are thoroughly investigated for biochemical imbalances and helped, through personalized nutrition and counseling support, to come back to life, instead of being imprisoned in the chemical straitjacket of the major tranquilizers. I also look forward to the day when the role of nutrition in mental health is on the curriculum of every medical school and every school of psychotherapy.

Humanity as a whole is having a hard time adapting to this extraordinary period of rapid change. The future is coming at us like a freight train. Time is compressing, demands are increasing. We are being stretched to our limits as a species. We need all the help we can get. Optimum nutrition isn't a luxury. It's a necessity if you want to stay healthy and happy and keep your mind intact in the twenty-first century.

Wishing you the best of health.

Patrick Holford

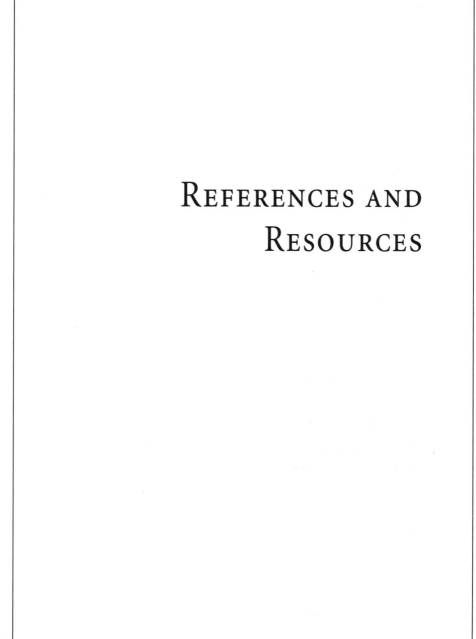

REFERENCES AND RESOURCES

References

Part 1: Food for Thought (Chapters 1–7)

1. World Health Organization, *The World Health Report 2001—Mental Health: New Understanding, New Hope.* See www.who.int/whr/2001/

2. D. Benton and G. Roberts, "Effect of vitamin and mineral supplementation on intelligence of school children," *Lancet,* Vol 1(8578), 1998, pp. 140–3

3. T. H. Crook et al., "Effects of phosphatidylserine in Alzheimer's disease," *Psychopharmacol Bull,* Vol 28, 1992, pp. 61–6

4. Survey by Dr. Bernard Rimland. See www.autism.com/ari

5. C. Birmingham et al., "Controlled trial of zinc supplementation in anorexia nervosa," *Int J Eat Disord,* Vol 15 (3), 1994, pp. 251–5

6. A. Hoffer, "Chronic schizophrenic patients treated ten years or more," *J Orthomolecular Medicine,* Vol 9, 1994, pp. 7–37 and *Vitamin B3 and Schizophrenia: Discovery, Recovery, Controversy,* Quarry Press (2000)

7. W. Poldinger et al., "A functional-dimensional approach to depression: serotonin deficiency and target syndrome in a comparison of 5-hydroxytryptophan and fluvoxamine," *Psychopathology,* Vol 24(2), 1991, pp. 53–81

8. B. Gesch, "Influence of supplementary vitamins, minerals and essential fatty acids on the antisocial behaviour of young adult prisoners," *Brit J Psychiatry,* Vol 181, 2002, pp. 22–8

9. A. Schauss, "Nutrition and behavior: complex interdisciplinary research," *Nutr Health,* Vol 3(1–2), 1984, pp. 9–37

10. D. Benton, "The impact of the supply of glucose to the brain on mood and memory," *Nutr Rev,* Vol 59(1 Pt 2), 2001, p. S20–1

11. R. G. Walton et al., "Adverse reactions to aspartame: double blind challenge in patients from a vulnerable population," *Journal of Biological Psychiatry,* Vol 34(1–2), 1993, pp. 13–7

12. S. E. Carlson et al., "Long-term feeding of formulas high in linolenic acid and marine oil to very low birth weight infants: phospholipid fatty acids," *Pediatr Res*, Vol 30, 1991, pp. 404–12

13. *New Scientist*, 26 June 1995

14. D. O. Rudin, "The major psychoses and neuroses as omega-3 essential fatty acid deficiency syndrome: substrate pellagra," *Biol Psychiatry*, Vol 16(9), 1981, pp. 837–50

15. D. Horrobin, "Essential fatty acids, prostaglandins and schizophrenia," *Proceedings of the World Congress of Psychiatry*, October 1989

16. D. Horrobin et al., "Essential fatty acids in plasma phospholipids in schizophrenia," *Biol Psychiatry*, Vol 25, 1989, pp. 562–8

17. C. Bates et al., "Fatty acids in plasma phospholipids and cholesterol esters from identical twins concordant and discordant for schizophrenia," *Schizophr Res*, Vol 6(1), 1991, pp. 1–7

18. H. Kaiya et al., "Essential and other fatty acids in plasma in schizophrenics and normal individuals from Japan," *Biol Psychiatry*, Vol 30(4), 1991, pp. 357–62

19. K. S. Vaddadi et al., "A double blind trial of essential fatty acid supplementation in patients with tardive dyskensia," *Psychiatric Res*, Vol 27, 1989, pp. 313–23

20. K. S. Vaddadi, "Use of gamma-linolenic acid in the treatment of schizophrenia and tardive dyskinesia," *Prostaglandins Leukot Essent Fatty Acids*, Vol 46(1), 1992, pp. 67–70

21. A. Glen et al., "Essential fatty acids and alcoholism," in D. Horrobin (ed), *Omega-6 Essential Fatty Acids: Pathophysiology and Roles in Clinical Medicine*, Alan Liss (1990), pp. 321–32

22. A. Glen et al., "The role of essential fatty acids in alcohol dependence and tissue damage," *Alcoholism Clin Exp Res*, Vol 11, 1987, pp. 37–41

23. A. Glen et al., "Possible pharmacological approaches to the prevention and treatment of alcohol-related CNS damage: results of a double blind trial of essential fatty acid," in Edwards et al. (eds), *Pharmacological Treatments for Alcoholism*, Croon Helm (1985), pp. 331–50

24. Skinner et al., "Repeated automated assessment of abstinent male alcoholics: essential fatty acid supplementation and age effects," *Alcohol Alcoholism*, Vol 24, 1989, pp. 129–139

25. A. Glen et al., "Essential fatty acids in the treatment of the alcohol dependence syndrome," in Birch and Lindlay (eds), *Alcoholic Beverages*, Elsevier (1985), pp. 203–21

26. F. M. Corrigan et al., "Essential fatty acids in Alzheimer's disease," *Ann N Y Acad Sci*, Vol 640, 1991, pp. 250–2

27. G. Pyapali et al., "Prenatal dietary choline supplementation," *Journal of Neurophysiology*, Vol 79(4), pp. 1790–6 and W. H. Meck et al., *Neuroreport*, Vol 8, 1998, 1997, pp. 2831–5

28. T. Crook et al., "Effects of phosphatidyl serine in age-associated memory impairment," *Neurology*, Vol 41(5), 1991, pp. 644–9

29. R. Alfin-Slater, reported at the International Congress of Nutrition in Kyoto, Japan, 1975

30. S. Y. Chung et al., "Administration of phosphatidylcholine increases brain acetylcholine concentration and improves memory in mice with dementia," *J Nutr*, Vol 125(6), 1995, pp. 1484–9

31. R. J. Wurtman and S. H. Zeisel, "Brain choline: its sources and effects on the synthesis and release of acetylcholine," *Aging*, Vol 19, 1982, pp. 303–13

32. D. J. Canty and S. H. Zeisel, "Lecithin and choline in human health and disease," *Nutr Rev*, Vol 52(10), 1994, pp. 327–39

33. S. Suzuki et al., "Oral administration of soybean lecithin transphosphatidylated phosphatidylserine improves memory impairment in aged rats," *J Nutr*, Vol 131(11), 2001, pp. 2951–6

34. T. H. Crook et al., "Effects of phosphatidylserine in Alzheimer's disease," 1992

35. J. Gindin et al., "The effect of plant phosphatidylserine on age-associated memory impairment and mood in the functioning elderly," Geriatric Institute for Education and Research, and Dept of Geriatrics, Kaplan Hospital, Rhovot, Israel (1995)

36. M. Maggioni et al., " Effects of phosphatidylserine therapy in geriatric subjects with depressive disorders," *Acta Psychiatr Scand*, Vol 81, 1990, pp. 265–70

37. W. Poldinger et al., "A functional-dimensional approach to depression: serotonin deficiency and target syndrome in a comparison of 5-hydroxytryptophan and fluvoxamine," 1991

38. J.B. Deijen et al., "Tyrosine improves cognitive performance and reduces blood pressure in cadets," *Brain Research Bulletin*, Vol 48 (2), 1999, pp. 203–9

39. I. S. Shiah and N. Yatham, "GABA functions in mood disorders: an update and critical review," *Nature Life Sciences*, Vol. 63(15) 1998, pp. 1289–1303

40. K. A. Smith et al, "Relapse of depression after rapid depletion of tryptophan," *Lancet*, Vol. 349, pp. 915–19

41. J.B. Deijen et al., "Tyrosine improves cognitive performance and reduces blood pressure in cadets," 1999

42. D. Benton and G. Roberts, "Effect of vitamin and mineral supplementation on intelligence of school children," *Lancet*, Vol 1(8578), 1998, pp. 140–3

43. A. Lucas, R. Morley, and T. Cole, "Randomised trial of early diet in preterm babies and later intelligence quotient," *BMJ*, Vol 317, 28 November 1998, pp. 1481–7

44. D. Benton et al., "The impact of long-term vitamin supplementation on cognitive functioning," *Psychopharmacology (Berl)*, Vol 117(3), 1995, pp. 298–305

45. D. Benton et al., "Thiamine supplementation mood and cognitive functioning," *Psychopharmacology (Berl)*, Vol 129(1), 1997, pp. 66–71

46. S. Loriaux et al., *Psychopharmacology*, Vol 87, 1985, pp. 390–5

47. G. Shor-Posner et al., "Impact of vitamin B_6 status on psychological distress in a longitudinal study of HIV-1 infection," *Int J Psychiatry Med*, Vol 24(3), 1994, pp. 209–22

48. P. Godfrey et al., *Lancet*, Aug 18, 1990, pp. 392–5

49. M. Carney, "Serum folate values in 423 psychiatric patients," *Brit Med Journal*, Vol 4, 1967, pp. 512–16

50. R. Carmel et al., "The frequently low cobalamin levels in dementia usually signify treatable metabolic, neurologic and electrophysiologic abnormalities," *Eur J Haemotol*, Vol 54(4), 1995, pp. 245–53

51. Swiecicki et al., *Psychiatria Polska*, Vol 26(5), 1992, pp. 399–409

52. M. Louwman et al., "Signs of impaired cognitive function in adolescents with marginal cobalamin status," *Am J Clin Nutr*, Vol 72, 2000, pp. 762–9

53. J. Greenblatt et al., *Progress in Neuro-Psychopharmacology and Biological Psychiatry*, Vol 18(4), 1994, pp. 647–60

54. G. Milner, *Brit J Psychiat*, Vol 109, 1963, pp. 294–9

55. K. Suboticanec et al., "Vitamin C status in chronic schizophrenia," *Biol Psychiatry*, Vol 28, 1990, pp. 959–66

56. H. Vandercamp, *Int J Neuropsychiatry*, 22 July 1965
57. P. Alexander, "Serum calcium and magnesium in schizophrenia: relationship to clinical phenomena and neuroleptic treatment," *Br J Psychiatry*, Vol 133, 1978, pp. 143–9
58. C. Pfeiffer and B. Barnes, *International Journal Environmental Studies*, Vol 17, 1981, pp. 43–7
59. C. Pfeiffer and D. Bacchi, "Copper, zinc, manganese, niacin and pyridoxine in the schizophrenias," *Journal of Applied Nutrition*, Vol 27(223), 1975, pp. 9–39
60. B. Aston, *Orthomolecular Psychiatry*, Vol 9, 1980, pp. 237–49

Part 2: Protecting Your Brain (Chapters 8–11)

1. S. Johnson, "Micronutrient accumulation and depletion in schizophrenia, epilepsy, autism and Parkinson's disease?," *Med Hypotheses*, Vol 56(5), 2002, pp. 641–5
2. S. Beratis et al., 2001, "Factors affecting smoking in schizophrenia," *Compr Psychiatry*,Vol 42(5), pp. 393–402
3. Z. Xu et al., "Fetal and adolescent nicotine administration: effects on CNS serotonergic systems," *Brain Res*, Vol 914(1/2), 2001, pp. 166–78
4. A. Corvin et al., "Cigarette smoking and psychotic symptoms in bipolar affective disorder," *British Journal of Psychiatry*, Vol 179, 2001, pp. 35–8
5. M. Ramirez-Lassepas "Stroke and the aging of the brain and the arteries," *Geriatrics*, Vol 53 Suppl 1, 1998, S44–8
6. A. J. Perkins et al., "Association of antioxidants with memory in a multiethnic elderly sample using the Third National Health and Nutrition Examination Survey," *Am J Epidemiol*, Vol 150(1), 1999, pp. 37–44
7. W. J. Perrig et al., "The relation between antioxidants and memory performance in the old and very old," *J Am Geriatr Soc*, Vol 45(6), 1997, pp. 718–24
8. R. T. Matthews et al., "Coenzyme Q_{10} administration increases brain mitochondrial concentrations and exerts neuroprotective effects," *Proc Natl Acad Sci*, Vol 95(15), 1998, pp. 8892–7
9. C. W. Shults et al., "Coenzyme Q_{10} levels correlate with the activities of complexes I and II/III in mitochondria from parkinsonian and nonparkinsonian subjects," *Ann Neurol*, Vol 42(2), 1997, pp. 261–4
10. S. N. Mattson et al., "Teratogenic effects of alcohol on brain and behaviour," *Alcohol Res Health*, Vol 25(3), 2001, pp. 185–91
11. R. M. Sapolsky, "Why stress is bad for your brain," *Science*, Vol 273(5276), 1996, pp. 749–50
12. J. D. Bremner, "Does stress damage the brain?," *Biol Psychiatry*, Vol 45(7), 1999, pp. 797–805
13. C. Kirschbaum et al., "Stress- and treatment-induced elevations of cortisol levels associated with impaired declarative memory in healthy adults," *Life Sci*, Vol 58(17), 1996, pp. 1475–83
14. J. W. Newcomer et al., "Decreased memory performance in healthy humans induced by stress-level cortisol treatment," *Arch Gen Psychiatry*, Vol 56(6), 1999, pp. 527–33
15. F. Giubilei et al., 2001, "Altered circadian cortisol secretion in Alzheimer's disease: clinical and neuroradiological aspects," *J Neurosci Res*, Vol 66(2), 2001, pp. 262–5
16. L. E. Carlson et al., "Relationships between dehydroepiandrosterone sulfate (DHEAS)

and cortisol (CRT) plasma levels and everyday memory in Alzheimer's disease patients compared to healthy controls," *Horm Behav* 35(3), 1999, pp. 254–63

17. O. M. Wolkowitz et al., "Dehydroepiandrosterone (DHEA) treatment of depression," *Biol Psychiatry*, Vol 41(3), 1997, pp. 311–8

18. A. G. Schauss, "Nutrition and behavior," *Journal of Applied Nutrition*, Vol 35(1), 1983, pp. 30–35 and MIT Conference Proceedings on Research Strategies for Assessing the Behavioural Effects of Foods and Nutrients, 1982

19. D. Benton et al., "Mild hypoglycaemia and questionnaire measures of aggression," *Biol Psychol*, Vol 14(1–2), 1982, pp. 129–35

20. A. Roy et al., "Monoamines, glucose metabolism, aggression toward self and others," *Int J Neurosci*, Vol 41(3–4), 1988, pp. 261–4

21. A. G. Schauss, *Diet, Crime and Delinquency*, Parker House (1980)

22. M. Virkkunen, "Reactive hypoglycaemic tendency among arsonists," *Acta Psychiatr Scand*, Vol 69(5), 1984, pp. 445–52

23. M. Virkkunen and S. Narvanen, "Tryptophan and serotonin levels during the glucose tolerance test among habitually violent and impulsive offenders," *Neuropsychobiology*, Vol 17(1–2), 1987, pp. 19–23

24. J. Yaryura-Tobias and F. Neziroglu F, "Violent behaviour, brain dysrhythmia and glucose dysfunction. A new syndrome," *J Ortho Psych*, Vol 4, 1975, pp. 182–5

25. M. Bruce and M. Lader, "Caffeine abstention and the management of anxiety disorders," *Psychol Med*, Vol 19, 1989, pp. 211–14

26. W. Wendel and W. Beebe, "Glycolytic activity in schizophrenia," in *Orthomolecular Psychiatry, treatment of schizophrenia*, (eds) D. Hawkins and L. Pauling (1973), W. H. Freeman, San Francisco

27. R. Prinz and D. Riddle, "Associations between nutrition and behaviour in 5 year old children," *Nutr Rev*, Vol 43, suppl., 1986

28. L. Christensen, "Psychological distress and diet—effects of sucrose and caffeine," *J Appl Nutr*, Vol 40(1), 1988, pp. 44–50

29. D. Fullerton et al., "Sugar, opionoids and binge eating," *Brain Res Bull*, Vol 14(6), 1985, pp. 273–80

30. L. Christensen, "Psychological distress and diet"

31. M. Colgan and L. Colgan L, "Do nutrient supplements and dietary changes affect learning and emotional reactions of children with learning difficulties? A controlled series of 16 cases," *Nutr Health*, Vol 3, 1984, pp. 69–77

32. J. Goldman et al., "Behavioural effects of sucrose on preschool children," *J Abnormal Child Psychol*, Vol 14(4), 1986, pp. 565–77

33. M. Lester et al., "Refined carbohydrate intake, hair cadmium levels and cognitive functioning in children," *Nutr Behav*, Vol 1, 1982, pp. 3–13

34. S. Schoenthaler et al., "The impact of low food additive and sucrose diet on academic performance in 803 New York City public schools," *Int J Biosocial Research*, Vol 8(2), 1986, pp. 185–95

35. F. G. Epstein, "Mechanisms of disease," *N Eng J Med*, Vol 334(6), 1996, pp. 374–381

36. N. J. Richardson, P. J. Rogers et al., "Mood and performance effects of caffeine in relation to acute and chronic caffeine deprivation," *Pharmacology, Biochemistry and Behavior*, Vol 52(2), 1995, pp. 313–320

37. K. Gilliland and D. Andress, "Ad lib caffeine consumption, symptoms of caffeinism,

and academic performance," *American Journal of Psychiatry*, Vol 138(4), 1981, pp. 512–4

38. See full references at http://www.doctoryourself.com/caffeine_allergy.html

39. S. Davies, Editorial, *J Nut Med*, Vol 2(3), 1991, pp. 227–247

40. C. Patterson, *An Alternative Perspective—Lead Pollution in the Environment*, Commission of Natural Resources Research Council, US National Acadamy of Sciences (1980)

41. H. L. Needleman and C. A. Gatsonis, "Low level lead exposure and the IQ of children," *JAMA*, Vol 263(5), 1990, pp. 673–78

42. Q. Yule and R. Lansdown et al., "The relationship between blood lead concentrations, intelligence and attainment in a school population: a pilot study," *Dev Med Child Neurol*, Vol 23(5), 1981, pp. 567–76

43. G. Winneke, "Neuropsychological studies in children with elevated tooth-lead concentrations. I. Pilot study," *Int Arch Occup Environ Health*, Vol 51(2), 1982, pp. 169–83

44. H. L. Needleman et al., "The long-term effects of exposure to low doses of lead in childhood. An 11-year follow-up report," *N Engl J Med*, Vol 332, 1990, pp. 83–8

45. P. Holford and C. Pfeiffer, *Mental Health and Mental Illness—The Nutrition Connection*, ION Press (1996). Also see www.mentalhealthproject/features for feature on copper and schizophrenia

46. S. Davies et al., "Age-related decreases in chromium levels in 51,665 hair, sweat, and serum samples from 40,872 patients—implications for the prevention of cardiovascular disease and type II diabetes mellitus," *Metabolism*, Vol 46(5), 1997, pp. 469–73, and unpublished data on toxic element accumulation with age

47. R. Goyer, "Nutrition and metal toxicity," *Am J Clin Nutr*, Vol 61 (3Suppl), 1995, pp. 646S–650S

48. R. Goyer and M. G. Cherian, "Ascorbic acid and EDTA treatment of lead toxicity in rats," *Life Sci*, Vol 24(5), 1979, pp. 433–8

49. E. J. O'Flaherty, "Modeling normal aging bone loss, with consideration of bone loss in osteoporosis," *Toxicol Sci*, Vol 55(1), 2000, pp. 171–88

50. N. I. Ward et al., *J Nutr Med*, Vol 10, 1990, pp. 415–31

51. T. Randolph, "Allergy as a causative factor of fatigue, irritability and behaviour problems of children," *J Pediatr*, Vol 31, 1947, p. 560

52. A. Rowe, "Allergic toxemia and fatigue," *Ann Allergy*, Vol 17, 1959, p. 9

53. F. Speer, ed., "Etiology: Foods," in *Allergy of the Nervous System*, Charles Thomas (1970)

54. M. Campbell, "Neurologic manifestations of allergic disease," *Ann Allergy*, Vol 31, 1973, p. 485

55. K. Hall, "Allergy of the nervous system: a review," *Annals of Allergy*, Vol 36, 1976, pp. 49–64

56. V. Pippere, "Some varieties of food intolerance in psychiatric patients," *Nutr Health*, Vol 3(3), 1984, pp. 125–136

57. C. Pfeiffer and P. Holford, *Mental Illness and Schizophrenia: The Nutrition Connection*, Thorsons (1989)

58. T. Tuormaa, *An Alternative to Psychiatry*, The Book Guild (1991)

59. J. Egger et al., "Controlled trial of oligoantigenic treatment in the hyperkinetic syndrome," the *Lancet*, 9 March 1985, pp. 540–5

60. J. Egger et al., "Is migraine a food allergy? A double-blind controlled trial of oligoanti-

genic diet treatment," *Lancet*, 15 October 1983, pp. 865–9

61. W. Philpott and D. Kalita, *Brain Allergies*, Keats Publishing (1980)

62. D. S. King, "Can allergic exposure provoke psychological symptoms? A double-blind test," *Biol Psychiatry* 16(1), 1981, pp. 3–19

63. B. Feingold, "Dietary management of behavior and learning disabilities," in *Nutrition and Behavior*, S. A. Miller (ed), Franklin Institute Press, (1981), p. 37

64. J. McGovern et al., *Ann Allergy*, Vol 47, 1981, p. 123

65. E. Young et al., "A population study of food intolerance," *Lancet*, Vol 343, 1994, pp. 1127–9

66. British Society for Allergy and Environmental Medicine, *Effective Allergy Practice*, (1984)

67. National Dairy Council, *Adverse Reactions to Food: Topical Update* (1994). Available from the National Dairy Council, 5–7 John Princes Street, London W1M 0AP

68. M. Hadjivassilou, "Idiopathic cerebellar ataxia associated with celia disease," *Neurology*, Vol 56, 1991, pp. 385–8

Part 3: Improving Your IQ, Memory, and Mood (Chapters 12–17)

1. A. L. Kubala and M. M. Katz, "Nutritional factors in psychological test behaviour," *J Genet Psychol*, Vol 96, 1960, pp. 343–52

2. D. Benton and G. Roberts G, "Effect of vitamin and mineral supplementation on intelligence of school children," *Lancet*, Vol 1(8578), 1988, pp. 140–3

3. S. J. Schoenthaler et al., "Controlled trial of vitamin-mineral supplementation: Effects on intelligence and performance," *Person Individ Diff*, Vol 12(4), 1991, pp. 351–2

4. M. Nelson et al., "Nutrient intakes, vitamin-mineral supplementation and intelligence in British schoolchildren," *Br J Nutr*, Vol 64(1), 1990, pp. 13–22

5. D. Benton et al., "The impact of long-term vitamin supplementation on cognitive functioning," *Psychopharmacology (Berl)*, Vol 117(3), 1995, pp. 298–305

6. W. Snowden, *Person Individ Diff*, Vol 22(1), 1997, pp. 131–4

7. P. Willatts et al., "Effect of long-chain polyunsaturated fatty acids in infant formula on problem solving at 10 months of age," *Lancet*, Vol 352(9129), 1998, pp. 688–91

8. C. Agostoni et al., "Developmental quotient at 24 months and fatty acid composition of diet in early infancy: a follow up study," *Arch Dis Child*, Vol 76(5), 1997, pp. 421–4

9. L. Horwood et al., *Pediatrics*, Vol 101, January 1998, pp. 1–13

10. C. Lanting et al., *Lancet*, Vol 344(13), 12 Nov 1994, pp. 9–22

11. D. Benton et al., "Mild hypoglycaemia and questionnaire measures of aggression," *Biol Psychol*, Vol 14(1–2), 1982, pp. 129–35

12. M. Colgan L. Colgan, "Do nutrient supplements and dietary changes affect learning and emotional reactions of children with learning difficulties? A controlled series of 16 cases," *Nutr Health*, Vol 3, 1984, pp. 69–77

13. J. Goldman et al., "Behavioural effects of sucrose on preschool children," *J Abnormal Child Psychol*, Vol 14(4), 1986, pp. 565–77

14. M. Lester et al., "Refined carbohydrate intake, hair cadmium levels and cognitive functioning in children," *Nutr Behav*, Vol 1, 1982, pp. 3–13

15. S. Schoentahler et al., "The impact of a low food additive and sucrose diet on academic performance in 803 New York City public schools," *Int J Biosocial Res*, Vol 8(2), 1986, pp. 185–95

16. C. S. Wallace, W. T. Greenough et al., "Increases in dendritic length in occipital cortex after 4 days of differential housing in weanling rats," *Behav Neural Biol*, Vol 58(1), 1992, pp. 64–8

17. R. M. Sapolsky, "Why stress is bad for your brain," *Science*, Vol 273(5276), 1996, pp. 749–50

18. J. P. Jones, H. S. Swartzwelder et al., "Choline availability to the developing rat fetus alters adult hippocampal long-term potentiation," *Brain Res Dev Brain Res*, Vol 118 (1–2), 1999, pp. 159–67

19. F. Safford and G. I. Krell (eds), *Gerontology for Health Professionals: A practice guide*, NASW Press (1997), p. 282

20. S. L. Ladd et al., "Effect of phosphatidylcholine on explicit memory," *Clin Neuropharmacol*, Vol 16(6), 1993, pp. 540–9

21. W. Dimpfel et al., "Source density analysis of functional topographical EEG: monitoring of cognitive drug action," *European Journal of Medical Research*, Vol 1(6), 1996, pp. 283–90

22. Cases published in Ward Dean, John Morgenthaler and Steven Fowkes, *Smart Drugs II: The next generation*, Smart Publications (1993), reproduced with their kind permission

23. T. H. Crook et al., "Effects of phosphatidylserine in Alzheimer's disease," *Psychopharmacol Bull*, Vol 28, 1992, pp. 61–66

24. H. Pilch and W. E. Muller, "Piracetam elevates muscarinic cholinergic receptor density in the frontal cortex of aged but not of young mice," *Psychopharmacology*, Vol 94(1), 1988, pp. 74–8

25. D. Ward and J. Morgenthaler, *Smart Drugs and Nutrients*, B&J Publications, 1990, pp. 42–3

26. S. Grioli et al., "Pyroglutamic acid improves the age associated memory impairment," *Fundam Clin Pharmacol*, Vol 4(2), 1990, pp. 169–73

27. Judy Shabert et al., *The Ultimate Nutrient—Glutamine*, Avery Publications (1990)

28. T. Ziegler et al., "Safety and metabolic effects of L-glutamine administration in humans," *J Parenter Enteral Nutr*, Vol 14(4supp), 1990, pp. 137S–146S

29. L. Young et al., "Patients receiving glutamine-supplemented intravenous feedings report an improvement in mood," *J Parenter Enteral Nutr*, Vol 17, 1993, pp. 422–7

30. J. Liu, T. M. Hagen, B. N. Ames et al., "Memory loss in old rats is associated with brain mitochondrial decay and RNA/DNA oxidation: Partial reversal by feeding acetyl-L-carnitine and/or R-alpha-lipoic acid," *Proc Natl Acad Sci U S*, Vol 99(4), 2002, pp. 2356–61

31. J. Kleijnin and P. Knipschild, "Ginkgo biloba," *Lancet*, Vol 340(8828), 1992, pp. 1136–9

32. P. L. Le Bars, "A placebo-controlled, double-blind, randomised trial on an extract of Ginkgo Biloba for dementia," *JAMA*, Vol 278(16), 1997, pp. 1327–32

33. I. Hindmarch et al., "Efficacy and tolerance of vinpocetine in ambulant patients suffering from mild to moderate organic psychosyndromes," *Int Clin Psychopharmacol*, Vol 6(1), 1991, pp. 31–43

34. R. Balestreri et al., "A double-blind placebo controlled evaluation of the safety and efficacy of vinpocetine in the treatment of patients with chronic vascular senile cerebral dysfunction," *J Am Geriatr Soc*, Vol 35(5), 1987, pp. 425–30

35. Z. Subhan and I. Hindmarch, "Psychopharmacological effects of vinpocetine in normal healthy volunteers," *Eur J Clin Pharmacol*, Vol 28(5), 1985, pp. 567–71

36. S. M. Loriaux et al., "The effects of nicotinic acid and xanthinol nicotinate on human memory in different categories of age. A double blind study," *Psychopharmacology (Berl)*, Vol 87(4), 1985, pp. 390–5

37. H. L. Newbold, *Meganutrients for Your Nerves*, Berkeley Books (1985)

38. S. Tsujimaru et al., "Vitamin B12 accelerates re-entrainment of activity rhythms in rats," *Life Sci*, Vol 50(24), 1992, pp. 1843–50

39. R. T. Bartus et al., "Profound effects of combining choline and piracetam on memory enhancement and cholinergic function in aged rats," *Neurobiology of Aging 2*, 1981, pp.105–111

40. S. Ferris et al., "Combination of choline/piracetam in the treatment of senile dementia," *Psychopharmacology Bulletin*, Vol 18, 1982, pp. 94–8

41. P. S. Godfrey et al., "Enhancement of recovery from psychiatric illness by methylfolate," *Lancet*, Vol 336, 1990, pp. 392–395

42. G. Milner, "Ascorbic acid in chronic psychiatric patients: A controlled trial," *Brit J Psychiat*, Vol 109, 1963, pp. 294–9

43. R. Jaffe and O. Kruesi, "The biochemical-immunology window: a molecular view of psychiatric case management," *Int Clin Nut Rev*, Vol 12(1), 1992, pp. 9–26

44. A. Dubini et al., "Do noradrenaline & serotonin differentially affect social motivation and behaviour?," *European Neuropsychopharmacology*, Vol 7(Suppl), 1997, pp. S49–S55

45. G. R. Heninger, "Serotonin, sex, psychiatric illness," *Proc Natl Acad Sci*, Vol 94 (4), 1997, pp. 823–4

46. K. A. Smith et al., "Relapse of depression after rapid depletion of tryptophan," *Lancet*, Vol 349, 1997, pp. 915–9

47. J. Shepherd, "Effects of oestrogen on cognition, mood and degenerative brain diseases," *J Am Pharm Assoc (Wash)*, Vol 41(2), 2001, pp. 221–8

48. K. A. Smith et al., "Relapse of depression after rapid depletion of tryptophan," *Lancet*, Vol 349, 1997, pp. 915–9

49. R. Wurtman and J. Wurtman, "Carbohydrates and depression," *Scientific American*, Vol 260(1), 1989, pp. 68–75

50. I. von Sano, "L-5-Hydroxytryptophan (L-5-HTP) therapie," *Folia Psychiatrica et Neurologica Japonica*, Vol 26(1), 1972, pp. 7–17

51. T. Nakajima et al., "Clinical evaluation of 5-Hydroxytryptophan as an antidepressant," *Folia Pychiatrica et Neurologica*, Vol 32(2), 1978, pp. 225ff

52. W. Poldinger et al., "A functional-dimensional approach to depression: serotonin deficiency and target syndrome in a comparison of 5-hydroxytryptophan and fluvoxamine," *Psychopathology*, Vol 24(2), 1991, pp. 53–81

53. A. Woggon and J. Schoef, "The treatment of depression with L-5-Hydroxytryptophan versus Imipramine," *Arch Psychiat Nervenkr*, Vol 224, 1977, pp. 175–186

54. T. Nakajima et al., "Clinical evaluation of 5-Hydroxy-L-Tryptophan as an antidepressant drug," *Folia Psychiatrisa et Neurologica Japonica*, Vol 32(2), 1978, pp. 223–230; H. M. van Praag et al., "A pilot study of the predictive value of the probnecid test in application of 5-Hydroxytryptophan as antidepressant," *Psychopharmacologica (Berl)*, Vol 25, 1972, pp. 14–21; M. Kaneko et al., "L-5-HTP treatment and serum 5-HT level after L-5-HTP loading on depressed patients," *Neuropsychobiology*, Vol 5, 1979, p232–240; L. J. van Heile, "L-5-Hydroxytryptophan in depression: the first substitution therapy in psychiatry?," *Neuropsychobiology*, Vol 6, 1980, pp. 230–40; and I. von Sano, "L-5-

Hydroxytryptophan (L-5-HTP) therapie," *Folia Psychiatrica et Neurologica Japonica,* Vol 26(1), 1972, pp. 7–17

55. H. Beckmann et al., "DL-phenylalanine versus imipramine: a double-blind controlled study," *Arch Psychiatr Nervenkr,* Vol 227(1), 1979, pp. 49–58

56. H. C. Sabelli et al., "Clinical studies on the phenylethylamine hypothesis of affective disorder: urine and blood phenylacetic acid and phenylalanine dietary supplements," *J Clin Psychiatry,* Vol (2), 1986, pp. 66–70

57. J. Mouret et al., "L-tyrosine cures, immediate and long term, dopamine-dependent depressions. Clinical and polygraphic studies," *C R Acad Sci III,* Vol 306(3), 1988, pp. 93–8 (in French)

58. J. B. Deijen et al., "Tyrosine improves cognitive performance and reduces blood pressure in cadets after one week of a combat training course," *Brain Research Bulletin,* Vol 48(2), 1999, pp. 203–9

59. H. Cass, "SAMe—the master tuner supplement for the 21st century," published on www.naturallyhigh.co.uk (2001)

60. B. L. Kagan et al., "Oral S-adenosylmethionine in depression: a randomized, double-blind, placebo-controlled trial," *Am J Psychiatry,* Vol 147(5), 1990, pp. 591–5

61. P. G. Janicak et al., "Parenteral S-adenosyl-methionine (SAMe) in depression: literature review and preliminary data," *Psychopharmacol Bull,* Vol 25(2), 1989, pp. 238–42

62. G. M. Bressa, "S-adenosyl-methionine as antidepressant: meta-analysis of clinical studies," *Acta Neurologica Scandinavian,* Vol 154(supp), 1994, pp. 7–14

63. J. R. Hibbeln, "Fish consumption and major depression," *Lancet,* Vol 351, 1998, pp. 1213

64. B. Nemets et al., "Addition of omega-3 fatty acid to maintenance medication treatment for recurrent unipolar depressive disorder," *Am J Psychiatry,* Vol 159, 2002, pp. 477–9

65. B. Puri et al., "Eicosapentaenoic acid in treatment-resistant depression," Letters to the Editor, *Archives of General Psychiatry,* Vol 59(1), 2002

66. G. E. Abraham, "Nutritional factors in the etiology of the premenstrual tension syndromes," *J Reprod Med,* Vol 28(7), 1983, pp. 446–64

67. M. G. Brush, M. Perry, "Pyridoxine and the premenstrual syndrome," *Lancet,* Vol 1(8442), 1985, p.1399

68. G. E. Abraham and M. D. Lubran, "Serum and red cell magnesium levels in patients with premenstrual tension," *Am J Clin Nutr,* Vol 34, 1981, pp. 1264–6

69. A. Nicholas, "Traitement du syndrome premenstrual et de la dysmenorrhee par l'ion magnesium," in J. Durlach (ed), *First Int Sympos on Magnesium Deficiency in Human Pathology,* Springer Verlag, 1983, pp. 261–3

70. D. F. Horrobin, "The role of essential fatty acids and prostaglandins in the pre-menstrual syndrome," *J Reprod Med,* Vol 28(7), 1983, pp. 465–8

71. G. A. Colditz et al., "The use of estrogens and progestins and the risk of breast cancer in postmenopausal women," *N Engl J Med,* Vol 332(24), 1995, pp. 1589–93

72. E. Barrett-Connor et al., "Bioavailable testosterone and depressed mood in older men: the Rancho Bernardo Study," *J Clin Endocrinol Metab,* Vol 84(2), 1999, pp. 573–7

73. O. M. Wolkowitz et al., "Dehydroepiandrosterone (DHEA) treatment of depression," *Biol Psychiatry,* Vol 41(3), 1997, pp. 311–8

74. NOP Poll, May 2001, *Panorama,* BBC, UK: see http://news.bbc.co.uk/hi/english/audiovideo/programmes/panorama/tranquillisers/newsid_1325000/1325909.stm

75. I. S. Shiah and N. Yatham, "GABA functions in mood disorders: An update and critical review," *Life Sciences*, Vol 63(15), 1998, pp. 1289–1303

76. G. Warnecke, "Psychosomatic dysfunctions in the female climacteric: clinical effectiveness and tolerance of kava extract WS 1490," *Fortschr Med*, Vol 109(4), 1991, pp. 119–22

77. H. P. Volz and M. Kieser, "Kava-kava extract WS 1490 versus placebo in anxiety disorders—A randomized placebo-controlled 25-week outpatient trial," *Pharmacopsychiatry*, Vol 30, 1997, pp. 1–5

78. T. F. Munte et al., "Effects of Oxazepam and an extract of kava root (*Piper methysticum*) on event-related potentials in a word-recognition task," *Neuropsychobiology*, Vol 27(1), 1993, pp. 46–53

79. H. Woelk et al., "Double blind study: Kava extract versus benzodiazepines in treatment of patients suffering from anxiety," *Z Allg Med*, Vol 69, 1993, pp. 271–7

80. D. Lindenberg et al., "Kavain in comparison with Oxazepam in anxiety disorders: a double blind study of clinical effectiveness," *Fortschr Med*, Vol 108, 1990, pp. 49–50

81. See www.patrickholford.com/kavaconcerns. For more in-depth information on kava, see Hyla Cass and Terrence McNally, *Kava: Nature's Answer to Stress, Anxiety, and Insomnia*, Prima Publishing (1998)

82. F. N. Pitts and J. N. McClure, "Lactate metabolism in anxiety neurosis," *New Engl J Med*, Vol 277, 1967, pp. 1328–1336

Part 4: What Is Mental Illness? (Chapters 18–21)

1. World Health Organization, *The World Health Report 2001—Mental Health: New Understanding, New Hope*, WHO, 2001. Available at www.who.int/whr/2001/

2. WHO, *The World Health Report 2001*

3. WHO, *The World Health Report 2001*

4. R. Hall et al., "Physical illness manifesting as psychiatric disease," *Arch Gen Psychiatry*, Vol 37, 1980, pp. 989–995

5. British National Formulary, tricyclic antidepressant side effects

6. J. Burne, "Antidepressants and suicide," *Medicine Today*, December 2001. Available at www.medicine-today.co.uk

7. See *Guardian* article "Murder, suicide: A bitter aftertaste for the 'wonder' depression drug" at www.guardian.co.uk/Archive/Article/0,4273,4201752,00.html

8. N. D. Volkow et al., "Therapeutic doses of oral methylphenidate significantly increase extracellular dopamine in the human brain," *J Neuroscience*, Vol 21(RC121), 2001, pp. 1–5

9. J. Baizer, *Annual Meeting of the Society for Neuroscience*, 11 November 2001

10. Department of Health, *Department of Health, UK, Prescription Cost Analysis* (1999)

11. DoH, *Department of Health, UK, Prescription Cost Analysis*

12. M. Lader, "Dependence on benzodiazapenes," *J Clin Psychiatr*, Vol 44, 1983, pp. 121–7

13. See http://news.bbc.co.uk and search under "tranquillisers."

14. A. Sohler and C. Pfeiffer, "A direct method for the determination of manganese in whole blood: patients with seizure activity have low blood levels," *Orthomolecular Psychiatry*, Vol 18, 1979, pp. 275–80

15. L. Adler et al., *Psychopharmacology Bulletin*, Vol 29(3), 1993, pp. 371–4

Part 5: Solving Depression, Manic Depression, and Schizophrenia (Chapters 22–25)

1. A. L. Miller, "St John's Wort: Clinical effects on depression and other conditions," *Alt Med Rev*, Vol 3(1), 1998, pp. 18–26

2. H. Woelk, "Comparison of St John's Wort and imipramine for treating depression: randomised controlled trial," *BMJ*, Vol 321(7260), 2000, pp. 536–539

3. K. Linde, "St John's wort for depression: an overview and meta-analysis of randomised clinical trials," *BMJ*, Vol 313(7052), 1996, pp. 253–8

4. U. Schmidt and H. Sommer, "St. John's wort extract in the ambulatory therapy of depression. Attention and reaction ability are preserved," *Fortschr Med*, Vol 111(19), 1993, pp. 339–42 (in German)

5. S. Bratman, *Beat Depression with St John's Wort*, Prima Publishing (1997)

6. H. Winterhoff et al., Nervenheilkunde 12, 1993, pp. 341–345

7. M. Fava et al., "Folate, vitamin B12 and homocysteine in major depressive disorder," *Am J Pysch*, Vol 154, 1997, pp. 426–8

8. P. S. Godfrey et al., "Enhancement of recovery from psychiatric illness by methylfolate," *Lancet*, Vol 336(8712), 1990, pp. 392–5

9. R. Crellin et al., "Folates and psychiatric disorders. Clinical potential," *Drugs*, Vol 45(5), 1993, pp. 623–636

10. M. Murray, *Encyclopaedia of Natural Supp*, 1996, Prima Pub

11. E. H. Reynolds et al., "Methylation and mood," *Lancet*, Vol 2(8396), 1984, pp. 196–8

12. B. Nemets et al., "Addition of omega-3 fatty acid to maintenance medication treatment for recurrent unipolar depressive disorder," *Am J Psychiatry*, Vol 159, 2002, pp. 477–479

13. J. R. Hibbeln, "Fish consumption and major depression," *Lancet*, Vol 351(9110), 1998, p. 1213

14. E. C. Suarez, "Relations of trait depression and anxiety to low lipid and lipoprotein - concentrations in healthy young adult women," *Psychosom*, Vol 61(3), 1999, pp. 273–9

15. T. Partonen et al., "Association of low serum total cholesterol with major depression and suicide," *British Journal of Psychiatry*, Vol 175, 1999, pp. 259–62

16. F. Dimeo et al., "Benefits from aerobic exercise in patients with major depression: a pilot study," *Br J Sports Med*, Vol 35(2), 2001, pp. 114–7

17. M. Babyak et al., "Exercise treatment for major depression: maintenance of therapeutic benefit at 10 months," *Psychosom Med*, Vol 62(5), 2000, pp. 633–8

18. D. Kritz-Silverstein et al., "Cross-sectional and prospective study of exercise and depressed mood in the elderly: the Rancho Bernardo study," *Am J Epidemiol*, Vol 153(6), 2001, pp. 596–603

19. A. Corvin et al., "Cigarette smoking and psychotic symptoms in bipolar affective disorder," *British Journal of Psychiatry*, Vol 179, 2001, pp. 35–38

20. G. N. Schrauzer et al., "Lithium in scalp hair of adults, students and violent criminals. Effects of supplementation and evidence for interactions of lithium with vitamin B_{12} and with other trace elements," *Biol Trace Elem Res*, Vol 34(2), 1992, pp. 161–76

21. A. Coppen et al., "Plasma folate and affective morbidity during long-term lithium therapy," *Br J Psychiatry*, Vol 141, 1982, pp. 87–9

22. A. L. Stoll et al., "Omega 3 fatty acids in bipolar disorder: a preliminary double-blind, placebo-controlled trial," *Arch Gen Psychiatry*, Vol 56(5), 1999, pp. 407–12

23. G. Chouinard et al., "A pilot study of magnesium hydrochloride (Magnesiocard) as a mood stabiliser for rapid cycling bipolar affective disorder patients," *Prog Neuropsychopharmacol Biol Psychiatry*, Vol 14(2), 1990, pp. 171–80

24. A. Heiden et al., "Treatment of severe mania with intravenous magnesium sulphate as a supplementary therapy," *Psychiatry Res*, Vol 89(3), 1999, pp. 239–46

25. C. J. Schorah et al., "Plasma vitamin C concentrations in patients in a psychiatric hospital," *Hum Nutr Clin Nutr*, Vol 37C, 1983, pp. 447–52

26. Z. A. Leitner and I. C. Church, "Nutritional studies in a mental hospital," *Lancet*, Vol 1, 1956, pp. 565–67

27. J. W. Maas, *Arch Gen Psychiatry*, Vol 4, 1961, p. 109

28. G. Milner, "Ascorbic acid supplementation in chronic psychiatric patients: A controlled trial," *Br J Psychiatry*, Vol 109, 1963, pp. 294–99

29. G. J. Naylor et al., "Tissue vanadium levels in manic depressive psychosis," *Physiological Medicine*, Vol 14, 1984, pp. 767–72

30. D. A. Dick, "Plasma vanadium concentration in manic-depressive illness," *Psychol Med*, Vol 12(3), 1982, pp. 533–7

31. B. J. Kaplan et al., "Effective mood stabilisation in open trials with a chelated mineral supplement: an open-label trial in bipolar disorder," *J Clin Psychiatry*, Vol 62(12), 2001, pp. 936–44

32. D. P. Cole et al., "Slower treatment response in bipolar depression predicted by lower pretreatment thyroid function," *American Journal of Psychiatry*, Vol 159, 2002, pp.116–121

33. G. D. Honey et al., *Proceedings of the National Academy of Sciences*, Vol 96, 1999, pp. 13418–23

34. D. F. Horrobin DF et al., "Fatty acid levels in the brains of schizophrenics and normal controls," *Biol Psychiatry*, Vol 30, 1991, pp. 795–805

35. D. F. Horrobin et al., "The membrane hypothesis of schizophrenia," *Schizophrenia Research*, Vol 13, 1994, pp. 195–207

36. P. E. Ward et al., "Niacin skin flush in schizophrenia: a preliminary report," *Schizophr Res*, Vol 29, 1998, pp. 269–74

37. S. H. Shah et al., "Unmedicated schizophrenic patients have a reduced skin response to topical niacin," *Schizophr Res*, Vol 43, 2000, pp. 163–4

38. C. Hudson, B. M. Ross et al., "Clinical subtyping reveals significant differences in calcium-dependent phospholipase A2 activity in schizophrenia," *Biol Psychiatry*, Vol 46(3), 1999, pp. 401–5

39. O. Christensen and E. Christensen, "Fat consumption and schizophrenia," *Acta Psychiatr Scand*, Vol 78, 1988, pp. 587–91

40. 50 patients given efas got better: A. Glen, personal communication, due for publication.

41. K. S. Vaddadi et al., "A double-blind trial of essential fatty acid supplementation in patients with tardive dyskinesia," *Psychiatry Res*, Vol 27(3), 1989, pp. 313–23

42. W. S. Fenton et al., "A placebo-controlled trial of omega-3 fatty acid (ethyl eicosapentaenoic acid) supplementation for residual symptoms and cognitive impairment in schizophrenia," *Am J Psychiatry*, Vol 158(12), 2001, pp. 2071–4

43. D. Shtasel et al., *Psychiatric Services*, Vol 46(3), March 1995, p. 293

44. G. Milner, *Brit J Psychiat*, Vol 109, 1963, pp. 294–99

45. K. Suboticanec et al., *Biol Psychiatry*, Vol 28, 1990, pp. 959–66 (see also Part 1, reference 56)

46. A. Hoffer, "Megavitamin B$_3$ therapy for schizophrenia," *Canad Psychiatric Ass J*, Vol 16,

1971, pp. 499–504

47. J. R. Wittenborn, "Niacin in the long term treatment of schizophrenia," *Arch Gen Psychiatry*, Vol 28, 1973, pp. 308–15

48. J. R. Wittenborn, "A search for responders to niacin supplementation," *Arch Gen Psychiatry*, Vol 31, 1974, pp. 547–52

49. M. W. Carney and B. F. Sheffield, "Serum folic acid and B_{12} in 272 psychiatric in-patients," *Psychol Med*, Vol 8(1), 1978, pp. 139–44

50. P. Godfrey et al., "Enhancement of recovery from psychiatric illness by methylfolate," *Lancet*, Vol 336(8712), 1990, pp. 392–5

51. B. Regland et al., "Homocysteinemia and schizophrenia as a case of methylation deficiency," *J Neural Transm Gen Sect*, Vol 98(2), 1994, pp. 143–52

52. P. O. O'Reilly et al., "The mauve factor: an evaluation," *Dis Nerv Syst*, Vol 26(9), 1965, pp. 562–8

53. L. Bender, "Childhood schizophrenia," *Psychiatric Quarterly*, Vol 27, 1953, pp. 3–81

54. H. Graff and A. Handford, "Celiac syndrome in the case history of five schizophrenics," *Psychiatric Quarterly*, Vol 35, 1961, pp. 306–13

55. F. C. Dohan et al., "Relapsed schizophrenics: more rapid improvement on a milk and cereal-free diet," *Brit J Psychiat*, Vol 115, 1969, pp. 595–6

56. D. S. King, "Can allergic exposure provoke psychological symptoms? A double-blind test," *Biol Psychiatry*, Vol 16(1), 1981, pp. 3–19

57. W. Philpott and D. Kalita, *Brain Allergies*, Keats Publishing (1980)

58. A. Hoffer, Megavitamin B_3 therapy for schizophrenia

59. H. Karlsson and R. H. Yolken et al., "Retroviral RNA identified in the cerebrospinal fluids and brains of individuals with schizophrenia," *Proc Natl Acad Sci*, Vol 98(8), 2001, pp. 4634–9

60. T. Soutzos, unpublished 2002 study of forty patients at Guy's and St. Thomas's Hospitals, London, in which 90 percent had high sulphite levels in their urine, compared with none of the healthy individuals used as controls, the majority of whom had none. See http://news.bbc.co.uk/hi/english/health/newsid_117000/117990.stm

61. B. F. El-Khodor and P. Boksa, "Birth insult increases amphetamine-induced behavioural responses in the adult rat," *Neuroscience*, Vol 87(4), 1998, pp. 893–904

Part 6: Mental Health in the Young (Chapters 26–33)

1. National Institutes of Health, Bethedsa, NIH Consensus Statement 1998, "Diagnosis and Treatment of ADHD"

2. A. Richardson, "Fatty acids in dyslexia, dyspraxia, ADHD and the autistic spectrum," *The Nutrition Practitioner*, Vol 3(3), 2001, pp. 18–24

3. A. Lucas, R. Morley, and T. Cole, "Randomised trial of early diet in preterm babies and later intelligence quotient," *BMJ*, Vol 317, 28 November 1998, pp. 1481–7

4. A. L. Kubala and M. M. Katz, "Nutritional factors in psychological test behaviour," *J Genet Psychol*, Vol 96, 1960, p. 343–52

5. A. Schauss, "Nutrition and behaviour," *J App Nutr*, Vol 35, 1983, p. 30–5

6. S. J. Schoenthaler et al., "The effect of randomised vitamin-mineral supplementation on violent and non-violent antisocial behaviour among incarcerated juveniles," *J Nut*

Env Med, Vol 7, 1997, pp. 343–52

7. S. J. Schoenthaler et al., "The effect of vitamin-mineral supplementation on the intelligence of American schoolchildren: a randomized, double-blind placebo-controlled trial," *J Altern Complement Med,* Vol 6(1), 2000, pp. 19–29

8. R. M. Carlton et al., "Rational dosages of nutrients have a prolonged effect on learning disabilities," *Altern Ther Health Med,* Vol 6(3), 2000, pp. 85–91

9. M. Colgan and L. Colgan, "Do nutrient supplements and dietary changes affect learning and emotional reactions of children with learning difficulties? A controlled series of 16 cases," *Nutr Health,* Vol 3, 1984, pp. 69–77

10. L. Rogers and R. Pelton, "Effects of glutamine on IQ scores of mentally deficient children," *Tex Rep Biol Med,* Vol 15, 1957, pp. 84–90

11. A. J. Richardson and J. Wilmer, "Association between fatty acid symptoms and dyslexic and ADHD characteristics in normal college students," paper given at British Dyslexia Association International Conference, University of York, April 2001

12. A. J. Richardson et al., "Fatty acid deficiency signs predict the severity of reading and related problems in dyslexic children," paper given at British Dyslexia Association International Conference, University of York, April 2001

13. C. M. Absolon et al., "Psychological disturbance in atopic eczema: the extent of the problem in school-aged children," *Br J Dermatol,* Vol 137(2), 1997, pp. 241–5

14. A. J. Richardson et al., "Abnormal cerebral phospholipid metabolism in dyslexia indicated by phosphorus-31 magnetic resonance spectroscopy," *NMR Biomed,* Vol 10, 1997, pp. 309–14

15. B. J. Stordy, "Dyslexia, attention deficit hyperactivity disorder, dyspraxia—do fatty acids help?," *Dyslexia Review,* Vol 9(2), 1997, pp. 1–3

16. B. J. Stordy, "Benefit of decosahexanoic acid supplements to dark adaptation in dyslexia," *Lancet,* Vol 346, 1995, p. 385

17. M. Colgan and L. Colgan, "Do nutrient supplements and dietary changes affect learning and emotional reactions of children with learning difficulties?," 1984

18. H. L. Needleman and C. A. Gatsonis, "Low level lead exposure and the IQ of children," *JAMA,* Vol 263(5), 1990, pp. 673–78

19. I. D. Capel et al., "Comparison of concentrations of some trace, bulk, and toxic metals in the hair of normal and dyslexic children," *Clin Chem,* Vol 27(6), 1981, pp. 879–81

20. N. D. Volkow et al., "Therapeutic doses of oral methylphenidate significantly increase extracellular dopamine in the human brain," *J Neuroscience,* Vol 21(RC121), 2001, pp. 1–5

21. Dr. Joan Baizer of the State University of New York at Buffalo at the Annual Meeting of the Society for Neuroscience, 11 November 2001

22. See www.blockcenter.com/articles2/ritalin_dea.htm and R. D. Ciaranello, "Attention deficit-hyperactivity disorder and resistance to thyroid hormone—a new idea?," *N Engl J Med,* Vol 328(14), 1993, pp. 1038–9

23. *NIH Consensus Statement: Diagnosis and Treatment of Attention Deficit Hyperactivity Disorder (ADHD),* National Institutes of Health, Bethesda (1998)

24. N. Lambert and C. Hartsough, "Prospective study of tobacco smoking and substance dependencies among samples of ADHD and non-ADHD participants," *Journal of Learning Disabilities,* Vol 31, 1998, pp. 533–44

25. A. Hoffer, "Vitamin B$_3$ dependent child," *Schizophrenia,* Vol 3, 1971, pp. 107–13

26. B. Starobrat-Hermelin and T. Kozielec, "The effects of magnesium physiological supplementation on hyperactivity in children with attention deficit hyperactivity disorder (ADHD). Positive response to magnesium oral loading test," *Magnes Res*, Vol 10(2), 1997, pp. 149–56

27. See the Optimal Wellness Centre website www.mercola.com/2001/jan/7/lendon_smith.htm, and www.smithsez.com/ADHDandADD.html

28. N. I. Ward, "Assessment of clinical factors in relation to child hyperactivity," *J Nutr Environ Med*, Vol 7, 1997, pp. 333–342

29. N. I. Ward, "Hyperactivity and a previous history of antibiotic usage," *Nutrition Practitioner*, Vol 3(3), 2001, p. 12

30. S. J. Schoenthaler et al., "The effect of randomised vitamin-mineral supplementation on violent and non-violent antisocial behaviour among incarcerated juveniles," *J Nut Env Med*, Vol 7, 1997, pp. 343–352

31. I. Colquhon and S. Bunday, "A lack of essential fatty acids as a possible cause of hyperactivity in children," *Medical Hypotheses*, Vol 7, 1981, pp. 673–9

32. L. J. Stevens et al., "Essential fatty acid metabolism in boys with attention-deficit hyperactivity disorder," *Am J Clin Nutr*, Vol 65, 1995, pp. 761–8

33. J. R. Burgess, "ADHD; observational and interventional studies," NIH workshop on omega-3 EFAs in psychiatric disorder, National Institutes of Health, Bethesda, 1998

34. A. J. Richardson et al., "Treatment with highly unsaturated fatty acids can reduce ADHD symptoms in children with specific learning difficulties: a randomised controlled trial," paper given at British Dyslexia Association International Conference, University of York, April 2001

35. A. Richardson and B. Puri, "A randomized double-blind, placebo-controlled study of the effects of supplementation with highly unsaturated fatty acids on ADHD-related symptoms in children with specific learning difficulties," *Prog Neuropsychopharmacol Biol Psychiatry*, Vol 26(2), 2002, pp. 233–9

36. A. Richardson and B. Puri, "A randomized double-blind, placebo-controlled study of the effects of supplementation with highly unsaturated fatty acids on ADHD," 2002

37. B. O'Reilly, paper given at Hyperactive Childrens Support Group Conference, June 2001, UK

38. N. I. Ward et al., "The influence of the chemical additive tartrazine on the zinc status of hyperactive children—a double-blind placebo controlled study," *J Nutr Med*, Vol 1, 1990, pp. 51–57

39. M. D. Boris and F. S. Mandel, *Annals of Allergy*, Vol 72, 1994, pp. 462–8

40. R. J. Theil, "Nutrition based interventions for ADD and ADHD," *Townsend Letter for Doctors and Patients*, April 2000, pp. 93–5

41. Swain et al., "Salicylates, oligoantigenic diet and behaviour," *Lancet*, Vol 2(8445), 1985, p. 41–2

42. R. J. Prinz et al., "Dietary correlates of hyperactive behaviour in children," *J Consulting Clin Psychol*, Vol 48, 1980, pp. 760–69

43. S. J. Schoenthaler et al., "The effect of randomised vitamin-mineral supplementation on violent and non-violent antisocial behaviour among incarcerated juveniles," 1997

44. L. Langseth and J. Dowd, "Glucose tolerance and hyperkinesis," *Fd Cosmet Toxicol*, Vol 16, 1978, p. 129

45. D. Papalos and J. Papalos, *The Bipolar Child*, Broadway Books (2000)

46. K. Blum and J. Holder, 2002, "The Reward Deficiency Syndrome," American College of Addictionology and Compulsive Disorders, pub. Amereon Ltd, Mattituck, NY

47. N. D. Volkow et al., "Therapeutic doses of oral methylphenidate significantly increase extracellular dopamine in the human brain," 2001

48. R. Huff, *US State Department of Developmental Services Report on Autism*, 1999

49. B. Rimland et al., "The effect of high doses of vitamin B_6 on autistic children: a double-blind crossover study," *Am J Psychiatry*, Vol 135(4), 1978, pp. 472–5

50. S. I. Pfeiffer et al., "Efficacy of vitamin B_6 and magnesium in the treatment of autism: a methodology review and summary of outcomes," *J Autism Dev Disord*, Vol 25(5), 1995, pp. 481–93

51. J. Martineau et al., "Vitamin B_6, magnesium, and combined B_6-Mg: therapeutic effects in childhood autism," *Biol Psychiatry*, Vol 20(5), 1985, pp. 467–78

52. S. Vancassel et al., "Plasma fatty acid levels in autistic children," *Prostaglandins Leukot Essent Fatty Acids*, Vol 65, 2001, pp. 1–7

53. J. G. Bell et al., "Red blood cell fatty acid compositions in a patient with autism spectrum disorder: a characteristic abnormality in neurodevelopmental disorders?," *Prostaglandins Leukot Essent Fatty Acids*, Vol 63(1–2), 2000, p21–5.

54. J. G. Bell, "Fatty acid deficiency and phospholipase A2 in autistic spectrum disorders," report given at research workshop on fatty acids in neurodevelopmental disorders, St Anne's College, Oxford, September 2001

55. M. Megson, "Is autism a G-Alpha protein defect reversible with natural vitamin A?," *Medical Hypotheses*, Vol 54(6), 2000, pp. 979–983

56. M. Megson, "The biological basis for perceptual deficits in autism: vitamin A and G-proteins," lecture given at Ninth International Symposium on Functional Medicine, May 2002

57. P. Whitely, the Sunderland University Autism Unit, talk given at the Autism Unravelled Conference, London, May 2001

58. P. Whitely et al., "A gluten free diet as an intervention for autism and associated disorders: preliminary findings," *Autism: International J of Research and Practice*, Vol 3, 1999, pp. 45–65

59. J. Robert Cade, University of Florida Department of Medicine and Physiology, at www.panix.com/~paleodiet/autism/cadelet.txt

60. Letter to the Editor, "Anti-fungal drugs more helpful than Ritalin in autistic children," *Townsend Letter for Doctors and Patients*, April 2001, p. 99

61. A. Wakefield et al., "Enterocolitis in children with developmental disorders," *Am J Gastroenterol*, Vol 95(9), 2000, pp. 2285–95

62. M. A. Brudnak, "Application of genomeceuticals to the molecular and immunological aspects of autism," *Med Hypotheses*, Vol 57(2), 2001, pp. 186–91

63. P. Varmanen et al., "S54X-prolyl dipeptidyl aminopeptidase gene (pepX) is part of the glnRA operon in *Lactobacillus rhamnosus*," *J Bacteriol*, Vol 182(1), 2000, pp. 146–54

64. Whitely et al., "A gluten free diet as an intervention for autism and associated disorders: preliminary findings," *Autism: International J of Research and Practice*, Vol 3, 1999, pp. 45–65

65. J. Robert Cade, University of Florida Department of Medicine and Physiology, at www.panix.com/~paleodiet/autism/cadelet.txt

66. M. Ash and E. Gilmore, "Modifying autism through functional nutrition," paper given at Allergy Research Group conference, January 2001

67. Dr. Rosemary Waring, University of Birmingham School of Biosciences, speaking at the Autism Unravelled Conference, London, May 2001

68. W. Walsh et al., *Metallothionein and Autism*, Pfeiffer Treatment Center, Naperville, Illinois (2001). See www.hriptc.org

69. A. J. Wakefield et al., "Ileal-lymphoid hyperplasia, non-specific colitis, and pervasive developmental disorder in children," *Lancet*, Vol 351, 1998, pp. 637–41

70. Andrew Wakefield, speaking at the Allergy Research Foundation conference, November 1999

71. F. E. Yazbak, "Autism—is there a vaccine connection?." See www.autisme.net/Yazbak1.htm

72. B. Rimland, *J Nut Env Med*, Vol 10, 2000, pp. 267–9

73. See ref 72 (B. Rimland). See also Ashcraft & Gerel (law firm), "Autism caused by childhood vaccinations containing Thimerosal or mercury," which considers the litigation of individual claims www.ashcraftandgerel.com/thimerosal.html

74. B. Rimland, "Parents' ratings of the effectiveness of drugs and nutrients," *Autism Research Review International*, October 1994

75. H. Turkel, et al., "Intellectual improvement of a retarded patient treated with the 'U' series," *J Orthomol Psychiatry*, Vol 13(4), 1984, pp. 272–6

76. R. F. Harrell et al., "Can nutritional supplements help mentally retarded children? An exploratory study," *Proc Natl Acad Sci*, Vol 78(1), 1981, pp. 574–8

77. T. Tuormaa, *An Alternative to Psychiatry*, The Book Guild Ltd (1991). Also see B. Rimland, "Parents' ratings of the effectiveness of drugs and nutrients," 1994

78. M. Pogribna et al., "Homocysteine metabolism in children with Down syndrome: in vitro modulation," *Am J Hum Genet*, Vol 69(1), 2001, pp. 88–95

79. Study reported on www.tri21.org/leichtman/

80. R. Bidder et al., "Multivitamins and minerals for children with downs syndrome," *Dev Med Child Neurol*, Vol 31, 1989, pp. 532–7

81. N. J. Lobaugh et al., "Piracetam therapy does not enhance cognitive functioning in children with Down syndrome," *Arch Paedatr Adolesc Med*, Vol 155(4), 2001, pp. 442–8

82. S. L. Black, "Piracetam therapy for Down syndrome: a rush to judgment?," Letter, *Archives of Paediatric and Adolescent Medicine*, 155(10), 2001

83. B. Gesch, "The SCASO project," *Int J Biosocial Med Res*, Vol 12(1), pp. 41–68

84. M. Virkunnen, "Reactive hypoglycemic tendency among habitually violent offenders," *Nutrition Reviews*, Vol 44(suppl), 1986, pp. 94–103

85. S. J. Schoenthaler, "The Northern California diet-behavior program: An empirical evaluation of 3,000 incarcerated juveniles in Stanislaus County juvenile hall," *Int J Biosocial Res*, Vol 5(2), 1983, pp. 99–106

86. S. J. Schoenthaler, "The Los Angeles probation department diet-behavior program: An empirical analysis of six institutional settings," *Int J Biosocial Res*, Vol 5(2), 1983, pp. 107–17

87. R. Freeman et al., *Lead Burden of Sydney Schoolchildren*, University of New South Wales (1979)

88. H. Needleman et al., 1979, "Deficits in psychological and classroom performance of children with elevated dentine lead levels," *New England J of Med*, Vol 300, pp. 689–95

89. G. Thomson et al., "Blood lead levels and children's behaviour: results from the Edinburgh lead study," *J Child Psychol Psychiatry*, Vol 30(4), 1989, pp. 515–28

90. R. Pihl and O. Ervin, "Lead and cadmium levels in violent criminals," *Psychol Rep*, Vol 66(3:1), 1990, pp. 839–44

91. G. Schauss, "Comparative hair mineral analysis results of 21 elements, in a randomly selected behaviourally 'normal' 19–59 year old population and violent adult offenders," *Int J Biosocial Res*, Vol 1(2), 1981, pp. 21–41

92. S. J. Schoenthaler, "The northern-California diet-behaviour program: An empirical evaluation of 3000 incarcerated juveniles in Stanislaus County Juvenile Hall," *Int J Biosocial Res*, Vol 5(2), 1983, pp. 107–17

93. S. J. Schoenthaler et al., "The effect of randomised vitamin-mineral supplementation on violent and non-violent antisocial behaviour among incarcerated juveniles," *J Nut Env Med*, Vol 7, 1997, pp. 343–52

94. T. Hamazaki et al., "The effect of docosahexaenoic acid on aggression in young adults: a placebo-controlled double-blind study," *J Clin Invest*, Vol 97, 1996, pp. 1129–33

95. I. Menzies, "Disturbed children: The role of food and chemical sensitivities," *Nutr Health*, Vol 3, 1984, pp. 39–45

96. J. Egger et al., "Controlled trial of oligoantigenic treatment in the hyperkinetic syndrome," *Lancet*, Vol 1(8428), 1985, pp. 540–5

97. A. G. Schauss and C. E. Simonsen, "A critical analysis of the diets of chronic juvenile offenders," Part 1, *J Orthomol Psychiatry*, Vol. 8(3), 1979, pp. 149–57

98. B. Gesch, SCASO pilot study data, unpublished

99. See ref. 85 (S. J. Schoenthaler, 1983) and features on www.mentalhealthproject.com

100. B. Gesch, "Influence of supplementary vitamins, minerals and essential fatty acids on the antisocial behaviour of young adult prisoners," *Brit J Psychiatry*, Vol 181, 2002, pp. 22–28

101. E. Noble, "The gene that rewards alcoholism," *Scientific American*, Science and Medicine, March/April 1996, pp. 52–61

102. U. D. Register et al., "Influence of nutrients in intake of alcohol," *J Am Diet Assoc*, Vol 61(2), 1972, pp. 159–62

103. A. F. Libby et al., "The junk food connection—alcohol and drug lifestyle adversely affect metabolism and behaviour," *Orthomolecular Psychiatry*, Vol 11(2), 1982, pp. 116–27

104. Personal communication with Dr. Abram Hoffer. See also W. E. Beebe and O. W. Wendel, *Preliminary Observations of Altered Carbohydrate Metabolism in Psychiatric Patients*, D. Hawkins and L. Pauling (eds), W. H. Freeman and Co. (1973), pp. 435–51

105. U. D. Register et al., "Influence of nutrients in intake of alcohol," 1972

106. W. Philpott and D. Kalita, *Brain Allergies*, Keats Publishing (1980)

107. Society for the Study of Addiction. See www.addiction-ssa.org/

108. M. R. Werbach, *Nutritional Influences on Mental Illness*, Third Line Press (1991)

109. B. Spittle and J. Parker, "Wernicke's encephalopathy complicating schizophrenia," *Aust and NZ J Psych*, Vol 27, 1993, pp. 638–52

110. K. Eriksson et al., "Effects of thiamine deprivation and antagonism on voluntary ethanol intake in rats," *J Nutr*, Vol 110, 1980, p. 937

111. L. L. Rogers et al., "Voluntary alcohol consumption by rats following administration of glutamine," *J Biol Chem*, Vol 220(1), 1956, pp. 321–3

112. H. Ikeda, "Effects of taurine on alcohol withdrawal," *Lancet*, Sept. 1977, Vol. 2(8036), p. 509

113. R. M. Guenther, "Role of nutritional therapy in alcoholism treatment," *Int J Biosocial Res*, Vol 4(1), 1983, pp. 5–18

114. R. F. Smith, "A five year field trial of massive nicotinic acid therapy of alcoholics in Michigan," *J Orthomolec Psych*, Vol 3, 1974, pp. 327–31

115. A. Hoffer and H. Osmond et al., "Treatment of schizophrenia with nicotinic acid and nicotinamide," *J Clin Exper Psychopathol*, Vol 18, 1957, pp. 131–58

116. A. F. Libby and I. Stone, "The Hypoascorbemia-Kwashiorkor approach to drug addiction therapy: pilot study," *Orthomolecular Psychiatry*, Vol 6(4), 1977, pp. 300–8

117. K. M. Hambidge and A. Silverman, "Pica with rapid improvement after dietary zinc supplementation," *Arch Dis Child*, Vol 48, 1973, pp. 567–8

118. R. Bakan, "The role of zinc in anorexia nervosa: etiology and treatment," *Med Hypotheses*, Vol 5(7), 1979, pp. 731–6

119. D. Horrobin et al., *Med Hyp*, Vol 6, 1980, pp. 277–296

120. Casper and Prasad, 1980, later confirmed by L. Humphries et al., "Zinc deficiency and eating disorders," *J Clin Psychiatry*, Vol 50(12), 1989, pp. 456–9

121. P. R. Flanagan, "A model to produce pure zinc deficiency in rats and its use to demonstrate that dietary phytate increases the excretion of endogenous zinc," *J Nutr*, Vol 114, 1984, pp. 493–502 and A. Grider et al., "Age-dependent influence of dietary zinc restriction on short-term memory in male rats," *Physiology and Behaviour*, Vol 72(3), 2001, pp. 339–48

122. A. Arcasoy, N. Akar, et al., "Ultrastructural changes in the mucosa of the small intestine in patients with geophagia (Prasad's syndrome)," *J Pediatr Gastroenterol Nutr*, Vol 11(2), 1990, pp. 279–82

123. D. Bryce-Smith and R. I. Simpson, "Case of anorexia nervosa responding to zinc sulphate," *Lancet*, Vol 2(8398), 1984, p. 350

124. Katz et al., *J Adol Health Care*, Vol 8, 1987, pp. 400–6

125. L. Humphries et al., "Zinc deficiency and eating disorders," *J Clin Psychiatry*, Vol 50(12), 1989, pp. 456–9

126. C. Birmingham et al., "Controlled trial of zinc supplementation in anorexia nervosa," *Int J Eat Disord*, Vol 15(3), 1994, pp. 251–55

127. N. F. Shay and H. F. Mangian HF, "Neurobiology of zinc-influenced eating behavior," *J Nutr*, Vol 130(5S Suppl), 2000, pp. 1493S–9S

128. R. Bakan et al., "Dietary zinc intake of vegetarian and non-vegetarian patients with anorexia nervosa," *Int J Eat Disord*, Vol 13(2), 1993, pp. 229–33

129. F. Askenazy et al., "Whole blood serotonin content, tryptophan concentrations, and impulsivity in anorexia nervosa," *Biological Psychiatry*, Vol 43(3), 1998, pp. 188–195

130. A. Favaro, "Tryptophan levels, excessive exercise, and nutritional status in anorexia nervosa," *Psychosomatic Medicine*, Vol 62(4), 2000, pp. 535–8

131. P. J. Cowen and K. A. Smith, "Serotonin, dieting, and bulimia nervosa," *Advances in Experimental Medicine and Biology*, Vol 467, 1999, pp. 101–4

132. W. H. Kaye et al., "Effects of acute tryptophan depletion on mood in bulimia nervosa," *Biol Psychiatry*, Vol 47(2), 2000, pp. 151–7

133. D. B. Smith and E. Obbens, "Antifolate-antiepileptic relationships," in M. I. Botez and E. H. Reynolds, eds, *Folic Acid in Neurology, Psychiatry and Internal Medicine*, Raven Press (1979)

134. F. B. Gibberd et al., "The influence of folic acid on the frequency of epileptic attacks," *Europ J Clin Pharmacology*, Vol 19(1), 1981, pp. 57–60

135. See ref 133

136. M. Nakazawa, "High dose vitamin B₆ therapy in infantile spasms—the effect of adverse reactions," *Brain and Development*, Vol 5(2), 1983, p. 193

137. J. Pietz et al., "Treatment of infantile spasms with high-dosage vitamin B₆," *Epilepsia*, Vol 34(4), 1993, pp. 757–63

138. A. Sohler and C. Pfeiffer, "A direct method for the determination of manganese in whole blood: patients with seizure activity have low blood levels," *J Orthomol Psychiat*, Vol 12, 1983, pp. 215–234

139. C. L. Dupont and Y. Tanka, "Blood manganese levels in children with convulsive disorder," *Biochem Med*, Vol 33(2), 1985, pp. 246–55

140. P. S. Papavasiliou et al., "Seizure disorders and trace metals: Manganese tissue levels in treated epileptics," *Neurology*, Vol 29, 1979, p. 1466

141. Y. Tanaka, "Low manganese level may trigger epilepsy," *JAMA*, Vol 238, 1977, p. 1805

142. C. Pfeiffer et al., "Zinc and manganese in the schizophrenias," *J Orthomol Psychiat*, Vol 12, 1983, pp. 215–34

143. Y. Shoji, "Serum magnesium and zinc in epileptic children," *Brain and Development*, Vol 5(2), 1983, p. 200

144. S. K. Gupta et al., "Serum magnesium levels in idiopathic epilepsy," *J Assoc Physicians India*, Vol 42(6), 1994, pp. 456–7

145. L. F. Gorges et al., "Effect of magnesium on epileptic foci," *Epilepsia*, Vol 19(1), 1978, pp. 81–91

146. *Pediatria Romania*, Vol 31(4), 1982, pp. 343–7

147. C. L. Zhang et al., "Paroxysmal epileptiform discharges in temporal lobe slices after prolonged exposure to low magnesium are resistant to clinically used anticonvulsants," *Epilepsy Res*, Vol 20(2), 1995, pp. 105–11

148. Y. Shoji, "Serum magnesium and zinc in epileptic children," 1983

149. A. Barbeau et al., "Zinc, taurine and epilepsy," *Arch Neurol*, Vol 30, 1974, pp. 52–8

150. M. I. Botez et al., "Thiamine and folate treatment of chronic epileptic patients: a controlled study with the Wechsler IQ scale," *Epilepsy-Res*, Vol 16(2), 1993, pp. 157–63, and A. Keyser, "Epileptic manifestations and vitamin B₁ deficiency," *Eur-Neurol*, Vol 31(3), 1991, pp. 121–5

151. V. T. Ramaeckers, "Selenium deficiency triggering intractable seizures," *Neuropediatrics*, Vol 25(4), 1994, pp. 217–23

152. I. R. Tupeev, "The antioxidant system in the dynamic combined treatment of epilepsy patients with traditional anticonvulsant preparations and an antioxidant—alpha-tocopherol," *Biull Eksp Biol Med*, Vol 116(10), 1993, pp. 362–4

153. S. Yehuda, "Essential fatty acid preparation (SR-3) raises the seizure threshold in rats," *Eur J Pharmacol*, Vol 254(1–2), 1994, pp. 193–8

154. S. Schlanger, M. Shinitzky, and D. Yam, "Diet enriched with omega-3 fatty acids alleviates convulsion symptoms in epilepsy patients," *Epilepsia*, Vol 43(1), 2002, pp. 103–4

155. E. S. Roach et al., "N,N-dimethylglycine for epilepsy," Letter to the Editor, *N Engl J Med*, Vol 307, 1982, pp. 1081–2

156. R. Huxtable et al., "The prolonged anticonvulsant action of taurine on genetically determined seizure-susceptibility," *Canadian J Neurol Sci*, Vol 5, 1978, p. 220

157. D. A. Richards et al., "Extracellular GABA in the ventrolateral thalamus of rats exhibiting spontaneous absence epilepsy: a microdialysis study," *J Neurochem*, Vol 65(4), 1995, pp. 1674–80

158. J. Schmidt, "Comparative studies on the anti-convulsant effectiveness of nootropic drugs in kindled rats," *Biomed Biochim Acta*, Vol 49(5), 1990, pp. 413–9

159. J. W. Crayton et al., "Epilepsy precipitated by food sensitivity: Report of a case with double-blind placebo-controlled assessment," *Clinical Electroencephalo*, Vol 12(4), 1981, p192–8

160. W. J. Rea and C. W. Suits, "Cardiovascular disease triggered by foods and chemicals," in J. W. Gerrard, *Food Allergy: New Perspectives*, Charles C. Thomas (1980)

Part 7: Mental Health in Old Age (Chapters 34–37)

1. V. L. Davidson and D. B. Sittman, *Biochemistry: The National Medical Series for Independent Study*, Harawl Publishing (1994), pp. 477–8

2. L. Fleming et al., "Parkinson's disease and brain levels of organochlorine pesticides," *Ann Neurol*, Vol 36(1), 1994, pp. 100–3

3. M. Thiruchelvam et al., "The Nigrostriatal Dopaminergic System as a preferential target of repeated exposures to combined paraquat and maneb: implications for Parkinson's Disease," *Journal of Neuroscience*, Vol 20(24), 2000, pp. 9207–14 and J. Corell et al., "The risk of Parkinson's disease with exposure to pesticides, farming, well water and rural living," *Neurology*, Vol 67, 1998, pp. 1210–1218

4. L. Leader, *Parkinson's Disease—The Way Forward*, Denor Press (2000), p. 77

5. W. Duan et al., "Dietary folate deficiency and elevated homocysteine levels endanger dopaminergic neurons in models of Parkinson's Disease," *J Neurochemistry*, Vol 80, 2002, pp. 101–10

6. L. Leader, *Parkinson's Disease—The Way Forward* (2001), p. 87, Optimizing Function by Nutritional Manipulation, p. 145, Liver Detoxification and Optimal Liver Function, Helen Kimber

7. G. B. Steventon et al., "Plasma cysteine and sulphate levels in patients with motor neurone, Parkinson's and Alzheimer's Disease," *Neurosci Letts*, Vol 110, 1990, pp. 216–20

8. S. Fahn, "A pilot trial of high dose alpha-tocopherol and ascorbate in early Parkinson's Disease," *Ann Neurol*, Vol 32(S), 1992, pp. 128–32

9. J. S. Bland and J. A. Bralley, "Nutritional upregulation of hepatic detoxification enzymes," *J Applied Nutrition*, Vol 4, 1992, pp. 3–15

10. R. B. D'Agostino et al., "Plasma homocysteine as a risk factor for dementia and Alzheimer's disease," *N Engl J Med*, Vol 346(7), 2002, pp. 476–83

11. W. Duan, M. P. Mattson et al., "Dietary folate deficiency and elevated homocysteine levels endanger dopaminergic neurons in models of Parkinson's disease," *J Neurochem*, Vol 80(1), 2002, pp. 101–10

12. G. Leader and L. Leader, *Parkinson's Disease—The New Nutritional Handbook*, Denor Press (1996/7), p. 96

13. *ABPI Compendium of Data Sheets and Summaries of Product Characteristics (1999–2000)*, pp. 371, 1333, Datapharm Publications Limited

14. *ABPI Compendium*, pp. 1105–6

15. G. Leader and L. Leader, *Parkinson's Disease—The New Nutritional Handbook*, p. 96

16. R. K. Chandra, "Effect of vitamin and trace-element supplementation on cognitive function in elderly subjects," *Nutrition*, Vol 17(9), 2001, pp. 709–12

17. I. R. Bell et al., "Brief communication. Vitamin B_1, B_2, and B_6 augmentation of tricyclic antidepressant treatment in geriatric depression with cognitive dysfunction," *J Am College of Nutrition*, Vol 11(2), 1992, pp. 159–63

18. W. J. Perrig et al., "The relation between antioxidants and memory performance in the old and very old," *J Am Geriatr Soc*, Vol 45(6), 1997, pp. 718–24

19. A. J. Perkins et al., "Association of antioxidants with memory in a multiethnic elderly sample using the Third National Health and Nutrition Examination Survey," *Am J Epidemiol*, Vol 150(1), 1999, pp. 37–44

20. J. W. Miller, "Vitamin E and memory: is it vascular protection?," *Nutr Rev*, Vol 58(4), 2000, pp. 109–11

21. D. Edwin et al., "Cognitive impairment in alcoholic and nonalcoholic cirrhotic patients," *Hepatology*, Vol 30(6), 1999, pp. 1363–7

22. R. Wurtman et al., "Effect of oral CDP-choline on plasma choline and uridine levels in humans," *Biochem Pharm*, Vol 60, 2000, pp. 989–92

23. S. Suzuki et al., "Oral administration of soybean lecithin transphosphatidylated phosphatidylserine improves memory impairment in aged rats," *J Nutr*, Vol 131(11), 2001, pp. 2951–6

24. J. Kleijnin and P. Knipschild, "Ginkgo biloba," *Lancet*, Vol 340(8828), 1992, pp. 1136–9

25. P. L. Le Bars, "A placebo-controlled, double-blind, randomised trial on an extract of Ginkgo Biloba for dementia," *JAMA*, Vol 278(16), 1997, pp. 1327–32

26. F. Huguet et al., "Decreased cerebral 5-HT1A receptors during aging: reversal by Ginkgo biloba extract," *J Pharm Pharmacol*, Vol 46, 1994, pp. 316–8

27. R. M. Sapolsky, "Why stress is bad for your brain," *Science*, Vol 273(5276), 1995, pp. 749–50

28. T. Satoh et al., "Walking exercise and improved neuropsychological functioning in elderly patients with cardiac disease," *J Intern Med*, Vol 238(5), 1995, pp. 423–8

29. Tom Warren, *Beating Alzheimer's*, Avery, 1997

30. G. Kempermann and F. Gage, "New nerve cells for the adult brain," *Scientific American*, 12(1), 2002, pp. 38–44

31. R. Itzhaki et al., "Herpes simplex virus type 1 in brain and risk of Alzheimer's disease," *Lancet*, Vol 349(9047), 1997, pp. 241–4

32. M. Morris et al., "Vitamin E and vitamin C supplement use and risk incident Alzheimer disease," *Alzheimer Dis and Assoc Disorders*, Vol 12, 1998, pp. 121–6

33. M. Morris et al., "Dietary intake of antioxidant nutrients and the risk of incident Alzheimer's disease," *JAMA*, Vol 284(24), pp. 3230–3237. Also see pp. 3223–61

34. M. Sano et al., "A controlled trial of selegiline, alpha tocopherol or both as treatment of Alzheimer's disease," *New Eng J Med*, Vol 336, 1997, pp. 1216–22

35. A. Hoffman et al., letter in *Lancet*, Vol 349, 1997, p. 151

36. R. M. Sapolsky, "Why stress is bad for your brain," 1996

37. R. M. Sapolsky and B. S. McEwen, "Stress, glucocorticoids, and their role in the aging hippocampus," in *Treatment Development Strategies for Alzheimer's Disease*, Mark Powley Associates (1986), pp. 151–71

38. I. Graham et al., "Plasma homocysteine as a risk factor for vascular disease," *JAMA*, Vol 277(22), 1997, pp. 1775–81

39. M. Toshifumi et al., "Elevated plasma homocysteine levels and risk of silent brain infarction in elderly people," *Stroke*, Vol 32, 2001, p. 1116

40. H. X. Wang et al., "Vitamin B(12) and folate in relation to the development of Alzheimer's disease," *Neurology*, Vol 56(9), 2001, pp. 1188–94

41. D. A. Snowdon et al., "Serum folate and the severity of atrophy of the neocortex in Alzheimer disease: findings from the Nun Study," *American Journal of Clinical Nutrition*, Vol 71(4), 2000, pp. 993–8

42. S. Seshadri et al., "Plasma homocysteine as a risk factor for dementia and Alzheimer's disease," *N Engl J Med*, Vol 346(7), 2002, pp. 476–483

43. S. L. Rifat et al., "Effect of exposure of miners to aluminium powder," *Lancet*, Vol 336(8724), 1990, pp. 1162–5

44. D. Wenstrup et al., "Trace element imbalances in isolated subcellular fractions of Alzheimer's disease patients," *Brain Research*, Vol 553, 1990, pp. 125–31

45. C. Hock et al., "Increased blood mercury levels in patients with Alzheimer's disease," *J Neural Transm*, Vol 105(1), pp. 59–68

46. C. C. Leong et al., "Retrograde degeneration of neurite membrane structural integrity of nerve growth cones following in vitro exposure to mercury," *Neuroreport*, Vol 12(4), 2001, pp. 733–7. See also www.commons.ucalgary.ca/mercury

47. P. Tariska and A. Paksy, "Cognitive enhancement effect of piracetam in patients with mild cognitive impairment and dementia," *Orv Hetil*, Vol 141(22), 2000, pp. 1189–93

48. H. Pilch and W. E. Muller, "Chronic treatment with piracetam elevates muscarinic cholinergic receptor density in the frontal cortex of aged mice," *Pharmacopsychiatry*, Vol 21(6), 1988, pp. 324–5

49. J. D. Elsworth et al., "Deprenyl administration in man: A selective MAO-B inhibitor without the 'cheese effect'," *Psychopharmacology (Berl)*, Vol 57(1), 1978, pp. 33–8

50. Knoll research reported in W. Dean et al., *Smart Drugs II—The Next Generation*, Health Freedom Publications (1993)

51. D. S. Khalsa, *Altern Ther Health Med*, Vol 4(6), 1998, pp. 38–43 and R. M. Wu et al., *Ann NY Acad Sci*, Vol 786, 1996, pp. 379–90

52. D. Ward and J. Morgenthaler, *Smart Drugs and Nutrients*, B and J Publications (1990), pp. 42–3

53. P. Mindus et al., "Piracetam-induced improvement of mental performance. A controlled study on normally aging individuals," *Acta Psychiat Scand*, Vol 54, 1976, pp. 150–60

54. L. Israel et al., "Drug therapy and memory training programs: a double-blind randomized trial of general practice patients with age-associated memory impairment," *Int Psychogeriatr*, Vol 6(2), 1994, pp. 155–70

55. L. S. Schneider and J. T. Olin, "Overview of clinical trials of hydergine in dementia," *Arch Neurol*, Vol 51(8), 1994, pp. 787–98

56. L. S. Schneider and J. T. Olin, "Overview of clinical trials of hydergine in dementia," 1994

57. D. Ward and J. Morgenthaler, *Smart Drugs and Nutrients*

58. I. Zhdanova et al., "Sleep-inducing effects of low doses of melatonin ingested in the evening," *Clinical Pharmacology and Therapeutics*, Vol 57(5), 1995, pp. 552–8

59. R. Nave et al., "Melatonin improves evening napping," *Eur J Pharmacol*, Vol 275(2), 1995, pp. 213–16

Recommended Reading

General

Holford, P., *The Optimum Nutrition Bible,* Crossing Press, 1999

Holford, P. and Cass, H., *Natural Highs,* Avery, 2001

Pfeiffer, C. C., *Mental and Elemental Nutrients,* Keats Publishing, 1975

Werbach, M., *Nutritional Influences on Mental Illness,* Third Line Press, 1991

Chapters 4 and 5—Smart Fats and Phospholipids

Schmidt, M. A., *Smart Fats,* Frog Ltd, 1997

Stoll, A. L. *The Omega 3 Connection,* Simon and Schuster, 2002

Chapter 6—Amino Acids

Braverman, E. R. et al., *The Healing Nutrients Within,* Basic Health Publishing, 2002

Chapter 12—Boosting Intelligence

Benton, D., *Food for Thought,* Penguin, 1996

Chapters 13, 35 and 36—Memory Enhancement, Preventing Memory Decline, and Alzheimer's Disease

Hoffer, A., *Smart Nutrients—A Guide to Nutrients That Can Prevent and Reverse Senility,* Avery Publishing, 1994

Khalsa, D. S. and Stauth, C., *Brain Longevity*, Warner Books, 1997
Lombard, J. and Germano, C., *The Brain Wellness Plan*, Kensington Books, 1997
Warren, T., *Beating Alzheimer's*, Avery, 1991

Chapters 14 and 22–Beating the Blues and Depression

Brown, M. and Robinson, J., *When Your Body Gets the Blues*, Rodale Press, 2002
Cass, H., *St John's Wort—Nature's Blues Buster*, Avery Publishing, 1998
Ross, J., *The Mood Cure*, Thorsons, 2003

Chapter 15–Hormonal Mood Swings

Carruthers, M., *The Testosterone Revolution*, Thorsons, 2001
Colgan, M., *Hormonal Health*, Apple Publishing Canada, 1996
Lee, J., *What Your Doctor Didn't Tell You About Menopause*, Warner Books, 1996

Chapter 16–Unwinding Anxiety

Cass, H. and McNally, T., *Kava—Nature's Answer to Stress, Anxiety, Insomnia*, Prima
Health, 1998

Chapters 23 to 25–Manic Depression and Schizophrenia

Dryden, W. and Gordon, J., *Think Your Way to Happiness—How to Help Yourself
with Cognitive Therapy*, Sheldon Press, 1990
Hoffer, A., *Vitamin B-3, Schizophrenia, Discovery, Recovery and Controversy*, Quarry
Health Books, 2000
Horrobin, D., *The Madness of Adam and Eve—How Schizophrenia Shaped Humanity*, Bantam Press, 2001
Lawson, V., *Inside Out*, 2001. This is a good, practical self-help guide for people
with manic depression, available from the Manic Depression Fellowship (call
020 7793 2600).

Chapter 27–Attention Deficit Disorders

ADHD—Hyperactive Children: A Parents' Guide, Hyperactive Children's Support
Group, 2002. To order, see www.hacsg.org.uk
Papolos, D. and M., *The Bipolar Child*, Broadway Books, 2000
Weintrub, S., *Natural Treatments for ADD and Hyperactivity*, Woodland Publish-
ing, 1997
Block, M., *No More ADHD*, Block Books, 2001

Chapter 28–Autism

Gillberg, C. and Coleman, M., *Biology of the Autistic Syndrome,* Mac Keith Press, 2000

McCandless, J., *Children with Starving Brains,* Bramble Books, 2002

Chapter 31–Beating Addictions

Holford, P., *Beat Stress and Fatigue,* Piatkus Books, 1999

Chapter 32–Eating Disorders

Woodman, M., *The Owl was a Baker's Daughter—Obesity, Anorexia Nervosa, and the Repressed Feminine,* Inner City Books, 1980

Chapter 34–Parkinson's Disease

Leader, G. and L., *Parkinson's Disease—The Way Forward,* Denor Press, 1999. See www.parkinsonsdisease-the-way-forward.com for more details.

Chapter 37–Smart Drugs and Hormones

Dean, W. and Morgenthaler, J., *Smart Drugs and Nutrients,* B&J Publications, 1990

Dean, W., Morgenthaler, J., and Fowkes, S. W., *Smart Drugs II—The Next Generation,* Health Freedom Publications, 1993

Useful Addresses

Addictions

Alcoholics Anonymous is a fellowship of men and women who share their experience, strength, and hope with each other so that they may solve their common problem and help others to recover from alcoholism using a 12-step program. The only requirement for membership is a desire to stop drinking. Alcoholics Anonymous is worldwide with A.A. meetings in almost every community. You can find times and places of local A.A. meetings or events by contacting a nearby central office, intergroup or answering service of U.S. and Canada. **Contact:** http://www.alcoholics-anonymous.org/default/en_contact. cfm?contype=central for a comprehensive list of locations throughout the United States. The General Service Office does not maintain local meeting information.

Narcotics Anonymous is a nonprofit society of recovering addicts who meet regularly to help each other stay clean. Recovery in NA focuses on the problem of addiction, rather than on any particular drug, using the same 12-step program as Alcoholics Anonymous. Membership is not limited to addicts who use one drug or another. Those who feel they may have a problem with any drugs-legal or illegal, including alcohol-are welcome in Narcotics Anonymous. **Contact:** Narcotics Anonymous, PO Box 9999, Van Nuys, CA 91409 / Tel: (818) 773-9999 / Fax: (818) 700-0700 / Website: www.nana.org

mentalhealthproject.com

The Mental Health Project, founded by Patrick Holford, exists to inform the public about the role of nutrition in mental health, to promote the nutrition connection to health professionals, policy makers and sufferers, and to provide resources to encourage more research and implementation of nutritional strategies.

Visit our website for:

- A FREE monthly e-letter on alternative approaches to mental health.

- The latest research on drug-free approaches to mental health.

- Your questions answered.

- Referral to clinical nutritionists near you.

- Mental health seminars and events near you.

- Mental health books, supplements, and other resources.

- Details on the Brain Bio Centre, Britain's only clinic specializing in the optimum nutrition approach to mental health (see page 366).

The website also contains features on:

- How to quit: smoking, stimulants, and alcohol.

- Coming off: tranquilizers, antidepressant drugs, and stimulant drugs.

- The optimum nutrition approach for: ADHD, Alzheimer's disease, anorexia, anxiety, autism, dementia, depression, Down's syndrome, dyslexia, dyspraxia, manic depression, Parkinson's disease, schizophrenia, sleeping problems, and much more.

Check yourself out on the Mental Health Questionnaire: a FREE online questionnaire that takes five minutes to complete and tells you instantly if you are likely to have any biochemical imbalances that are affecting your mental health. If you would like to support the Mental Health Project by volunteering or making a donation, call +44 20 8871 2949 or visit the website. www.mentalhealthproject.com

ADHD/Hyperactivity

The **Feingold Association of United States** is an organization of families and professionals, dedicated to helping children and adults apply proven dietary techniques for better behavior, learning and health. **Contact:** The Feingold Association, 127 East Main Street, #106, Riverhead, NY 11901 / Tel: (800) 321-3287 / Fax: (631) 369-2988 / Website: www.feingold.org / E-mail: Help@feingold.org

Children and Adults with Attention-Deficit/Hyperactivity Disorder (CHADD) is a national non-profit organization providing education, advocacy, and support for individuals with AD/HD. In addition to its informative website, CHADD also publishes a variety of printed materials to keep members and professionals current on research advances, medications and treatments affecting individuals with AD/HD. **Contact:** CHADD, 8181 Professional Place, Suite 150, Landover, MD 20785 / Tel: (800) 233-4050 / Fax: (301) 306-7090 / Website: www.chadd.org

Allergies

Practical Allergy Research Foundation for public awareness, research, products, teaching aids, books, audio, videotapes. **Contact:** Practical Allergy Research Foundation, PO Box 60, Buffalo, NY 14223 / Tel: (716) 875-0398

Food allergy testing is available through your clinical nutritionist or doctor.

York Nutritional Laboratories, Inc. specialize in testing for allergies and intolerances offering a FoodScan test that tests you for IgG sensitivity to a wide range of foods. It involves a home kit that enables you to send a pinprick of blood that is then used to test your food intolerances, giving you a clear indication of your food intolerances. They also test for IgE sensitivity. **Contact:** York Nutritional Laboratories, Inc., 2700 North 29th Avenue, Suite # 205, Hollywood, FL 33020 / Tel: (888) 751-3388 / Website: www.yorkallergiesusa.com

Autism

The **Autism Society of America** was founded in 1965 by a small group of parents working on a volunteer basis out of their homes. Over the last 35 years, the Society has developed into the leading source of information and referral on autism. Today, over 20,000 members are connected through a working network of over 200 chapters in nearly every state. Membership in ASA continues to grow as more and more parents and professionals unite to form a collective voice representing the autism community. **Contact:** The Autism Society of America, 7910 Woodmont Avenue, Suite 300, Bethesda, MD 20814-3067 / Tel: (301) 657-0881 / Website: www.autism-society.org

Center for the Study of Autism (CSA) provides information about autism to parents and professionals, and conducts research on the efficacy of various therapeutic interventions, in collaboration with the Autism Research Institute in San Diego, CA. Contact: CSA, PO Box 4538, Salem, OR 97302 / Website: www.autism.org

Autism Research Institute (ARI), founded by Bernard Rimland Ph.D., is the hub of a worldwide network of parents and professionals concerned with autism. The only organization of its kind, ARI was founded in 1967 to conduct and foster scientific research designed to improve the methods of diagnosing, treating, and preventing autism. ARI also disseminates research findings to parents and others all over the world that are seeking help. The ARI data bank, the world's largest, contains nearly 25,000 detailed case histories of autistic children from more than sixty countries. ARI publishes *Autism Research International.* Contact: ARI, 4182 Adams Avenue, San Diego, CA 92116 / Tel: (619) 563-6840 / Website: www.autism.com/ari

Depression

The **Depression and Bipolar Support Alliance (DBSA)** is the nation's leading patient-directed organization focusing on the most prevalent mental illnesses-depression and bipolar disorder. The organization fosters an understanding about the impact and management of these life-threatening illnesses by providing up-to-date, scientifically based tools and information written in language the general public can understand. DBSA supports research to promote more timely diagnosis, develop more effective and tolerable treatments, and discover a cure. The organization works to ensure that people living with mood disorders are treated equitably. **Contact:** Depression and Bipolar Support Alliance (DBSA), 730 North Franklin Street, Suite 501, Chicago, IL 60610-7204 / Tel: (800) 826-3632 / Fax: (312) 642-7243

Down's Syndrome

Friends of Trisomy 21 Research is a voluntary support group set up by parents of children with Down's syndrome to back the **Trisomy 21 Research Foundation**. The Friends aim to raise the necessary funding for research into Down's syndrome and nutrition intervention, and to improve the availability of information for parents and caregivers so they are able to make informed choices about treatment and care. They publish a newsletter for members packed with invaluable information and advice. **Contact:** Friends of Trisomy 21 Research, 11718 Barrington Court, #511, Los Angeles, CA 90049 / Tel: (310) 472-8778 / **Also contact:** The Trisomy 21 Research Foundation, 933 First Colonial Road, Suite 109, Virginia Beach, VA 23454 / Tel: (310) 425-1969 / Website: www.tri21.org. Also see some good articles on The Down's Syndrome Page at www.ceri.com/downhome.htm

Dyslexia

The **International Dyslexia Association (IDA)** was established to continue the pioneering work of Dr. Samuel T. Orton, a neurologist who was one of the first to identify dyslexia as a neurological difference and, along with Anna Gillingham, develop effective teaching approaches. For over 50 years it has fought for the rights of people with dyslexia while fending off critics who said that there was no such thing as dyslexia-that children who exhibited signs of dyslexia and other learning disabilities were lazy, stupid or worse, developmentally disabled, and therefore incapable of learning. During this time the organization has tested and tutored hundreds of thousands of children so that they would grow up to lead productive and fulfilling lives. Nowhere else can a person discover such a full range of useful information, practices, and research about dyslexia than through The International Dyslexia Association. **Contact:** IDA, Chester Building, Suite 382, 8600 LaSalle Road, Baltimore, MD 21286-2044 / Tel: (410) 296-0232 / Fax: (410) 321-5069 / Voice Message Requests for Information: 1 (800) ABCD123

Eating Disorders

National Eating Disorders Association (NEDA) is the largest not-for-profit organization in the United States working to prevent eating disorders and provide treatment referrals to those suffering from anorexia, bulimia and binge eating disorder and those concerned with body image and weight issues. **Contact:** National Eating Disorders Association, 603 Stewart Street, Suite 803, Seattle, WA 98101 / Tel: (206) 382-3587 / E-mail: info@NationalEatingDisorders.org

Laboratory Testing

Laboratory tests are becoming increasingly available for measuring a person's status for vitamins, essential fats, hormones, and even neurotransmitters. An up-to-date list of the best laboratories is on www.mentalhealthproject.com

Great Smokies Diagnostic Laboratory is a full-service testing company dealing with digestion, nutrition, detoxification, oxidative stress, immunology, allergy, hormones and endocrine regulation, and cardiovascular function. Client services are available 8 AM to 8 PM EST. **Contact:** Great Smokies Diagnostic Laboratory, 63 Zillicoa Street, Asheville, NC 28801 / Tel: (828) 253-0621 / Fax: (828) 252-9303 / Website: www.greatsmokieslab.com

Diagnostech is the UK agent for Diagnos-Techs, Inc, clinical research laboratory in Washington state. They offer salivary tests for DHEA, melatonin, oestrogen, progesterone, and testosterone, among other tests. A nutritionist can arrange for you to have these tests. **Contact:** Diagnos-Techs, Inc., 6620 South 192nd Place, Building J, Kent, WA 98032 / Tel: (800) 878-3787 / Fax: (425) 251-0637 / E-mail: diagnos@diagnostechs.com

BioLab carry out blood tests for essential fats, urine tests for pyroluria, chemical sensitivity panels, toxic element screens, and more. Only available through qualified practitioners. **Contact:** BioLab, 3100 North Hillside Avenue, Witchita, KS 67219 / Tel: (316) 684-7784 / (800) 494-7785 / Fax: (316) 82-2062 [MISSING #]

Trace Elements, Inc., a leading laboratory for hair mineral analysis for health-care professionals worldwide. **Contact:** Trace Elements, Inc., 4501 Sunbelt Drive, Addison, TX 75001 / Tel: (972) 250-6410 / (800) 824-2314 (United States and Canada) / Fax: (972) 248-4896 / Website: www.traceelements.com / E-mail: teilab@traceelements.com

Doctor's Data, Inc. is an independent reference laboratory providing data on levels of toxic and essential elements in hair, and elements, amino acids, and metabolites in blood and urine. DDI uses ICP-MS, HPLC, [SHOULD WE KNOW WHAT THESE ARE?]and photometric analyses to measure elements, amino acids and metabolites. DDI's specialized instrumentation can detect ultratrace levels of analytes. **Contact:** Doctor's Data, Inc., PO Box 111, West Chicago, IL 60186 / Tel: (800) 323-2784 / or (630) 377-8139 / Fax: (630) 587-7860 / Website: www.doctorsdata.com / E-mail: inquiries@doctorsdata.com

Vitamin Diagnostics, Inc. performs an up-to-19-item assay of vitamins and micronutrients in their metabolically available forms. Includes vitamins A, B_1, B_2, B_3, B_5, B_6, B_{12}, C, E, beta-carotene, biotin, lipoate, biopterin, carnitine, acyl-carnitine, folic acid, free and total choline, and inositol. **Contact:** Vitamin Diagnostics, Inc., Route 35 & Industrial Drive, Cliffwood Beach, NJ 07735 / Tel: (732) 583-7773 / Fax: (732) 583-7774 / Website: www.vitamindiagnostic.com / E-mail: vitamindia@aol.com

York Nutritional Laboratories Inc. specialize in testing for allergies and intolerances offering a FoodScan test that tests you for IgG sensitivity to a wide range of foods. It involves a home kit that enables you to send a pinprick of blood that is then used to test your food intolerances, giving you a clear indication of your food intolerances. They also test for IgE sensitivity. **Contact:** York Nutritional Laboratories, Inc., 2700 North 29th Avenue, Suite # 205, Hollywood, FL 33020 / Tel: (888) 751-3388 / Website: www.yorkallergiesusa.com

Memory

Cognitive Enhancement Research Institute (CERI) is the best way to keep up to date on mind and memory boosters. This website has many interesting features, and international listings for suppliers of smart drugs and nutrients, and will keep you updated on topical issues. **Contact:** CERI, PO Box 4029, Menlo Park, CA 94026 / Tel: (650) 321-CERI (2374) / Fax: (650) 323-3864 / Website: www.ceri.com / For books and products: www.smart-publications.com

Mental Health General

The **International Society of Orthomolecular Medicine** exists to further the advancement of orthomolecular medicine throughout the world, and to unite the many and various groups already operating in eighteen countries. Ortho-molecular Medicine describes the practice of using the most appropriate nutrients, including vitamins, minerals, and other essential compounds, in the most therapeutic amounts, according to an individual's particular biochemical requirements to establish optimum health.

The Society serves to educate health professionals and the public in the benefits and practice of orthomolecular medicine through publications, including the *Journal of Orthomolecular Medicine,* formerly the *Journal of Orthomolecular Psychiatry.* **Contact:** www.orthomed.org

National Alliance of the Mentally Ill, founded in 1979, is a nonprofit, grassroots, self-help, support and advocacy organization of consumers, families, and friends of people with severe mental illnesses, such as schizophrenia, schizoaffective disorder, bipolar disorder, major depressive disorder, obsessive-compulsive disorder, panic and other severe anxiety disorders, autism and pervasive developmental disorders, attention deficit/hyperactivity disorder, and other severe and persistent mental illnesses that affect the brain. **Contact:** NAMI, Colonial Place Three, 2107 Wilson Boulevard, Suite 300, Arlington, VA 22201-3042 / Tel: (703) 524-7600 / Fax: (703) 524-9094 / TDD: (703) 516-7227 / Member Services: (800) 950-NAMI

National Institute of Mental Health's mission is to reduce the burden of mental illness and behavioral disorders through research on mind, brain, and behavior. This public health mandate demands that we harness powerful scientific tools to achieve better understanding, treatment, and eventually, prevention of these disabling conditions that affect millions of Americans. **Contact:** NIMH Office of Communications, 6001 Executive Boulevard, Room 8184, MSC 9663, Bethesda, MD 20892-9663 / Tel: (301) 443-4513 or (866) 615-NIMH (6464) / Toll-free TTY: (301) 443-8431 / Fax: (301) 443-4279 / Fax: (301) 443-5158 / Website: http://www.nimh.nih.gov / E-mail: nimhinfo@nih.gov

The National Mental Health Association is the country's oldest and largest nonprofit organization addressing all aspects of mental health and mental illness. With more than 340 affiliates nationwide, NMHA works to improve the mental health of all Americans, especially the 54 million people with mental disorders, through advocacy, education, research and service. **Contact:** The National Mental Health Association, 2001 N. Beauregard Street, 12th Floor, Alexandria, Virginia 22311 / Tel: (703) 684-7722 / or (800) 969-NMHA (6642) / Fax: (703) 684-5968

Safe Harbor Project collects and distributes information on non-pharmaceutical approaches to mental disorders via their website, www.alternativementalhealth.com, which is full of useful information and articles. You can also subscribe to their free e-newsletter. **Contact:** Alternative Mental Health, 1718 Colorado Boulevard, Los Angeles, CA 90041 / Tel: (323) 257-7338 / Fax: (323) 257-7014 / Website: www.AlternativeMentalHealth.com

Nutritional Treatment

The **Pfeiffer Treatment Center** (PTC) is a private, non-profit clinic providing extensive biochemical analysis and individualized nutrient-based treatment to both children and adults for over 20 years. PTC specializes in treating learning and behavior problems, such as ADD and ADHD, and developmental disorders, such as autism, as well as depression, bipolar disorder and schizophrenia. PTC is staffed by a team of physicians, chemists, and other professionals who specialize in the effects of biochemistry on behavior, thought, or mood. The individualized biochemical treatment that PTC provides, based on the fact that each person has unique biochemistry, is a result of extensive research and has been shown to be effective through many outcome studies. **Contact:** PTC, 4575 Weaver Parkway, Warrenville, IL 60555-4039 / Tel: (630) 505-0300 / Fax: (630) 836-0667 / Website: www.hriptc.org

The **Brain Bio Centre** is a UK-based treatment center, set up by the Mental Health Project, putting the optimum nutrition approach into practice for those with mental health problems, including depression, learning difficulties, dyslexia, ADHD, autism, schizophrenia, dementia and Alzheimer's. **Contact:** Website: www.mentalhealthproject.com

Parkinsons Disease

Dr. Geoffrey Leader and **Lucille Leader** have specialized in the nutritional support of Parkinson's disease and have written *Parkinson's Disease: The Way Forward.* **Contact:** www.parkinsonsdisease-the-way-forward.com

Schizophrenia

International Schizophrenia Foundation works for improved diagnosis, treatment, preventative work and research into schizophrenia and related disorders. Research in alternative medicine has led to the positive treatment of degenerative illnesses such as diabetes, cancer, allergies and learning problems as well. Research papers are available for a fee. The Foundation sponsors an annual conference called "NUTRITION MEDICINE TODAY." **Contact:** International

Schizophrenia Foundation, 16 Florence Avenue, North York, Ontario M2N 1E9, Canada / Tel: (416) 733-2117 / Fax: (416) 733-2352 / Website: www.orthomed.org / E-mail: centre@orthomed.org

Well Mind Association Seattle distributes information on current research and promotes alternative therapies for mental illness and related disorders. WMA believes that physical conditions and treatable biochemical imbalances are the causes of many mental, emotional and behavioral problems. **Contact:** Well Mind Association Seattle, 4649 Sunnyside Avenue North, #344, Seattle, WA 98103 / Tel: (206) 547-6167 / Website: www.speakeasy.org/~wma/

National Alliance for Research on Schizophrenia and Depression is a private, not-for-profit public charity 501(C)(3) [SHOULD WE HAVE MORE OF AN EXPLANATION OF WHAT 501 C 3 is?]organized for the purpose of raising and distributing funds for scientific research into the causes, cures, treatments, and prevention of severe psychiatric brain disorders, such as schizophrenia and depression. **Contact:** NARSAD, 60 Cutter Mill Road, Suite 404, Great Neck, NY 11021 / Tel: (516) 829-0091 / Research Grants Program: (516) 829-5576 / Fax: (516) 487-6930

The **World Fellowship for Schizophrenia and Allied Disorders (WFSAD)** is the only global organization dedicated to lightening the burden of schizophrenia and allied disorders for sufferers and their families. **Contact:** WFSAD, 124 Merton Street, Suite 507, Toronto, Ontario, M4S 2Z2, Canada / Tel: (416) 961-2855 / Fax: (416) 961-1948 / Website: http://www.world-schizophrenia.org/

Information for Health Professionals

Health masterclasses. The nutritional approach to mental health problems is sadly lacking from most curricula within medicine, psychiatry, and psychotherapy. For this reason the Mental Health Project offers one- and two-day mental health master classes for doctors, psychiatrists, nutritionists, psychotherapists, and counselors. The aim of these master classes is, first, to enable health professionals to know when a person has a biochemical imbalance that may respond to nutritional intervention, and second, to learn how to provide nutritional support to maximize a person's mental health. For details about these training sessions, **Contact:** www.mentalhealthproject.com/professional

Referrals. The Mental Health Project also aims to establish a network of informed practitioners throughout the United Kingdom, and abroad, who can help those who wish to explore the nutritional approach to restoring mental health.

If you are involved in the nutritional treatment of mental health and would like to be on our contacts list, please go to the "Consultation" section of the website www.mentalhealthproject.com. Alternatively, email your details to info@mentalhealthproject.com

INDEX

abnormal behavior 153–4
acetyl-l-carnitine (ALC) 100
acetylcholine
  in action 95, 95
  for age-related memory decline
      296–7
  and Alzheimer's disease 95, 308–9
  boosting with choline 35
  boosting with DMAE 95
  boosting with phosphatidyl choline
      96
  boosting with pyroglutamate 99
  boosting with smart drugs 314, 315
  boosting with vitamin B_5 102
  functions 38
  and mental health problems 167
acetylcholine receptors 96–7
acid-alkali balance 269
adaptive capacity 145–6
addiction 263–71
  genetic factors 265
  how to quit 268–71
  mechanisms of 266–8
  and mental health problems 158–60
  prevalence 264
  symptoms 264
additives 75–6
adenochrome 210
adenosine 64
adrenal exhaustion 125–6, 305
adrenal imbalance 165–6, 316
Adrenal Stress Index 166

adrenaline 63
  composition 10
  and depression 108–9, 114–15
  functions 37
  and mental health problems 165–6
  and stimulants 64–5
adrenaline re-uptake inhibitors 108
age-related memory decline,
      prevention 5, 33, 93, 98–9,
      293–300, 319
aggressive behavior 6
  see also juvenile delinquency
alcohol
  as antinutrient 267–8
  and the brain 58–9
  and GABA 127–8
  how to quit 268
  and pregnancy 58–9
alcoholism 265–6, 266
alginic acid 75
allergens 80, 82
allergies
  see also food allergies
  chemical 160
  definition 80–2
  inhalant 193
  and mood 107
alpha lipoic acid 100
alphalinolenic acid 27, 28, 195
aluminum 72, 75, 232, 307–8
Alzheimer's disease 301–11
  and acetylcholine 95, 308–9

and cortisol 59–60
prevention and reversal plan 309–11
risk factors 302–3
smart drugs for 313–14, 319
amino acids 8, 10, 37–44, 100, 328
    see also specific amino acids
    calming 129
    Check 12–13
    for epilepsy 281–2
    essential 41
    free-form 43
    for manic depression 197–8
    and neurotransmitters 37–40, 39
    and Parkinson's disease 291
    and proteins 40–2
    sulphur-containing 75
    supplementation 42–4
amygdala 308
andropause 121, 124–5
anger, depression as 106–7
anorexia nervosa 5, 272–6, 277
anthocyanidins 57
antibiotics 229, 242–3
antibodies see immunoglobulin
    type E; immunoglobulin type G
antidepressants 108, 111, 169–70,
    179–83, 269–70
anti-inflammatories 304
antinutrients 68–76, 267–8
antioxidants
    see also specific antioxidants
    for age-related memory decline
        295–6
    for Alzheimer's disease 304
    mechanisms of action 56–8, 57
    and Parkinson's disease 289
    for schizophrenia 207
antipsychotic medications 173–5,
    202, 203
antisocial foods 260–1
anxiety 2, 127–8, 129–34
apathy/lack of motivation 2, 114–15
apolipoprotein E (ApoE) 302, 303,
    304
arachidonic acid (AA) 30, 231

arginine pyroglutamate 99, 104
Aricept (donepezil) 314
artificial sweeteners 20–1
aspartame 20–1
attention deficit hyperactivity
    disorder (ADHD) 97, 153–4,
    170–1, 220–1, 224, 226–37
autism 238–49
    and food allergies 241–6
    incidence 238, 239
    and the MMR vaccine 246–7
    natural approaches to 247–9
    and nutrient deficiencies 240–1
    onset 238, 239, 247
    symptoms 238

baby milk 46, 91
Baizer, Joan 171, 227
Benton, David 15, 45, 46, 89
benzodiazepines 128, 172
beta-amyloid 304
beta-carotene 57
binge foods 277
biochemical imbalance
    and antisocial behavior 261–2
    and mental illness 155–6, 157–68,
        205–18
Biolab 73
Birmingham, Carl 5, 274–5
blushing reaction 206, 207, 212
borage oil (see starflower oil)
brain
    "agers" 54–60
    and alcohol consumption 58–9
    anatomy 8–10, 9
    boosters 8–13, 88
    circulation aids 100–2
    dependence on fats 22, 23–4, 28,
        29, 54–5, 90–1, 206, 224
    and food allergies 77–84
    Food Check 10–13
    intelligent nutrients for 45–9,
        326–7, 328–9
    memory 94–5
    and oxidants 54–6, 55

phospholipids for 33, 35–6
and pollution 68–76, 224–5
protection for 53–84, 294–300
regeneration 98–9
in schizophrenia 204–5
and stress 59–60
and sugar 14, 15, 61–7
brain drain 93
brain-body connection 22
see also mind-body connection
brain-gut connection 13, 80
Braly, James 81, 84
breast milk 91
breast tenderness 122
Broda Barnes Temperature Test 161
Bryce-Smith, Derek 59, 274
bulimia nervosa 272–4, 275, 276, 277

cadmium poisoning 68, 71, 74–5,
    163, 259
caffeine 4, 64–5, 270
calcium 49–50
    and blood sugar levels 67
    chelating effects of 75
    for histadelia 186
    and sleep 140
candidiasis 84
carbohydrates **16**, 326
    see also glucose; sugar
    complex 14–21, **16**, 234
    fast-releasing 15–17
    refined 14–16, 62, 234, 326
    slow-releasing 15–17, 20, 21
    and tryptophan 112
cardiovascular disease 303–4, 306
carnitine 100
casein 217, 242, 243–4, 244
catecholamine pathway 114
CDP choline (citicholine) 297, 298
celiac disease 216
chelation 74–5
children
    see also juvenile delinquency
    ADHD 97, 153–4, 170–1, 220–1,
    224, 226–37

autism 238–49
Down's syndrome 250–5
essential fats 22–3
food allergies 77–8
intelligent nutrients for 45, 89–90
IQ boosters 89–90
lead poisoning 69–71, **70**
learning difficulties 220–5
manic depression in 235
chlorpromazine 173–4
chocolate 65, 66
cholesterol 23, 34, 120, 183
choline
    and Down's Syndrome 254
    and memory enhancement 33, 35,
    96–7, 103
chromium 67
circulation 100–2, 294, 298–9
citicholine 297, 298
coenzyme NAD 307
coenzyme-Q_{10} 57
coffee 64–6
cognitive behavioral therapy (CBT)
    199, 323
cola 65, 66
Colgan, Michael 223
concentration difficulties 2
convulsions 278–83
copper 72–3, 225
    and ADHD 232
    and autism 245–6
    and mental health problems 163
    and PMS 123
    and stress/anxiety 133
cortisol 63, 95, 102
    and age-related memory loss 299
    and Alzheimer's disease 59–60, 305
    effect of estrogen on 123
    and insomnia 138–9
Cowen, Philip 111, 276
criminal behavior 256–62
Crook, Thomas 5, 33, 98
cross-culturalization 3
cystine 75

D2 dopamine receptor gene 265
dairy produce
    allergies to 83, 84, 242, 243–4, 277
    and autism 242, 243–4
    as binge food 277
Deanor/Deanol *see* DMAE
delusions 201
dendrites 9, 95, 299
deprenyl (Selegiline) 291, 303, 313,
    319
depression 2, 6
    see also manic depression
    and 5-HTP 113–14, 115
    amino acid supplements for 43
    anatomy of 107–9
    as anger 106–7
    Check for 105–6
    combating 105–18, 178–89
    and fats 116
    and food allergies 79
    and histamine 183–7
    and light exposure 110, 117–18
    menopausal 124
    natural remedies for 179–83
    prevalence 105
    recommended foods for 118
    and SAMe **109**, 115–16, 118
    symptoms 178
    and the thyroid gland 187–8
    and TMG **109**, 115, 116, 118
    and tryptophan 107, 109, 110,
        111–12, 114, 118
    and tyrosine 107, 114–15, 118
    in women 109–10, 124
detox
    for addictions 270–1
    for Alzheimer's disease 305
    for autistic children 245
    overload 167–8
DHA *see* docosahexaenoic acid
DHEA (dehydroepiandrosterone) 60,
    119, 125–6
    for Alzheimer's disease 305
    as smart hormone 316, 319
    supplementation 126

tests for 125, 126
diabetes 62
*Diagnostic and Statistical Manual of
    Mental Disorders* (DSM-IV)
    150–1, 152
digestion
    age-related decline in 294
    and Alzheimer's disease 305
    in autistic children 242–3
    brain-gut connection 13, 80
Dilantin (phenytoin) 186, 279,
    315–16, 319
DMAE (Deanor/Deanol) 96, 97–8,
    103, 104
    for antipsychotic side effects 175
    for epilepsy 282
    for reward deficiency syndrome
        236
DMG (di-methyl glycine) 282
docosahexaenoic acid (DHA) 27, 28,
    30–2
    for ADHD 231
    for age-related memory decline 296
    and alcohol consumption 58
    and intelligence 90–1
    for manic depression 194–5
    for memory enhancement 104
donepezil 314
L-dopa 286, **287**, 287–8, 291, 292
dopamine 10, 37, 38, **287**
    and depression 108, 114, 115
    and Parkinson's disease 286, 288–9,
        290, 313
    and reward deficiency syndrome
        236
    and stimulants 64–5
Down's Syndrome 250–5
    genetic basis 250–1
    health problems involved with 250
    megavitamin therapy 251–5
dreaming 135–6
drugs 4
    see also addiction
    of abuse 127–8, 171
    interactions 175–6, 198

mechanisms of action 40
prescription drugs 269–70
side effects 169–77
smart drugs 293, 309, 312–16, 318–19
dysbiosis 245
dysglycemia 61, 62, 122, 158, 266
see also glucose, imbalances
dyslexia 220–5
dyspraxia 220–5

E101 (vitamin B$_2$) 76
E102 (tartrazine) 75–6, 233
E160 (carotene, vitamin A) 76
E300–304 (vitamin C) 76
E306–309 (tocopherols) 76
E322 (lecithin) 76
E375 (niacin) 76
E440 (pectin) 76
eating disorders 5, 272–7
EDTA 74
eggs 34–6, 96, 327
eicosapentaenoic acid (EPA) 27–8, 30–2, 194–5, 231, 296
ELISA IgG test 81, 83, 160, 233
emotional intelligence (EQ) 22
endorphins 217, 242
energy drinks 65, 66
enkephalins 217
environment, impact of 147, 148
eosonophilia myalgia syndrome 112
epilepsy 278–83
ergoloid mesylate *see* Hydergine
Erhlich's reagent 213
essential oils 189
estrogen
deficiency 110, 119, 122, 124, 316
excess (estrogen dominance) 119, 122–4
ethyl-EPA 116
evening primrose oil (EPO) 29, 123, 232, 328
exorphins 242, 243, 277
Experimental World Inventory (EWI) 185

fatigue 2
fats 22–32
see also omega-3 fats; omega-6 fats
Check 11–12
deficiency 25
essential 8, 10, 22–3
for ADHD 231–2
for age-related memory decline 296
antidepressant effects 182–3
for autism 240
for the brain 224
Check 25
for delinquents 259–60
for epilepsy 281
and hormone production 120
and mental health problems 162–3
and mood 107
and schizophrenia 206–7
and intelligence 90–1
monounsaturated 23
mood-boosting 116
polyunsaturated 26, 28
recommended intake 25–6
saturated 23, 24, 25, 26, 28
trans fats 54–5
unsaturated 24, 28
United States intake 55
Feingold diet 233–4
fetal alcohol syndrome 58
"fight-or flight" syndrome 127
fish
choline from 35
essential fats from 28, 30, 31, 32, 91
mercury levels in 72
as part of a balanced diet 326–7
fish oil 31–2, 194–5, 328
fits 278–83
fluphenazine 173, 174
folic acid (folate) 47, 48–9, 186
for Alzheimer's disease 306–7
antidepressant effects 181, 182
and Down's Syndrome 252–3
for epilepsy 279

and mental health problems 161–2
and mood 107–8, 115
for Parkinson's disease 290
recommended intake 328
for schizophrenia 212
food additives 75–6
food allergies **81**
and addiction 266–7
and ADHD 232–4
and autism 241–6
and the brain 77–84
and criminal behavior 260–1
delayed 81–2
and epilepsy 282–3
and manic depression 192–3
and mental health problems 160
and Parkinson's disease 290
and schizophrenia 216–17
testing for 83, 160, 233
top ten 82–3
free radicals 289
see also oxidants
fried food 54, 55, 327
fructose 15
fruit 15–16, 326
full-spectrum lighting 117
functional magnetic resonance
imaging (fMRI) 204–5

GABA (gamma-amino-butyric acid)
37, 43, 99, 309
and alcohol consumption 58
effects of tranquilizers on 172
for epilepsy 282
relaxing properties 127–8, 129–30
gamma-linolenic acid (GLA) 29,
30–2, 231
genes, impact of 147, 148
Gesch, Bernard 6, 256–8, 261
ginkgo biloba 96, 100–1, 104, 298–9
ginkgo flavone glycosides 101, 298
Glaxo Pharmaceuticals 293
gliadin 82
Gliadorphin-7 242
glucose 8, 14

and the brain 14, 15, 62, 102
Check 11
imbalances 61–4, **63**, 67
and addiction 266, 269
and ADHD 234
and delinquency 257–8
and manic depression 192
and mental health problems 158
and mood 107, 258
and PMS 122
symptoms of 14, 158
and intelligence 91
maintaining even levels 16–20, 91
from refined carbohydrates 16
glutamine 43, 96, 99–100, 104, 309
L-glutamine 223, 243
glutathione 57
gluten allergies 82–3, 84, 160
and autism 242, 243–4, **244**
and schizophrenia 216–17
glycation 62
glycemic index (GI) 16–17, **17**, **18–19**
glycogen 15
glycosylated hemoglobin 158
gut
-brain connection 13, 80
in autistic children 242–3

hair mineral analysis 72–4
halfway houses 324–5
hallucinations 201, 210
haloperidol 173, 174
heavy metal toxicity 68, 69–75
and ADHD 232
and Alzheimer's disease 307–8
and autism 245–6
and delinquency 258–9
detoxification of 74–5
and learning difficulties 224–5
and mental health problems 163
heroin addiction 263, 269
herpes simplex virus 302–3
hippocampus 95, 308
histadelia 183–7, 265
histamine 82, 133

and anxiety 133
and depression 183–7
and hallucinations 210
and mental health problems 164–5
and schizophrenia 217–18
Hoffer, Abram 5, 47, 156, 174, 194,
    197, 203, 205, 208, 209–10,
    228–9, 268
Hoffer-Osmond Diagnostic (HOD)
    test 155
homocysteine 161–2, 305–6
hops 129, 132, 141
hormones
    and cholesterol **120**
    and mood swings 119–26
    smart 313, 316–19
    steroid 120, **120**
hospitals 324
Huperzia serrata 314, 319
Hydergine (ergoloid mesylate) 315,
    319
hydrogen peroxide 252
hyperactivity 5, 170–1, 221, 228
see also attention deficit hyperactivity
    disorder
hypericin 181
hyperventilation 134
IAG 242
immune system 80–2, **81**
immunoglobulin type E (IgE) 80–1,
    82, 83
immunoglobulin type G (IgG) 81,
    81, 82, 83
indigestion 83–4
inflammation 167–8, 294, 295,
    303–5
inositol 212
insomnia 2, 135–42, 198
insulin 112
insulin resistance 61
intelligence 28, 90–4
    see also intelligence quotient
intelligence quotient (IQ) 5, 22, 23
    and complex carbohydrates 14–15
    in Down's syndrome 251–2

improving 45, 46, 90–4, 222–3,
    251–2
and lead levels 69–71, 224–5
and refined carbohydrates 62
scores 90
intelligent nutrients 8, 10, 13, 45–51
intestinal permeability 289
Inuit people 28
iodine 188
ions, negative 188–9

Japan 26, 30
jet lag 140, 316–17, 318
juvenile delinquency 230–1, 256–62

kava kava
    for insomnia 141
    for manic depression 198
    relaxing properties 129, 130–1
    side effects 131
kavalactones 131

lactic acid 133–4
lead poisoning 68, 69–71, 70
    and ADHD 232
    and delinquency 258–9
    detoxification of 74, 75
    and IQ 69–71, 224–5
    and mental health problems 163
Leader, Geoffrey 286–9, 290
Leader, Lucille 286–9, 290
leaky gut syndrome 84, 243
learning difficulties 220–5
lecithin 35, 36, 76, 96
    HiPC 96, 103, 328
lifestyle, happy 188–9
light exposure 110, 117–18, 188
lighting, full-spectrum 117
limbic system 308
linoleic acid 29
linseed (flaxseeds) 28, 30
lipoic acid 57
lithium 193–4
liver
    in autistic children 245

and the brain 295–6
kava kava toxicity 131
and Parkinson's disease 289
locus coeruleus 102
low sugar diets 256, 257–8, **257**

magnesium 47, 49–50
for ADHD 229
for autism 240
and blood sugar imbalance 67
and breast tenderness 122
for epilepsy 280, 281
for manic depression 195
for menopause 124
and mood 107
and PMS 123
recommended intake 328
relaxing properties 129, 132, 140
male menopause 121, 124–5
malnutrition, affluent xii
manganese 47, 50, 175
for epilepsy 280, 281
for histadelia 186
recommended intake 328
manic depression (bipolar disorder)
in children 235
combating 190–9
diagnosis 154
understanding 191–2
Manic Depression Fellowship (MDF)
(UK) 198
mast cells 80
mauve factor 213
melatonin 119, 119
and jet lag 140, 316–17, 318
and mood 118
and sleep 139–40
as smart hormone 316–18
memory 2
age-related decline 5, 33, 93, 98–9,
293–300, 319
Check 93–4
effects of stress 59–60
enhancing 93–104
and evening primrose oil 29

how it works 94–5
and phospholipids 33–6
and vitamin B$_5$ 48
menopause
female 121, 124
male 121, 124–5
mental health 145
model of 146–8, **146**
Mental Health Act 1983 (UK) 144
Mental Health Questionnaire 157
mental illness
see also specific conditions
and biochemical imbalance 155–6,
157–68
diagnosis 150–6
differentiation from abnormal
behavior 153–4
problems of diagnosis 144, 151–2
rise of 3, 148–9
understanding 144–9
mercury 72, 75, 247, 308
metallothionein 245–6
metals *see* heavy metal toxicity
methionine 75, 186
methylation 48, 107–8, 161, 181–2
milk 216–17
mind frames 147
mind-body connection 4–6, 145–8,
322
see also brain-body connection
minerals
see also specific minerals
intelligent 45, 47, 49–51
MMR vaccine 246–7
monosodium glutamate (MSG) 99,
309
monoamine oxidase inhibitors
(MAOIs) 108, 169, 313
mood swings 2
combating 190–9
hormonal 119–26
record keeping and self-
management 198–9
motivation 107–8
MSB Plus Version 4 254–5

MSM 253
multinutrients 328
    for age-related memory decline
        294–5
    for delinquency 259
    for giving up alcohol 268
    for IQ 5
    for manic depression 197
music 189
myelin sheath 24, **24**, 33

National Health Service (NHS) 149,
    301
Needleman, Herbert 69–71, 225, 258
nervous breakdowns 191
net protein usability (NPU) 41–2
neural networks 8, 9, 90, 94–5
neuroleptic malignant syndrome
    175
neurons 8, 9, 23, 38
    age-related decline 297
    dependence on fats 24
    dopaminergic 288
    myelin sheath 24, **24**
neurotics 150
Neurotransmitter Screening Tests
    165, 166, 167
neurotransmitters 10, **10**, 24, 37–8
    see also specific neurotransmitters
    calming 129
    and depression 108–14, **109**
    how they work 38–40, **38**
    key types 37–8, **39**
    protein consumption 41
    smart drugs 313–14
niacin see vitamin B$_3$
niacinamide 212
nootropics 314–16
noradrenaline 37, 108, 109, 114–15, 229
noradrenaline re-uptake inhibitors
    (NARIs) 108
nutritional psychiatry xi–xii
nutritionists, finding 323
NuTriVene formula 253, 254–5
nuts 327

Nystatin 257

oats 83
old age
    see also smart drugs; smart
        hormones
    age-related memory decline 5, 33,
        93, 98–9, 293–300, 319
    Alzheimer's disease 301–11
    Parkinson's disease 286–92
omega-3 fats 22–4, 26–9, **27**, 55
    for age-related memory decline 296
    for Alzheimer's disease 304
    antidepressant effects 182–3
    for autism 240
    for delinquents 260
    for epilepsy 281
    and intelligence 90–1
    for manic depression 194–5
    mood-boosting effects 116
    prevention of inflammation 167
    recommended intake 26
    and schizophrenia 207
    sources 30–2, 34, 326–7, 328
omega-6 fats 22–4, 29–32, **29**
    recommended intake 26
    and schizophrenia 207
    sources 30–2, 328
organ meats 34, 36
Osmond, Humphrey 47, 208, 209,
    230, 268
ovulation 121–22
oxidants
    see also antioxidants
    and Alzheimer's disease 304
    and the brain 54–7, **55**, **57**
    and Parkinson's disease 289
    and schizophrenia 207

pace of living 2–3
panic attacks 133–4
Parkinson's disease 286–92, 313
passion flower 129, 132, 141
Pauling, Linus 89, 296
pectin 75, 76

pellagra 208
penicillamine 74
Pfeiffer, Carl 50, 62, 74, 133, 183, 184, 185, 192, 196, 205, 213, 215, 280
phenylalanine 43, 114–15, 118
phenytoin (Dilantin) 186, 279, 315–16, 319
Philippines 26
Philpott, William 78, 82, 216, 267
phosphatidyl choline (PC)
   for age-related memory decline 297–8
   for antipsychotic side effects 175
   and memory function 33, 35, 96–7, 97, 103, 104
   as part of a balanced diet 328
phosphatidyl serine (PS)
   for age-related memory decline 298
   and memory function 33, 35–6, 98, 104
   as part of a balanced diet 328
phospholipidase A2 (PLA2) 206, 207
phospholipids 8, 10, 33–6, **297**
   see also specific phospholipids
   for age-related memory decline 297–8
   Check 12
   for epilepsy 281–2
   and the myelin sheath 24
   sources 34–5
physical exercise 188
physical intelligence (PQ) 22
phytoestrogens 122–3
Pilch, H. 98–9, 309
pineal gland 316–17
piracetam 98–9, 103, 254, 309, 314–15, 319
plaques 304
Poldinger, Dr. 5–6, 113
pollution 55, 68–76
polyethylene glycol (PEG 400) 289
porphyria 163–4
premenstrual syndrome (PMS) 121–24
pregnancy

and alcohol consumption 58–9
and the B vitamins 48–9
and choline 96–7
pregnenolone 316, **317**, 319
prescription drugs, addiction to 269–70
progesterone
   deficiency 119, 122, 124, 316
   natural creams 123
prostaglandins 27, 231
protein 40–2
   see also amino acids
   and L-dopa 290–1
   and Parkinson's disease 290–2
   and slow-releasing carbohydrates 20, 326
   sources 41–2
Prozac 170
psycho-neuro-immuno-endocrinology 80
psychoanalysis 203
psychotherapists, finding 323–4
psychotherapy 4, 6, 147, 189, 323–4
psychotics 150
   see also manic depression; schizophrenia
pyridoxine 161–2
pyroglutamate 98–9, 103, 104
pyroluria 163–4, 196, 211–15, 240
pyrroles 213

raisins 17
rapid eye movement (REM) sleep 135–6
reactive hypoglycemia 258
receptors 10, **10**, 24, 38
relaxants, natural 127–34
reward deficiency syndrome 236, 265
Rimland, Bernard 5, 97, 229, 230, 240, 247
Ritalin 170–1, 220, 226–7, 229
   and autism 247
   and biopolar children 235
   and reward deficiency syndrome 236

side effects 227
RNA (ribonucleic acid) 95, 102, 296, 308
Roberts, Gwillym 45, 89

St. John's wort 141, 179–81, 198
salicylates 233–4
salt 122
SAMe (s-adenosyl methionine) **109**
   antidepressant effects 115–16, 118, 181, 182
   and Down's syndrome 252–3
   for epilepsy 282
Sapolsky, Robert 59, 95, 299, 305
Schauss, Alex 252, 259, 260–1
schizoaffective patients 191
schizophrenia 5, 182
   and biochemical imbalance 205–18
   combating 204–18
   demystification 200–3
   diagnosis 152, 154–5, 156, 199, 203
   diagnostic difficulties 152, 199, 203
   and food allergies 79, 216–17
   and histadelia 185
   and manic depression 191
   and omega-6 fats 29
   prevalence 154, 202
   and pyroluria 213–15
   stigma of 154
Schoenthaler, Stephen 89, 222, 230–1, · 258, 259
seasonal affective disorder (SAD) 105, 117–18, 189, 318
secretin 247
seed oils 31, 32, 327
seeds
   essential fats from 28, 30–1, 32, 327
   protein intake 41
   zinc intake 103
selective serotonin re-uptake inhibitors (SSRIs) 6, 108, 113, 170
selegiline (deprenyl) 291, 303, 313, 319
selenium 57, 75, 188, 303
self-medicating, for stress/anxiety 127
serine 35

serotonin 10, 38, 40, 211
   and criminal behavior 262
   and depression 108–14, 116, 117, 179, 181
   functions 37
   menopausal deficiencies in 124
   and mental health problems 165
   and sleep 139–40
Seroxat 170
Showa Denko 112
sleep
   deprivation 136–7
   natural aids 140–2
   problems 2, 135–42, 198
smart drugs 293, 309, 312–16, 318–19
smart hormones 313, 316–19
smoking 55–6, 192, 267, 269
social deprivation 149
spiritual awakenings 202
starflower (borage) oil 29, 31, 328
steroid hormones 120, **120**
stimulants 169
   addiction to 62–7, 158–60, 270
   and insomnia 139
   kicking the habit 65–7
   and mental health problems 158–60
   side effects 170–1
stress
   and age-related memory loss 299
   and Alzheimer's disease 305
   and the brain 59–60
   danger substances 133–4
   effects on memory 95, 299
   and insomnia 138–9
   and mood 110
   natural relaxants 127, 129–33, 134
   and Parkinson's disease 290
sugar
   and ADHD 234
   as binge food 277
   and the brain 61–7
   low sugar diets 256, 257–8, 257
   refined 14–16, 62, 234, 326
suicide 178, 185–6
sulphation 245, 289

sulphite oxidase 245
superoxide dimutase (SOD) 252
synapses 9, 9, 38, 297
synergy 103–4

tardive dyskinesia 175
tartrazine (E102) 75–6, 233
taurine 43, 129, 130, 197–8, 282
tea 65, 66
tension fatigue syndrome 260
terpene lactones 101, 298
testosterone
    deficiency 119, 122, 124
    excess 119
Thailand 26
theobromine 65–6
theophylline 65–6
thimerosal 247
Thorazine 173–4
thyroid gland 252
    overactive 161
    underactive 161, 187–8
thyroxine 119, 120, 188
TMG (tri-methyl-glycine) 109,
    115–16, 118, 181, 282
tocopherols 76
    see also vitamin E
tranquilizers 127–9
    addictive nature of 172–4, 270
    major 169, 171–2, 173–5, 202, 203
    minor 169
    side effects 169, 171–4
transpersonal therapy 323–4
tricyclic antidepressants 108, 113,
    115, 179
Trisomy 21 Research Foundation 252,
    253, 255
tryptamines 38
tryptophan 37, 40, 43
    and criminal behavior 262
    and Down's Syndrome 253
    and eating disorders 275–7
    and mood 107, 109, 110, 110–11,
        114, 118
    recommended intake 111

and sleep 139
5-hydroxy-tryptophan (5-HTP) 6, 43,
    113–14, 115
    for depression 179
    for manic depression 197
    recommended intake 113, 118
    and sleep 139, 140, 141
L-tryptophan 197
tyramine 291
tyrosine, and mood 37, 40, 43, 107,
    114–15, 118, 179, 188
L-tyrosine 197

valerian 129, 131–2, 141
Valium 172–4, 198
vanadium 196–7
vegans 28, 30
vegetables 326
vegetarians 41, 195, 275
vigilance 198–9
vinpocetine 96, 101–2, 104, 282
visual defects 240–1
vitamin A (retinol) 76, 240–1
vitamin B$_1$ (thiamine) 46, 47, 96, 134,
    307
vitamin B$_2$ 76
vitamin B$_3$ (niacin) 47–8, 76
    for Alzheimer's disease 307
    for manic depression 196
    and memory function 102, 104
    and mental health problems 161–2
    and mood 107, 115, 182
    nonblushing formulation 212
    for post-addiction detox 271
    for schizophrenia 5, 182, 208–12,
        211
    tests for 206, 207
vitamin B$_5$ (pantothenic acid) 47, 48,
    96, 102, 103, 104
vitamin B$_6$ 47, 48–9
    for ADHD 229
    for Alzheimer's disease 306–7
    antidepressant effects 181, 182
    for autism 240
    and blood sugar levels 67

and breast tenderness 122
for epilepsy 279–80, 281
for histadelia 186
for menopause 124
and mood 107, 115
for Parkinson's disease 291
and PMS 123
for pyroluria 214, 215
and sleep 136, 139
vitamin B$_{12}$ 47, 48–9
for Alzheimer's disease 307
and memory function 96, 102, 104
and mental health problems 161–2
and mood 107, 115
recommended intake 328
for schizophrenia 212
vitamin B group 46–9
and blood sugar levels 67
and memory function 96, 102, 104
and sleep 140
and sugar consumption 61
vitamin C 47, 49
for age-related memory decline 296
antioxidant effects 56–7
for autism 240
and blood sugar levels 67
chelating effects of 74
for histadelia 186
and intelligence 89–90
for manic depression 196
and memory function 96
and mood 107, 108
for schizophrenia 5, 207
vitamin E (d-alpha tocopherol)
for age-related memory decline 296
for Alzheimer's disease 303
antioxidant effects 56, 57, 58
for antipsychotic side effects 175

vitamins
see also specific vitamins
intelligent nutrients 45–9
Volkow, Nora 171, 226–7

Ward, Neil 75–6, 229, 233
Wernicke-Korsakof syndrome 307
wheat allergies 82, 84, 160
and autism 242, 243–4
and binging 277
and schizophrenia 216–17
whole foods 326
withdrawal 268–71
women
depression 109–10
menopause 121, 124
premenstrual blues 121–23
World Health Organization (WHO)
3, 28, 206
Wurtman, Richard 35, 112

zinc 47, 51, 188
chelating effects 74
and delinquency 258, 259
and digestion 84
and dream recall 136
and eating disorders 5, 273–5
effects of smoking on 55–6
for epilepsy 280–1
for histadelia 186
and memory function 102–3
for the menopause 124
and mood 107
and PMS 123
and pyroluria/porphyria 163, 164
recommended intake 328
for schizophrenia 213–15
tartrazine's effects on 76

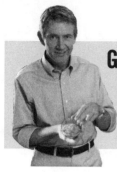

Get Patrick Holford's Recommendations for Optimum Health and Natural Healing at holfordhealth.com

- **FREE HEALTH E-LETTER:** Sign-up for Patrick's free e-letter that gives you the latest updates on optimum nutrition for your body & mind.

- **NUTRIENT FACTS:** Learn about the essential vitamins and minerals you need to achieve optimum health.

- **HEALTH FAQ's:** Get Patrick's answers to your commonly asked health questions.

- **SHOP ONLINE:** Order nutritional supplements specifically formulated by Patrick, with secure online ordering and a 100% satisfaction guarantee.

- **MONTHLY NEWSLETTER:** Subscribe to Patrick's monthly newsletter, *Wellness Advisor*, dedicated to bringing you nutritional therapies and breakthroughs to help you achieve superhealth.